FIRST AID FOR THE

EMERGENCY MEDICINE clerkship

THE STUDENT TO STUDENT GUIDE

SERIES EDITORS:

LATHA G. STEAD, MD
Assistant Professor of Emergency Medicine
Mayo Medical School
Rochester, Minnesota

S. MATTHEW STEAD, MD, PhD
Class of 2001
State University of New York—Downstate Medical Center
Brooklyn, New York

MATTHEW S. KAUFMAN, MD
Resident in Internal Medicine
Long Island Jewish Medical Center
Albert Einstein College of Medicine
New Hyde Park, New York

McGraw-Hill
Medical Publishing Division

New York   Chicago   San Francisco   Lisbon   London   Madrid
Mexico City   Milan   New Delhi   San Juan   Seoul
Singapore   Sydney   Toronto

McGraw-Hill

A Division of The McGraw-Hill Companies

First Aid for the Emergency Medicine Clerkship

4 5 6 7 8 9 0 VFM/VFM 0 9 8 7 6 5 4

ISBN 0-07-136426-9

Notice

Medicine is an ever-changing science. As new research and clinical experience broaden our knowledge, changes in treatment and drug therapy are required. The authors and the publisher of this work have checked with sources believed to be reliable in their efforts to provide information that is complete and generally in accord with the standards accepted at the time of publication. However, in view of the possibility of human error or changes in medical sciences, neither the authors nor the publisher nor any other party who has been involved in the preparation or publication of this work warrants that the information contained herein is in every respect accurate or complete, and they disclaim all responsibility for any errors or omissions or for the results obtained from use of the information contained in this work. Readers are encouraged to confirm the information contained herein with other sources. For example and in particular, readers are advised to check the product information sheet included in the package of each drug they plan to administer to be certain that the information contained in this work is accurate and that changes have not been made in the recommended dose or in the contraindications for administration. This recommendation is of particular importance in connection with new or infrequently used drugs.

This book was set in Goudy by Rainbow Graphics.
The editor was Catherine A. Johnson.
The production supervisor was Lisa Mendez.
Project management was provided by Rainbow Graphics.
The index was prepared by Oneida Indexing.
Von Hoffman Graphics was the printer and binder.

This book is printed on acid-free paper.

Library of Congress Cataloging-in-Publication Data

First aid for the emergency medicine clerkship / series editors, Latha Stead, S. Matthew
Stead, Matthew S. Kaufman.
    p. ; cm.
    Includes index.
    ISBN 0-07-136426-9 (alk. paper)
    1. Emergency medicine–Outlines, syllabi, etc. 2. Clinical clerkship–Outlines, syllabi,
etc. I. Stead, Latha. II. Stead, S. Matthew. III. Kaufman, Matthew S.
    [DNLM: 1. Emergencies. 2. Clinical Clerkship. WB 105 F527 2001]
RC86.92 .F57 2001
616.02′5–dc21

                            2001030744

Contributing Authors

THOMAS M. BOYD, MD
Resident in Emergency Medicine
Jacobi-Montefiore EM Residency
Albert Einstein College of Medicine
Bronx, New York
Hematologic and Oncologic Emergencies, Head and Neck Emergencies

HYUN CHUNG, MD
Attending Physician, Emergency Medicine
Hudson Valley Hospital Center
Cortland Manor, New York
Gastrointestinal Emergencies

MICHAEL R. EDWARDS, MD
Attending Physician
Department of Emergency Medicine
Beebe Medical Center
Lewes, Delaware
Section I, "How to Succeed in the Clerkship," Cardiovascular Emergencies, EMS and Disaster Medicine, Dermatologic Emergencies, Environmental Emergencies

FRANK A. ILLUZZI, MD
Chief Resident in Emergency Medicine
Long Island Jewish Medical Center
Albert Einstein College of Medicine
New Hyde Park, New York
Resuscitation

BARBARA G. LOCK, MD
Attending Physician in Emergency Medicine
Columbia Presbyterian Medical Center
New York, New York
Emergency Toxicology, Environmental Emergencies, Ethics, Medico-Legal and Evidence-Based Medicine

BONNIE McGEE, PT, MD
Resident in Emergency Medicine
Jacobi-Montefiore EM Residency
Albert Einstein College of Medicine
Bronx, New York
Musculoskeletal Emergencies

RUSSELL W. RASKIN, MD
Resident in Emergency and Internal Medicine
Long Island Jewish Medical Center
Albert Einstein College of Medicine
New Hyde Park, New York
Trauma

LEON D. SANCHEZ, MD, MPH
Attending Physician, Beth Israel Deaconess Medical Center
Harvard Affiliated Emergency Medicine Residency (HAEMR)
Boston, Massachusetts
Respiratory Emergencies

NIRAV N. SHAH, MD
Attending Physician in Emergency Medicine
Kaiser Permanente
Walnut Creek, California
Section I, "How to Succeed in the Clerkship," Gynecologic Emergencies, Obstetric Emergencies, Emergency Toxicology, Endocrine Emergencies

SACHIN J. SHAH, MD
Resident in Emergency Medicine
Jacobi-Montefiore EM Residency
Albert Einstein College of Medicine
Bronx, New York
Diagnostics, Immunologic Emergencies

WEYLIN SING, DO
Resident in Emergency Medicine
Jacobi-Montefiore EM Residency
Albert Einstein College of Medicine
Bronx, New York
Neurologic Emergencies

RYAN JAY ZAPATA, MD
Resident in Emergency and Internal Medicine
Long Island Jewish Medical Center
Albert Einstein College of Medicine
New Hyde Park, New York
Renal and Genitourinary Emergencies

Contents

Introduction

This clinical study aid was designed in the tradition of the *First Aid* series of books. It is formatted in the same way as the other books in the series; however, a stronger clinical emphasis was placed on its content. You will find that rather than simply preparing you for success on an exam, this resource will also help guide you in the clinical diagnosis and treatment of many of the problems seen by emergency physicians.

The content of the book is based on the American College of Emergency Physicians (ACEP) and Society of Academic Emergency Medicine (SAEM) recommendations for the Emergency Medicine curriculum for fourth-year medical students. It also contains information derived from the Core Curriculum, an outline developed by the Residency Review Committee, which details the information that EM residents are expected to learn and will ultimately be responsible for on their oral and written board exams. Each of the chapters contains the major topics central to the practice of EM and has been specifically designed for the medical student learning level. In addition, special chapters such as Emergency Medical Services, Diagnostics, and Procedures have been included to emphasize the more clinical nature of EM.

The content of the text is organized in the format similar to other texts in the *First Aid* series. Topics are listed by bold headings, and the "meat" of the topic provides essential information. The outside margins contain mnemonics, diagrams, exam and ward tips, summary or warning statements, and other memory aids. Exam tips are marked by 🖍 and ER tips by the symbol 🩺.

Acknowledgments

We would like to thank the following faculty for their help in reviewing the manuscript for this book:

William A. Gluckman, DO, EMT-P
Assistant Professor of Surgery, Division of Emergency Medicine
University Hospital (UMDNJ)
Newark, New Jersey

Terry J. Mengert, MD
Associate Professor of Emergency Medicine
University of Washington School of Medicine
Seattle, Washington

How to Succeed in the Emergency Medicine Clerkship

WHAT TO BRING

There is very little you will need to have on your person while working in the department. A basic list of equipment to carry with you includes:

1. Several black pens
2. Stethoscope
3. Trauma shears
4. Small notepad to track patients and record important teaching points
5. Penlight
6. A pocket-sized drug reference (e.g., Tarascon's *Pharmacopeia*)
7. EMRA's *Guide to Antibiotic Use in the Emergency Department* or Sanford's *Guide to Antimicrobial Therapy*

WHAT TO EXPECT

EM is a specialty with many unique aspects, which makes this clerkship a popular favorite. These include:
- A large variety of presenting complaints
- Being the first one to see a patient, which means being the first one to come up with a diagnosis
- Opportunity to do a number of procedures
- Opportunity to function as a real member of the resuscitation teams
- Opportunity for close interaction with attendings
- Constant ongoing teaching, with the opportunity to pick up many "pearls"

Many of the things that make EM so enjoyable may also pose a challenge at times:
- For many, the emergency department (ED) is the only place to obtain care, so what they perceive as an emergency may not be what you perceive as one. Often, eliciting the underlying issue requires a little finesse and remaining nonjudgmental. For example, the patient who presents with a rash of 3 weeks' duration at 4 A.M. may actually be a victim of domestic violence. The patient who presents multiple times with a complaint of pain with negative workup may be drug seeking. Because so many patients who present to the ED have underlying social and psychological issues, history taking can be quite challenging. It is important to remain nonjudgmental and provide the best possible care under sometimes less-than-optimal circumstances.
- The 24-hour open door policy of the ED, long waiting times, and uncomfortable waiting environment, along with the stress of high-acuity complaints, predispose to violence in the ED. Students should be aware of their environment and practice personal safety behavior as they would in any other potentially dangerous environment.
- While resuscitations are an exciting opportunity for students to learn and practice procedures, students often forget about universal precautions because of all the excitement, putting themselves at risk for needlestick injury. Remember, ALWAYS wear gloves, NEVER recap needles. Report any exposure to body fluids to the ED attending immediately.

HOW TO DRESS

Every ED will have a dress code. It is in your best interest to find out prior to your first shift what you are expected to wear. If for some reason this is not possible, men should wear any color shirt with tie, pants (not jeans), shoes (not sneakers), and a short white med-student coat. Women should also wear professional attire with the short white coat (no jeans, no sneakers). Although most people wear scrubs, it is not a universal rule that one can wear scrubs in the ED!

However, most departments are usually relaxed about what is acceptable and do allow scrubs, and sneakers/clogs.

WHAT TO DO (HOW TO BEHAVE)

There are a few things we can say about what makes a medical student look good. Generally, a medical student who can handle a resident's/intern's workload in the ED already demonstrates his or her value to the department at an early stage. However, not having the extra year or two of clinical experience a resident may have, this presents a challenge.

It is best to try to emulate an efficient and thorough resident that you may work beside. Every institution has its particular procedures for assigning patients, charting, "starting up" patients, admitting and discharging patients, and ordering labs or radiologic studies. Your efficiency in the department will be markedly improved if you can familiarize yourself with these administrative hurdles early on.

A few general pointers:
- Punctuality speaks for itself. Be the first one to arrive for sign-over rounds, codes, lectures, and grand rounds.
- Know all the important numbers for the department (door and copier codes, pager numbers, etc.).
- Ask the nurses for their help should you need it. They can be valuable allies and generally have the ear of the attendings.
- Be thorough in your history and physical, but presentations should include only the essentials (quick bullet).
- Show an interest in what you are doing (fecal disimpactions can be fun!!).
- Charting: "The chart is your life raft in a sea of litigation!" We guarantee if your document includes these things, you are already ahead of the game:
  - Times of initial evaluation, all orders, repeat exams, radiology/lab results, discharge instructions
  - Chief complaint and a good history *with review of systems*
  - Exam (don't forget the neuro/mental status/rectal exams) and *repeat* exam data as things change
  - Orders must be countersigned by a resident or attending.
  - *Write* the lab, radiology, and electrocardiogram results on the chart.
  - Discharge instructions must include *follow-up* arrangements and instructions for what to *return* for.
  - If a patient wants to sign out against medical advice, notify the attending.

WHAT NOT TO DO

- Be late
- Make up an answer to a question you might not know (just say you don't know)
- Look sloppy
- Seem uninterested
- Turn down the opportunity to do a procedure (even if you've done it before)

WHAT TO READ

Most EDs have a small collection of texts (usually locked up in a rack). If you have the time to read (i.e., the ED isn't that busy), you can read a little in one of the texts on each patient you see. However, *this book* should ultimately be the only one you'll need for the clerkship. If you feel the inevitable need to pore through page after page of medical minutia, you should do it when you are not working in the department. We advise that you write a little bit about each patient you see during your shift and then read up about them when you get home or at the library.

Suggested resources include:
- *Emergency Medicine (A Comprehensive Study Guide)*, 5th ed., Judith Tintinalli, 2127 pages. Designed as board review for residents
- *Pediatric Emergency Medicine (A Comprehensive Study Guide)*, 1st ed., Gary Strange, 728 pages. Designed as board review for residents
- *Clinical Procedures in Emergency Medicine*, 3rd ed., Roberts/Hedges, 1297 pages. A how-to for nearly all procedures you might be doing within the department
- *Emergency Medicine (Concepts and Clinical Practice)*, 4th ed., Rosen/Barkin, 2930 pages. A text resource for reading on the pathophysiology as well as clinical aspects of disease

THE EXAM

The last hoop you will need to jump through before finishing the clerkship will be the exam. Many departments will have their own exam designed for the fourth-year medical student rotator (almost always multiple guess). Some will use a "shelf exam" or one that is almost identical to the one used for resident yearly "in-service" exams. These are sometimes more difficult, but expectations of your performance are a bit lower. Some programs will further torture you by giving you an oral exam. This is a lot like taking the oral board exam as a graduating resident, only less strenuous and with less at stake.

The best strategy for doing well on the written, multiple-choice exam is to do A LOT of practice questions beforehand. *PEER VI* is a collection of questions put out by the ACEP as a board preparation (most like the shelf exam). This is probably your best source of questions as they are written by EM physicians for EM physicians, cover the specialty in appropriate scope and detail, and contain extensive explanations for each question. Your best bet to obtain a copy of *PEER VI* is to ask the residents in the program; someone is bound to have a copy you may borrow. There are a number of commercially published question-and-answer texts that are available but not as good. However, going through this many resources is probably overkill, as this book, *First Aid for the Clinical Clerkship in Emergency Medicine*, will have all the facts you need for both the test and the clerkship.

Seeing as many patients as possible and presenting cases to the attendings and senior residents is the best form of preparation for the oral exam.

A WORD ABOUT RESIDENCIES

ED attendings, residency directors, and department chairpersons will be observing you as a potential resident. You are, in a sense, auditioning for a position in the match. Residents you may work with can be your allies and help you "look good" to the attendings and ultimately attain a residency position (if this is your goal).

You are generally expected to do a rotation in your home hospital's department (the one affiliated with your medical school). Outside of that, it is always a good idea to do a rotation in the hospital you would most like to do your residency. Fall is the best season for this, as it is the beginning of interview season. You will most likely get an interview, barring any medical disasters you may precipitate or gross personality conflicts with the staff. Interviewing after your rotation usually is more of a formality since most of the attendings have already worked with you and know you (see the advantage?).

OK, good luck . . . enjoy the book.

Michael R. Edwards, MD,
Nirav N. Shah, MD,
and the FACC series editors

NOTES

High-Yield Facts

Resuscitation

BASIC LIFE SUPPORT (BLS) (ADULT)

Goal of BLS: Increasing the survival rates of cardiac and respiratory arrest through the training of laypersons to:
- Recognize the symptoms of inadequate circulation or respiration.
- Immediately activate the Emergency Medical Services (EMS).
- Support the circulation and respiration via cardiopulmonary resuscitation (CPR) and rescue breathing.

BLS Protocol (3As)
- **A**ssessment: Determine unresponsiveness of the patient.
- **A**ctivate the EMS system immediately by calling 9-1-1.
- **A**BCs of CPR (airway, breathing, and circulation)

Airway with C-Spine Control

- Position the patient supine on a flat surface using "logroll" technique.
- Open the airway using head tilt–chin lift maneuver or the jaw thrust maneuver.

Breathing

- Look, listen, and feel for breaths (approximately 3 to 5 seconds).
- Perform **rescue breathing** (mouth-to-mouth, etc.):
  - Give two initial breaths 1.5 to 2 seconds.
  - Deliver 10 to 12 breaths per minute.

Circulation

- Determine pulselessness by checking carotid artery pulse. If there is no pulse, begin chest compressions:
  - Proper hand position is on the lower half of the sternum.
  - Sternum should be depressed 1.5 to 2 inches for an adult.
  - Rate of chest compressions should be 80 to 100 per minute.
  - For one-rescuer CPR, ratio is 15 compressions to 2 breaths.
  - For two-rescuer CPR, ratio is 5 compressions to 1 breath.

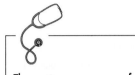

The most common cause of sudden cardiac death in adults is ventricular fibrillation (V-fib).

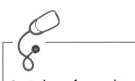

Survival rates from cardiac arrest are highest when BLS is initiated within 4 minutes and advanced cardiac life support (ACLS) is initiated within 8 minutes.

The **tongue** is the most common cause of airway obstruction in the unconscious victim.

Foreign body airway obstruction should be considered in any victim who suddenly becomes cyanotic and stops breathing, especially children.

In adults, poorly chewed meat is the most common cause of foreign body obstruction.

The **Heimlich maneuver** is the recommended method of expelling a foreign object from the airway.

A **finger sweep** should be attempted only in an unconscious victim, and never attempted in a seizure patient.

Risk Factors

- Large, poorly chewed pieces of food
- Excessive alcohol intake
- Dentures
- Children swallowing small objects (toys, beads, marbles, thumbtacks)
- Children eating foods that require adequate chewing (hot dogs, peanuts, popcorn, candy)
- Children running/playing while eating

Management of Partial Airway Obstruction

Do not interfere with any choking victim who is able to cough or speak. Coughing is the most effective way to clear a foreign body from the airway, and the ability to speak indicates that adequate ventilation is still occurring.

Signs of Complete Airway Obstruction

- High-pitched, stridorous sounds during inhalation
- Weak and ineffective coughing
- Respiratory distress
- Inability to speak
- Cyanosis

Heimlich Maneuver

In a Standing (Conscious) Victim
- Stand behind victim and wrap arms around waist.
- Make fist and place thumb of fist slightly above the navel of the victim's abdomen.
- Grasp fist with the other hand and quickly thrust inward and upward into victim's abdomen.
- Repeat until object is dislodged or patient becomes unconscious.

In an Unconscious Victim
- Lay victim supine.
- Straddle victim, place heel of palm just above navel (well below the xiphoid), and deliver quick inward and upward abdominal thrusts (up to five).
- Open the mouth of the unconscious victim and perform a **finger sweep** using a hooking motion of the index finger along the base of the tongue to dislodge the foreign body.
- Reposition the head and attempt rescue breathing.
- Repeat the sequence of the Heimlich maneuver, finger sweep, and rescue breathing attempts until victim resumes breathing or definitive help arrives.

Goals

To provide rapid assessment and definitive management of the cardiac arrest situation using cardiac monitoring equipment, advanced airway management, as well as electrical and pharmacologic therapy

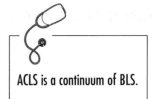

ACLS is a continuum of BLS.

Primary Survey

Focus on the ABCs of CPR and keep in mind defibrillation.

First "A-B-C-D"
- Airway—open the airway (maintaining C-spine control).
- Breathing—assess breathlessness and provide rescue breathing.
- Circulation—give chest compressions (CPR).
- Defibrillation—shock ventricular fibrillation and pulseless ventricular tachycardia.

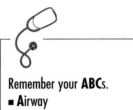

Remember your **ABC**s.
- ■ **A**irway
- ■ **B**reathing
- ■ **C**irculation
Don't forget to **D**efibrillate.

Secondary Survey

Secondary survey of ACLS focuses on the same ABCs in more detail: Establishing a definitive airway, establishing access to the circulation, assessing cardiac rhythms, pharmacologic interventions, etc.

Second "A-B-C-D"
- Airway—perform endotracheal intubation.
- Breathing—assess bilateral chest rise and bilateral breath sounds.
- Circulation—establish intravenous (IV) access, determine the cardiac rhythm, and give the appropriate medication for that rhythm.
- Differential diagnosis—why did the arrest occur? Are there any causes that are reversible and have a specific therapy?

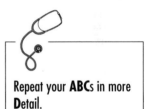

Repeat your **ABC**s in more Detail.

Airway

- **Nasal airway**—rubber nasal trumpet inserted into the nostril and passed into the posterior pharynx keeps the tongue from falling back and obstructing the airway.
- **Oral airway**—curved rigid airway, inserted using a tongue blade so that the distal edge prevents the tongue from falling backward. Often *incorrectly* used as a "bite block." Should be used only in unconscious patients with absent gag reflexes (i.e., it will cause gagging if any gag reflex remains).
- **Endotracheal intubation**—establishes a definitive airway that also protects against aspiration of blood, vomit, and pharyngeal secretions. Several cardiac medications can be given directly through the endotracheal tube (ETT). Usual ETT dose is 2 to 2.5 times the IV dose followed by 10 mL of normal saline flush and several ventilations by bag-valve ventilation.

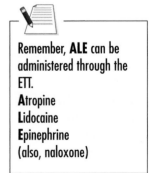

Remember, **ALE** can be administered through the ETT.
Atropine
Lidocaine
Epinephrine
(also, naloxone)

11

Breathing

- Assess the status of ventilations after intubation (listen for equal breath sounds over both lung fields and make sure there are no sounds of gastric insufflation) and adjust the tube as necessary.
- Assess the movement of the chest wall with ventilations.
- If in a hospital setting, obtain a STAT portable chest x-ray (CXR).
- If available, confirm ETT placement with an end-tidal CO_2 monitor.
- If there is any doubt of placement, consider extubation and reintubation under direct visualization with a laryngoscope.

Circulation

- Establish IV access (easiest access is usually the antecubital vein).
- *Normal saline* is the fluid of choice in the resuscitation setting.
- Determine cardiac rhythm.

Differential Diagnosis

- Continually ask yourself, "What caused this arrest?"
- Examine the rhythm and consider all the possible causes.
- Treat each of those possible causes that are reversible and/or have a specific therapy.

Classification of Therapeutic Interventions

2000 National Conference on CPR and Emergency Cardiovascular Care (ECC)

- **Class I**—a therapeutic option that is usually indicated, always helpful; considered useful and effective
- **Class II**—a therapeutic option that is acceptable, is of uncertain efficacy; may be controversial:
  - **Class IIa**—a therapeutic option for which the weight of evidence is in favor of its usefulness and efficacy
  - **Class IIb**—a therapeutic option that is not well established by evidence but may be helpful and probably not harmful
- **Class III**—a therapeutic option that is inappropriate, is without specific supporting data, and may be harmful

VENTRICULAR FIBRILLATION OR PULSELESS VENTRICULAR TACHYCARDIA (VF/VT)

VF and Pulseless VT Algorithm

Remember, a "shock" is administered after each medication given, and CPR is continued.

- It is essential to remember that early defibrillation is the most important therapy for this rhythm. (See Figures 2-1 and 2-2.)
- Defibrillation should take precedence over establishing IV access, intubation, or the administration of any drug!
- ABCs (always begin with assessing your ABCs!!!)
- Initiate and continue CPR until defibrillator is attached.
- Defibrillate (shock) × 3 (200J, 300J, 360J).

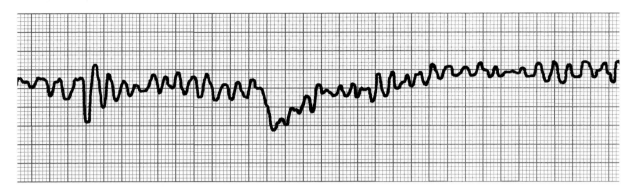

FIGURE 2-1. Ventricular fibrillation.

- **Epinephrine** 1 mg IV q 3–5 minutes or **vasopressin** 40 U IV × 1
- **Amiodarone** 150 mg IV
- **Lidocaine** 1 to 1.5 mg/kg IV; can repeat once
- **Magnesium sulfate** 1 to 2 g IV
- **Procainamide** 30 mg/min, max total dose 17 mg/kg
- **Sodium bicarbonate** 1 mg/kg IV ("1 amp")

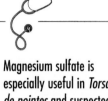

Magnesium sulfate is especially useful in *Torsade de pointes* and suspected hypomagnesemia; it should be given whenever these etiologies are suspected.

PULSELESS ELECTRICAL ACTIVITY (PEA)

Definition

- Any arrhythmia other than VF or VT in which there is an undetectable pulse
- The differential diagnosis for PEA is key because certain etiologies of PEA have specific treatments and therefore the arrhythmia may be easily reversible.

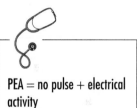

PEA = no pulse + electrical activity
(just like it sounds)

PEA Algorithm

1. ABCs, O$_2$, IV access, cardiac monitor, pulse oximetry, ECG, portable CXR
2. Confirm pulselessness by Doppler ultrasound (if available).
3. CPR

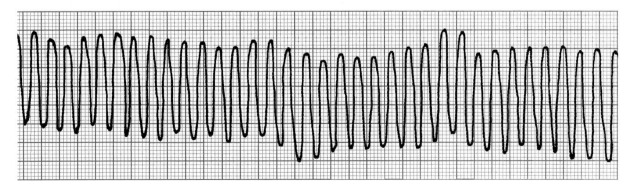

FIGURE 2-2. Ventricular tachycardia.

4. Consider possible causes of PEA (and specific treatments).
5. Epinephrine 1 mg IV, repeat q 3–5 minutes
6. Atropine 1 mg IV, repeat q 3 minutes, max total dose 0.03 to 0.04 mg/kg

Remember that cute lab partner in gross anatomy?
HOT MATCH MD
- **H**ypovolemia (volume — normal saline infusion)
- Hyp**o**xia (oxygen, intubation, ventilation)
- Hypo**t**hermia (warmed normal saline infusion)
- **M**assive pulmonary embolism (thrombolytics)
- **A**cidosis (sodium bicarbonate)
- **T**ension pneumothorax (needle decompression)
- **C**ardiac tamponade (pericardiocentesis)
- **H**yperkalemia (calcium sodium bicarbonate)
- Massive acute **M**yocardial infarction (percutaneous transluminal coronary angioplasty, thrombolysis)
- **D**rug overdose from tricyclic antidepressants (TCAs), digoxin, beta blockers, calcium channel blockers

ASYSTOLE

Definition

- A "flatline" rhythm is indicative of the absence of any electrical activity of the heart.
- The most common cause of a flatline tracing on ECG is a detached lead or malfunctioning equipment, not asystole; therefore, always confirm asystole in more than one lead!
- Asystole is always pulseless.
- Never shock asystole (no matter what you see on TV).

Asystole Algorithm

1. ABCs, O_2, IV access, cardiac monitor, pulse oximetry, ECG, portable CXR
2. CPR
3. Consider possible causes.
4. Consider immediate transcutaneous pacing (Class IIb).
5. **Epinephrine** 1 mg IV push q 3–5 minutes. If this fails, intermediate-dose epi (2 to 5 mg IV q 3–5 minutes), escalating-dose epi (1 mg, 3 mg, 5 mg IV 3 minutes apart), high-dose epi (0.1 mg/kg IV push q 3–5 minutes)—all Class IIb therapies.
6. **Atropine** 1 mg IV push q 3–5 minutes
7. Consider **sodium bicarbonate** (1 mEq/kg) if known preexisting bicarbonate-responsive acidosis, if TCA overdose suspected, or if attempting to alkalinize urine for appropriate drug overdoses.
8. Consider termination of efforts.

Asystole = no pulse + no electrical activity.
Always confirm flatline in more than one lead.
Never shock asystole.

BRADYCARDIA

Definition

- Defined as heart rate < 60 beats per minute
- It is considered symptomatic or "unstable" when accompanied by hypotension, shock, congestive heart failure (CHF), pulmonary edema, shortness of breath, cyanosis, lethargy, or chest pain.

Bradycardia Algorithm

- ABCs, O_2, IV access, cardiac monitor, pulse oximetry, ECG, portable CXR
- Call for transcutaneous pacer to bedside earlier rather than later.

Treatment of Unstable Bradycardia

1. **Atropine** 0.5 to 1 mg IVP q 3–5 minutes, max dose 0.04 mg/kg (remember that transplanted hearts are *denervated* and will not respond to atropine, go straight to pacing)
2. **Transcutaneous pacing (TCP)** (this is *painful,* use sedation and/or analgesia as needed) verifying electrical capture and mechanical contractions
3. **Dopamine** 5 to 20 μg/kg/min—titrate to acceptable heart rate (HR) and blood pressure (BP).
4. **Epinephrine** 2 to 10 μg/min—titrate to acceptable HR and BP.
5. Prepare for **transvenous pacing.**

TACHYCARDIA

Definition

- Any rhythm in which the heart is beating faster than 100 times per minute
- As with bradycardia, treatment of tachydysrhythmia is largely dictated by the severity of the signs and symptoms.
- If serious signs and symptoms are present, you should ask whether the tachycardia is causing the symptoms or is an underlying symptom causing the tachycardia.

ATRIAL FIBRILLATION AND ATRIAL FLUTTER

See Figures 8-7 and 8-8 (cardiovascular emergencies chapter) for ECGs of atrial fibrillation and atrial flutter.

Atrial Fibrillation/Flutter Algorithm

1. ABCs, O$_2$, IV access, cardiac monitor, pulse oximetry, ECG, portable CXR
2. Decide if *stable* or *unstable.*
3. If unstable, administer **synchronized cardioversion** (start at 50J for atrial flutter, 100J, 200J, 300J, 360J).
4. If stable, pharmacologic interventions include:
   - **Diltiazem** 0.25 mg/kg IV slowly over 2 minutes
   - Wait 15 minutes.
   - **Diltiazem** 0.35 mg/kg IV slowly over 2 minutes
   - Wait 15 minutes.
   - If no result, consider short-acting beta blocker (cautiously use beta blockers only after enough time has passed since last dose of calcium channel blockers):
     - **Metoprolol** 5 mg IV q 5 minutes × 3
     - **Esmolol** 500 μg/kg IV over 1 minute (loading dose), then 50 to 200 μg/kg/min infusion
     - **Atenolol** 2.5 to 5.0 mg IV over 2 minutes

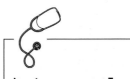

Presence of second- or third-degree heart block with bradycardia also makes it "unstable."

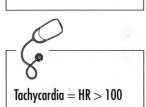

Atropine may convert Type II second-degree block into complete heart block; thus, TCP is indicated.

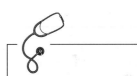

Tachycardia = HR > 100

Awake patients should be sedated prior to synchronized cardioversion with opiates and/or benzodiazepines.

- **Digoxin** 0.5 mg IV or PO × 1
- **Verapamil** 5 to 10 mg IV, wait 30 minutes, may repeat
- **Procainamide** 20 to 30 mg/min IV, max dose 17 mg/kg
- **Quinidine** 200 to 400 mg IV or PO
- Anticoagulation

PAROXYSMAL SUPRAVENTRICULAR TACHYCARDIA (PSVT)

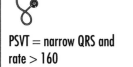

PSVT = narrow QRS and rate > 160

Definition

- Heart rate usually > 160 beats per minute
- Usually demonstrates a narrow QRS complex (< 0.10 second) on ECG (see Figure 2-3)

PSVT Algorithm

1. ABCs, O$_2$, IV access, cardiac monitor, pulse oximetry, ECG, portable CXR
2. Decide if *stable* or *unstable*.
3. If unstable, synchronized cardioversion (50J, 100J, 200J, 300J, then 360J)
4. If stable, proceed as follows:
   - **Vagal maneuvers:** Valsalva; carotid massage (listen first for bruits); ice water bath (not if history of MI)

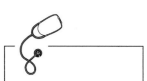

Avoid *carotid massage* if bruits present.
Avoid *ice bath* if history of myocardial infarction (MI).
Push adenosine *rapidly* with an immediate saline flush.
The biggest mistake when using adenosine is it is *not pushed rapidly enough*.

Adenosine feels like a *mule kick* to the chest—warn patients prior to giving it.

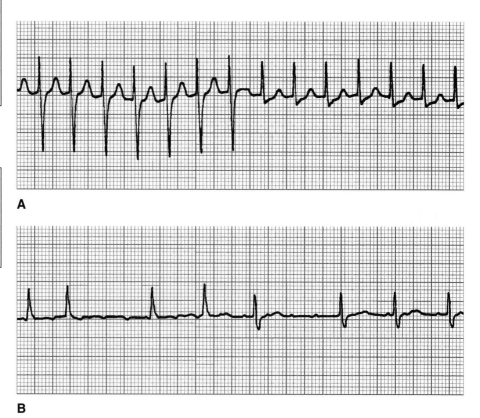

FIGURE 2-3. Paroxysmal supraventricular tachycardia. **A.** PSVT with 1:1 conduction. **B.** PSVT with variable conduction.

- **Adenosine** 6 mg *rapid* IV push
- Important: Wait 1 to 2 minutes.
- **Adenosine** 12 mg rapid IV push, repeat after 1 to 2 minutes
5. If tachycardia persists, analyze QRS complex on ECG and rhythm strip:
    - If **wide complex tachycardia** (and patient remains stable):
        - **Lidocaine** 1.0 to 1.5 mg/kg IV push
        - Lidocaine 0.5 to 0.75 mg/kg IV push q 5 minutes, max total dose 3 mg/kg
        - Procainamide 20 to 30 mg/min, max total 17 mg/kg
        - Synchronized cardioversion (50J, 100J, 200J, 300J, 360J)
    - If **narrow complex tachycardia** (and patient remains stable):
        - **Verapamil** 2.5 to 5.0 mg IV
        - Wait 15 to 30 minutes.
        - Verapamil 5 to 10 mg IV
        - Consider short-acting beta blockers, digoxin, diltiazem as in the atrial fibrillation algorithm.
6. If at any time the patient becomes unstable, proceed directly to synchronized cardioversion.

Definition

- Rate > 100 beats per minute
- **Widened QRS** complex
- Readily converts to ventricular fibrillation (BAD!)
- If pulseless VT, proceed immediately with defibrillation (remember VF/pulseless VT algorithm).

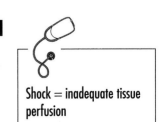

VT = wide QRS + rate > 100

VT with Pulse Algorithm

1. ABCs, O_2, IV access, cardiac monitor, pulse oximetry, ECG, portable CXR
2. Decide if stable or unstable.
3. If unstable, immediate synchronized cardioversion (100J, 200J, 300J, 360J)
4. If stable:
    - **Amiodarone** 150 mg IV bolus over 10 minutes or **lidocaine** 0.5 to 0.75 mg/kg IVP q 3–5 minutes (total max dose 3 mg/kg)
    - Procainamide 20 to 30 mg/min (max dose 17 mg/kg) may be used in patients with normal ejection fraction only.
    - Synchronized cardioversion (100J, 200J, 300J, 360J)

HYPOTENSION AND SHOCK

Shock = inadequate tissue perfusion

Definitions

- **Hypotension** is generally defined as an SBP < 100 and a DBP < 60.
- **Shock** is defined as inadequate tissue perfusion.

HIGH-YIELD FACTS

Resuscitation

These topics will be covered elsewhere, but they are included in the ACLS course and will therefore be discussed (briefly).

Causes

In order to rapidly assess a hypotensive patient, it is often helpful to divide the causes of shock into three etiologies.

Rate Problems
- Bradyarrhythmias:
  - Sinus bradycardia
  - Second- and third-degree heart block
  - Pacemaker failures
- Tachyarrhythmias:
  - Sinus tachycardia
  - Atrial flutter
  - Atrial fibrillation
  - PSVT
  - Ventricular tachycardia

Pump Problems
- Primary pump failure:
  - Myocardial infarction
  - Myocarditis
  - Cardiomyopathies
  - Ruptured chordae or papillary muscle damage
  - Aortic or mitral regurgitation/failure
  - Septal defect/damage
- Secondary pump failure:
  - Cardiac tamponade
  - Pulmonary embolism
  - Superior vena cava syndrome
  - Cardiodepressant drugs

Volume Problems
- Volume loss:
  - Blood loss
  - Gastrointestinal (GI) losses (vomiting, diarrhea, etc.)
  - Urine output
  - Third-space losses
- Decreased vascular resistance:
  - Central nervous system (CNS) or spinal injury
  - Sepsis
  - Vasodilatory drugs
  - Adrenal insufficiency

ADVANCED AIRWAY MANAGEMENT

Rapid Sequence Intubation Algorithm

1. Prepare the necessary equipment:
   - IV access, cardiac monitor, pulse oximetry
   - Bag-valve mask (Ambu bag)

- Suction equipment (make sure it works!)
- Laryngoscope with blade (check lightbulb!)
- ETT (7.0 adult female/8.0 adult male)
- Insert ETT stylet (if desired).
- Medications
- Prepare adjunct airway (laryngeal mask airway, cricothyroidotomy tray, etc.) in case ETT is unsuccessful.

2. Pretreat:
   - Lidocaine for head injury patients (decreases intracranial pressure)
   - Atropine for children (prevents bradycardia)

3. Position the patient:
   - Raise bed to height appropriate for intubation.
   - Place head in "sniffing position" with neck extended (except when C-spine injury suspected).

4. Preoxygenate the patient:
   - Bag-valve mask with 100% oxygen
   - Pulse oximetry should read 100%.
   - Hyperventilate patient to accomplish nitrogen washout.

5. Pressure on cricothyroid cartilage:
   - Sellick maneuver compresses esophagus to limit risk of aspiration.

6. Sedation: Many agents are available including:
   - Etomidate (does not cause hypotension, quite safe)
   - Thiopental (barbiturate, can cause hypotension)
   - Midazolam (benzodiazepine, quite safe)

7. Paralyze the patient:
   - Succinylcholine (1.5 mg/kg IVP) onset 45 to 60 seconds, duration 5 to 10 minutes. Do not use in hyperkalemia, crush injuries, or history of neuromuscular diseases.
   - Vecuronium (0.1 mg/kg IVP) onset 2 to 3 minutes, duration 25 to 30 minutes

8. Place the tube:
   - Open the mouth and displace the jaw inferiorly.
   - Holding the laryngoscope in the left hand, insert the blade along the right side of the tongue, and the tongue is swept toward the left.
   - If using a curved (Macintosh) blade, the tip should be inserted to the vallecula (the space between the base of the tongue and the epiglottis).
   - If using a straight (Miller) blade, the tip is inserted beneath the epiglottis.
   - The laryngoscope is the used to *lift* the tongue, soft tissues, and epiglottis to reveal the vocal cords (remember, it is a *lifting* motion, not a *rocking* motion).
   - Upon direct visualization of the cords, the tube is directed through the cords, the stylet (if used) is removed, the tube is connected to an oxygen source, and it is secured after proper placement is confirmed.

9. Confirm position of the tube by two methods:
   - Bilateral breath sounds (check both apical lung fields!)
   - Absence of breath sounds in abdomen
   - End-tidal carbon dioxide detection
   - Portable CXR
   - Condensation in ETT corresponding to bag-valve mask breaths

Prepare = equipment
Pretreat = drugs
Position = sniffing position
Preoxygenate = pulse oximetry of 100%
Pressure = Sellick maneuver
Paralyze = drugs
Placement of the tube
Position of tube = confirm by two methods

Resuscitation

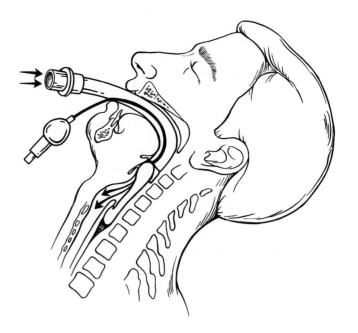

FIGURE 2-4. Laryngeal mask airway.

(Reproduced, with permission, from Tintinalli JE, Kelen GD, Stapczynski JS. *Emergency Medicine: A Comprehensive Study Guide,* 5th ed. New York: McGraw-Hill, 2000.)

LARYNGEAL MASK AIRWAY

- The **laryngeal mask airway** is an airway tube fitted with an inflatable cuff that acts as a mask when fitted directly over the larynx (see Figure 2-4).
- It is an effective adjunct when faced with a difficult airway in which endotracheal intubation was unsuccessful.
- It is inserted blindly into the hypopharynx and is advanced downward against the larynx.
- The cuff is then inflated, forming a seal over the larynx and permitting positive pressure ventilation.
- Since this airway merely rests on top of the larynx, it is not considered a secure airway; air leaks often occur (especially with rapid or forced ventilation, or with repositioning of the patient), and it does not prevent aspiration.
- However, it is an easy technique to learn, and it provides a very useful temporizing measure until a more definitive airway can be established.

NEEDLE CRICOTHYROIDOTOMY

Definition

- Temporizing measure to provide oxygen to a patient emergently after a failed or impossible endotracheal intubation
- The procedure entails inserting a large-bore angiocatheter through the cricothyroid membrane (see Figure 2-5) and providing oxygen through the catheter.
- It is important to note that while oxygen delivery can be established

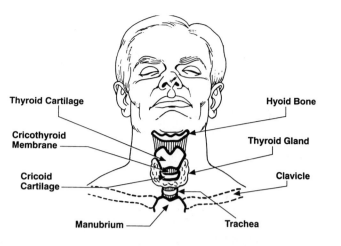

FIGURE 2-5. Anatomical landmarks for needle and surgical cricothyroidotomy.

with this procedure, adequate elimination of carbon dioxide is not achieved.

Needle Cricothyroidotomy Algorithm

1. Prep area with alcohol and povidone–iodine (Betadine).
2. Hyperextend neck (if no C-spine injury is suspected).
3. Identify cricothyroid membrane.
4. Insert 14-gauge angiocatheter on a syringe at 45° angle (toward feet) through cricothyroid membrane.
5. Advance with negative pressure until air is freely aspirated.
6. Remove needle and advance angiocatheter.
7. Use a syringe to verify placement in trachea.
8. Attach adapter from ETT and ventilate with bag-valve delivery system.

SURGICAL CRICOTHYROIDOTOMY

Definition

- Allows for rapid establishment of an airway once endotracheal intubation has failed or is impossible (e.g., severe facial trauma, burns, impacted obstruction)
- Permits both oxygen delivery and ventilation for elimination of carbon dioxide

Indications and Contraindications

Indications
- Whenever unable to obtain an airway by orotracheal or nasotracheal intubation due to anatomic distortion, massive hemorrhage, or severe aspiration
- When severe maxillofacial trauma renders other airways impossible

- Upper airway obstruction due to foreign body
- Massive upper airway edema

Contraindications
- Age under 5 to 10 years, depending on child's size
- Significant injury to larynx or cricoid
- Tracheal transection
- Expanding hematoma over the cricothyroid membrane
- Preexisting laryngeal pathology

Surgical Cricothyroidotomy Algorithm

1. Prep area with alcohol and povidone–iodine (Betadine).
2. Hyperextend neck (if no C-spine injury is suspected).
3. Identify cricothyroid membrane.
4. Holding a #10 scalpel at the hub of the blade, make a horizontal stab through the skin and cricoid membrane (hold at the hub to ensure the stab incision does not go too deep!).
5. Enlarge the stab incision to approximately 1.5 to 2.0 cm with a horizontal motion of the scalpel.
6. Keeping the scalpel in place, insert a tracheal hook next to the scalpel and retract the larynx.
7. Remove the scalpel.
8. Using the scalpel handle, or a dilator, dilate the surgical opening.
9. Place a tracheostomy tube into the opening, secure the airway, and ventilate with bag-valve oxygen delivery system.

Complications

Esophageal perforation, hemorrhage, subcutaneous emphysema, vocal cord injury

Diagnostics

LABORATORY TESTS

- Laboratory examinations are perhaps the most variable aspect of Emergency Medicine.
- The labs ordered for a patient differ greatly from one physician to another.
- In general, in the emergency department (ED), a test should not be ordered unless it will change your management of a patient.

Electrolytes

CALCIUM

- Over 99% of the calcium in the body is found in the bony skeleton.
- Remaining calcium is either protein bound (albumin, etc.), polyvalent (bound to phosphate, etc.), or ionized.
- Parathyroid hormone and calcitonin are counterregulatory hormones that respond to levels of ionized Ca.
- Vitamin D metabolites (calcitriol) are synthesized in liver/kidney in response to decreased calcium levels.

IONIZED CALCIUM

- Is most important physiologically
- Hypoalbuminemia will decrease total calcium, but ionized calcium is unaffected.
- Acid–base disorders (alkalosis) will decrease ionized calcium.

Hypercalcemia

SIGNS AND SYMPTOMS

- Neurologic: Weakness, fatigue, ataxia, altered mental status, seizures (rare)
- Gastrointestinal (GI): Decreased motility (constipation), vomiting
- Renal: Osmotic diuresis (polyuria), polydipsia, nephrolithiasis, potassium/magnesium losses
- Cardiovascular: Bradycardia, heart blocks, shortened QT interval, potentiates digoxin

Signs of hypercalcemia:
- Bones (bony pain)
- Stones (kidney stones)
- Groans (abdominal pain)
- Psychiatric overtones (change in mental status)

Chvostek's sign: Tapping facial nerve below zygomatic arch induces tetany of facial muscles.

Trousseau's sign: Inflating blood pressure (BP) cuff above systolic BP for 3 minutes induces carpal spasm.

TREATMENT

Aimed at correcting dehydration and promoting urinary excretion of calcium:
- Rehydrate with large amounts of intravenous (IV) saline until volume status is restored.
- Furosemide to promote diuresis once volume status is restored is controversial.
- Electrolytes must be monitored carefully (hypokalemia/hypomagnesemia).
- Dialysis in the setting of renal failure

Hypocalcemia

CAUSES

- Hypoalbuminemia (cirrhosis, nephrotic syndrome)
- Hypoparathyroidism (intrinsic or post-thyroid surgery), malnutrition (rickets/osteomalacia)
- Pancreatitis (saponification)
- Drugs (cimetidine)

PATHOPHYSIOLOGY

Neuronal membranes become more excitable secondary to increased sodium permeability.

SIGNS AND SYMPTOMS

- Perioral and digital paresthesias
- Decreased myocardial contractility (relaxation is inhibited) can predispose to congestive heart failure (CHF).

DIAGNOSIS

Electrocardiogram (ECG) characteristically shows prolonged QT intervals (see Figure 3-1).

TREATMENT

Supplement calcium:
- Asymptomatic patients should be given oral calcium (with or without vitamin D).

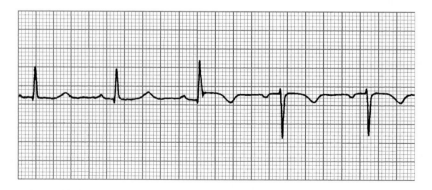

FIGURE 3-1. Prolonged QT.

- Symptomatic patients should be treated with IV calcium (Ca gluconate or Ca chloride).

Potassium

- Potassium is the intracellular cation (98% of total body potassium is intracellular).
- Intracellular K = 110 to 150, extracellular K = 3.5 to 5.0; gradient is critical for normal function.
- Potassium is excreted primarily in urine (small amount in feces, sweat).
- Renin–angiotensin–aldosterone axis regulates potassium secretion in distal tubules.

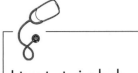

Interpret potassium levels in the context of serum pH: Acidosis causes potassium shift into serum; alkalosis causes potassium shift into cells.

Hypokalemia

CAUSES AND PATHOPHYSIOLOGY

Three mechanisms for decreased potassium:
- Intracellular shifts (alkalotic states, administration of insulin and glucose)
- Reduced intake (malnutrition)
- Increased losses (renal—diuretics, hyperaldosteronism; GI—vomiting, diarrhea, fistulas)

SIGNS AND SYMPTOMS

- Muscle weakness
- Hyporeflexia
- Intestinal ileus
- Respiratory paralysis
- Nephrogenic diabetes insipidus
- Dehydration

DIAGNOSIS

Hypokalemia results in hyperpolarization of cell membrane potential leading to:
- Cardiac abnormalities on ECG include flattened T waves, U waves (see Figure 3-2), low-voltage QRS, and prolonged QT and PR.
- Hypokalemia potentiates digitalis and increases likelihood of digitalis toxicity (arrhythmias and atrioventricular blocks).

TREATMENT

Supplement potassium:
- Mild hypokalemia: Potassium-rich foods or oral KCl supplements
- Severe hypokalemia: Treat with IV KCl (10 mEq/hr, max 40 mEq/hr)

Hyperkalemia

CAUSES

- Lab error: Hemolysis, thrombocytosis, leukocytosis, polycythemia
- Decreased excretion: Oliguric renal failure, angiotensin-converting enzyme inhibitors, K-sparing diuretics, type IV renal tubular acidosis

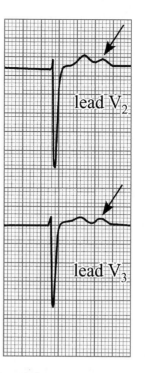

FIGURE 3-2. U waves (arrows) of hypokalemia.

- Increased release: Metabolic acidosis, trauma, burns, rhabdomyolysis, tumor lysis, succinylcholine
- Increased intake: Iatrogenic, dietary, salt substitutes

SIGNS AND SYMPTOMS

- GI: Nausea, vomiting, diarrhea
- Neurologic: Muscle cramps, weakness, paresthesias, paralysis, areflexia, tetany, focal neurologic deficits, confusion
- Respiratory insufficiency
- Cardiac arrest

DIAGNOSIS

ECG Findings
- At K = 5.0 to 6.0, rapid repolarization causes peaked T waves (most prominent in precordium) (see Figure 3-3).
- At K = 6.0 to 6.5, decrease in conduction causes prolonged PR and QT intervals.
- At K = 6.5 to 7.0, P waves are diminished and ST segment may be depressed.
- At K = 7.0 to 8.0, P waves disappear, QRS widens, and irregular idioventricular rhythm appears.
- At K = 8.0 to 10.0, QRS merges with T wave to produce classic sine wave.
- At K = 10.0 to 12.0, ventricular fibrillation and diastolic arrest occur.

TREATMENT

- Calcium gluconate: Stabilizes cardiac membrane, onset of action 1 to 3 minutes

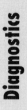

Patients on digitalis should be given calcium only in emergencies; calcium in the setting of digitalis toxicity may induce tetany and "stone heart."

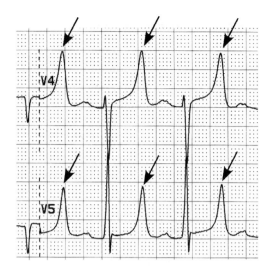

FIGURE 3-3. Peaked T waves (arrows) of hyperkalemia.

- Sodium bicarbonate: Alkalosis shifts potassium into cells, onset 5 to 10 minutes.
- Insulin and glucose: Insulin drives potassium and glucose into cells, onset 30 minutes.
- Lasix: Promotes renal excretion of potassium, onset with diuresis
- Kayexalate: Cation exchange resin (potassium for sodium in GI tract), onset 1 to 2 hours
- Dialysis: Peritoneal or hemodialysis removes potassium at time of dialysis.
- Dialysis is indicated for patients in renal failure with hyperkalemia that does not respond to above.

Sodium

- Ninety-eight percent of total body sodium is in extracellular fluid.
- Sodium is the major contributor to serum osmolarity.
- $S_{osm} = 2(Na) + (glucose/18) + (BUN/2.8)$
- Balance between sodium, water, and osmolarity is regulated by kidney (excretion and reabsorption of sodium and water), posterior pituitary (secretion of antidiuretic hormone), and the hypothalamus (thirst center).
- Understanding the relationship between osmolarity (tonicity) and volume is essential:
    - Volume status is a clinical diagnosis.
    - Tonicity is a laboratory diagnosis.
- Understanding where you are in terms of volume and tonicity allows you to guide therapy appropriately (see Table 3-1).

Hyponatremia

CAUSES

Hyponatremia is subdivided into three categories based on the serum osmolarity:

1. **Hypotonic hyponatremia** is further subdivided into three categories:

> The most common cause of hyponatremia is hemodilution.

TABLE 3-1. Sodium Balance: Volume vs. Tonicity

Volume	Tonicity		
	Hypertonic	**Isotonic**	**Hypotonic**
Hypervolemic	Iatrogenic	Early CHF, cirrhosis, nephrotic syndrome (no ADH stimulus)	Late CHF, cirrhosis, nephrotic syndrome (with ADH stimulus)
Euvolemic	Early stages of "dehydration"	Normal	Psychogenic polydipsia, SIADH "reset osmostat"
Hypovolemic	Late stages of "dehydration" (H_2O loss > salt loss)	Acute volume loss (i.e., burns, bleeding) (no ADH stimulus)	Chronic volume loss (with ADH stimulus) diuretics, Addison's

- Isovolemic/hypotonic hyponatremia: Renal failure, syndrome of inappropriate antidiuretic hormone (SIADH), glucocorticoid deficiency (hypopituitarism), hypothyroidism, and medications
- Hypovolemic/hypotonic hyponatremia:
  - Renal losses (diuretics, partial urinary tract obstruction, salt-wasting nephropathies)
  - Extrarenal losses (vomiting, diarrhea, extensive burns, third spacing, pancreatitis, peritonitis)
  - Hypervolemic/hypotonic hyponatremia: CHF, nephrotic syndrome, cirrhosis
2. **Isotonic hyponatremia** (normal serum osmolarity):
  - Pseudohyponatremia (discussed later)
  - Isotonic infusions (glucose, mannitol)
3. **Hypertonic hyponatremia** (increased serum osmolarity):
  - Hyperglycemia: Each 100 mL/dL increase in serum glucose above normal decreases plasma sodium concentration by 1.6 mEq/L.
  - Hypertonic infusions: Mannitol, glucose

PATHOPHYSIOLOGY

Severity is dependent on both the magnitude and rapidity of the fall in serum sodium:
- Initial response to low serum sodium is to shift water across blood–brain barrier into the central nervous system (CNS).
- CNS responds by shifting sodium and other osmotic agents from brain into cerebrospinal fluid to systemic circulation.
- If hyponatremia is corrected too quickly, CNS loses its ability to retain water (loss of osmotic agents).
- Brain rapidly becomes dehydrated, leading to osmotic demyelination syndrome, also known as central pontine myelinolysis (seen days after therapy; presents with bulbar dysfunction, quadriparesis, delirium, death).

SIGNS AND SYMPTOMS

- Early: Nonspecific headache, vomiting
- Late: Confusion, seizures, coma, bradycardia, or respiratory arrest

TREATMENT

- In symptomatic patients with severe (< 120 mEq/L) hyponatremia, consider hypertonic (3%) saline. Usually, normal saline is good enough.

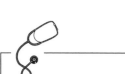

Pseudohyponatremia is present when glucose levels are elevated. Correct 1.6 mEq/L for every 100 mg/dL over 200.

Pseudohyponatremia is caused by:
- Hyperglycemia
- Hyperlipidemia
- Hyperproteinemia
The serum osmolarity will be normal or high in these cases.

- Patients with acute hyponatremia should be corrected no faster than 1.0 mEq/L/hr.
- Patients with chronic hyponatremia should be corrected no faster than 0.5 mEq/L/hr.
- Electrolytes must be checked every 1 to 2 hours; never correct above Na = 120 mEq/L.
- Furosemide should be given with 3% saline to blunt ADH stimulus (maintain negative H_2O balance).

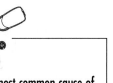

Correcting the sodium too quickly can result in central pontine myelinolysis, seizures, and cerebral edema.

Hypernatremia

CAUSES

- GI losses: Vomiting, diarrhea, decreased thirst
- Renal losses: Diabetes insipidus, osmotic diuretics, adrenal/renal disease
- Insensible losses: Respiratory, skin, hyperthermia

The most common cause of hypernatremia is decrease in total body water (i.e., dehydration).

SIGNS AND SYMPTOMS

- Early signs (Na > 158 mEq/L) include irritability, lethargy, anorexia, and vomiting.
- As serum osmolarity rises (350 to 400), begin to see ataxia, tremulousness, hypertonicity, and spasms.
- At serum osmolarity > 430, death usually ensues.

TREATMENT

- First step is to address fluid status: Hydrate with normal saline (NS) until volume is restored.
- Once perfusion is established, hydrate with hypotonic (0.45%) saline.
- Monitor urine output (0.5 mL/kg/hr) and check electrolytes every few hours.
- Target should be to correct sodium over 48 to 72 hours (max rate of 0.5 mEq/L/hr).

SIADH

PATHOPHYSIOLOGY

- Thirst mechanism and ADH work together to control intake/excretion of water.
- Both mechanisms are usually impaired before SIADH becomes clinically apparent (excess ADH → water retention, thirst → increased fluid intake).

CAUSES

CNS
- Head trauma, tumors, abscesses, meningitis, subarachnoid hemorrhage

Tumors
- Lung, pancreas, ovaries, lymphoma, thymoma

Pulmonary
- Pneumonia, chronic obstructive pulmonary disease (COPD), tuberculosis, cystic fibrosis, abscess

Drugs
- Opiates, nonsteroidal anti-inflammatory drugs, monoamine oxidase inhibitors, tricyclic antidepressants

Other
- Hypothyroidism, adrenal insufficiency, porphyria, idiopathic

DIAGNOSIS

SIADH is a diagnosis of exclusion (must rule out other causes of hyponatremia):
- Serum Na < 135 and serum osmolarity < 280
- Urine is not maximally diluted (urine osmolarity > 100).
- No evidence of dehydration, edema, hypotension
- No evidence of renal, cardiac, thyroid, or adrenal dysfunction

TREATMENT

- Treatment generally consists of fluid restriction. (Remember, clinical manifestations of SIADH usually become apparent only when the thirst mechanism leads to increased fluid intake!)
- Hypertonic (3%) saline is appropriate only for patients with neurologic symptoms of hyponatremia.

Acid–Base Disorders

Assess the acid–base disorder step by step (Figure 3-4):
- Is the primary disorder an acidosis (pH < 7.40) or alkalosis (pH > 7.40)?
- Is the disorder respiratory (pH and P_{CO_2} move in opposite directions)?
- Is the disorder metabolic (pH and P_{CO_2} move in same direction)?
- Is the disorder a simple or mixed disorder?

Use the following general rules of thumb for acute disorders:
- Metabolic acidosis: P_{CO_2} drops ~1.5 (drop in HCO_3)
- Metabolic alkalosis: P_{CO_2} rises ~1.0 (rise in HCO_3)
- Respiratory acidosis: HCO_3 rises ~0.1 (rise in P_{CO_2})
- Respiratory alkalosis: HCO_3 drops ~0.3 (drop in P_{CO_2})

Compensation beyond above parameters suggests mixed disorder.

METABOLIC ACIDOSIS

Two varieties: Anion gap and nonanion gap

Calculating the Anion Gap
$AG = Na - [Cl + HCO_3]$
Normal $AG = 10$

METABOLIC ALKALOSIS

Two mechanisms:
- Loss of H^+:
    - Renal: Mineralocorticoid excess, diuretics, potassium-losing nephropathy
    - GI: Vomiting, gastric drainage, villous adenoma of colon
- Gain HCO_3: Milk–alkali syndrome, exogenous $NaHCO_3$

Neither respiratory (12 hours) nor metabolic compensation (24 to 48 hours) will return pH completely to normal.

Causes of elevated anion gap metabolic acidosis:
MUDPILES
Methanol, metabolism (inborn errors)
Uremia
Diabetic ketoacidosis
Paraldehyde
Iron, isoniazid
Lactic acidosis
Ethylene glycol
Salicylates, strychnine

Causes of normal anion gap metabolic acidosis:
HARD UP
Hyperparathyroidism
Adrenal insufficiency, anhydrase (carbonic anhydrase) inhibitors
Renal tubular acidosis
Diarrhea

Ureteroenteric fistula
Pancreatic fistulas

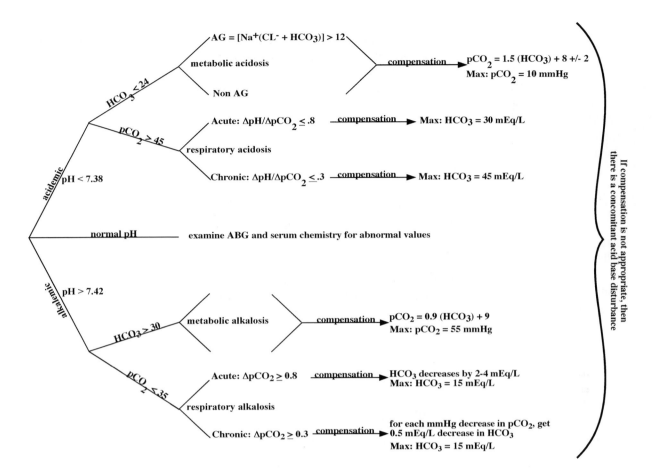

FIGURE 3-4. Acid–base algorithm.

(Reproduced, with permission, from Stead L. *BRS Emergency Medicine.* Philadelphia, PA: Lippincott Williams & Wilkins, 2000.)

The figure contains the following labeled content:

$AG = [Na^+(Cl^- + HCO_3)] > 12$

metabolic acidosis / Non AG

compensation → $pCO_2 = 1.5\,(HCO_3) + 8 \pm 2$
Max: $pCO_2 = 10$ mmHg

$HCO_3 \leq 24$

$pCO_2 \geq 45$

acidemic / pH < 7.38

Acute: $\Delta pH/\Delta pCO_2 \leq .8$ — compensation → Max: $HCO_3 = 30$ mEq/L

respiratory acidosis

Chronic: $\Delta pH/\Delta pCO_2 \leq .3$ — compensation → Max: $HCO_3 = 45$ mEq/L

normal pH — examine ABG and serum chemistry for abnormal values

alkalemic / pH > 7.42

$HCO_3 \geq 30$

metabolic alkalosis — compensation → $pCO_2 = 0.9\,(HCO_3) + 9$
Max: $pCO_2 = 55$ mmHg

$pCO_2 \leq 35$

Acute: $\Delta pCO_2 \geq 0.8$ — compensation → HCO_3 decreases by 2-4 mEq/L
Max: $HCO_3 = 15$ mEq/L

respiratory alkalosis

Chronic: $\Delta pCO_2 \geq 0.3$ — compensation → for each mmHg decrease in pCO_2, get 0.5 mEq/L decrease in HCO_3
Max: $HCO_3 = 15$ mEq/L

If compensation is not appropriate, then there is a concomitant acid base disturbance

RESPIRATORY ACIDOSIS

Hypercapnia secondary to one of two mechanisms:

- Hypoventilation (brain stem injury, neuromuscular disease, ventilator malfunction)
- Ventilation–perfusion (V/Q) mismatch (COPD, pneumonia, pulmonary embolism, foreign body, pulmonary edema)

RESPIRATORY ALKALOSIS

- Hyperventilation secondary to anxiety, increased intracranial pressure (ICP), salicylates, fever, hypoxemia, systemic disease (sepsis), pain, pregnancy, CHF, pneumonia, asthma, liver disease
- Alkalosis causes decrease in serum K and ionized Ca, resulting in paresthesias, carpopedal spasm, and tetany.

Vitamin Disorders

WATER-SOLUBLE VITAMINS

Thiamine

- Deficiency primarily seen in chronic alcoholics
- "Dry beriberi"—sensorimotor neuropathy

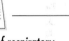

Cause of respiratory alkalosis: **MIS[HAP]³S**
- **M**echanical overventilation
- **I**ncreased ICP
- **S**epsis
- **H**ypoxemia, **H**yperpyrexia, **H**eart failure
- **A**nxiety, **A**sthma, **A**scites
- **P**regnancy, **P**ain, **P**neumonia
- **S**alicylates

- "Wet beriberi"—high-output cardiac failure
- Wernicke's encephalopathy—confusion, ataxia, altered mental status
- Korsakoff's syndrome—impaired memory with intact cognition, psychosis

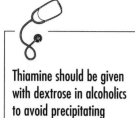

Thiamine should be given with dextrose in alcoholics to avoid precipitating Wernicke's encephalopathy.

Three doctors drank a nice Pellegrino.

Riboflavin (B_2)

- Cofactor for oxidation/reduction reactions
- Deficiency leads to angular stomatitis and cheilosis.

Niacin (B_3)

- Cofactor for oxidation/reduction reactions
- Deficiency leads to pellagra (3 Ds—diarrhea, dementia, dermatitis).

Pyridoxine (B_6)

- Deficiency leads to convulsions.
- Excess leads to neuropathy (usually sensory).

Cobalamin (B_{12})

Produced by microorganisms, binds to intrinsic factor in stomach, absorbed in ileum

Causes of Deficiency
- Pernicious anemia—macrocytic anemia with mean corpuscular volume > 100 and hypersegmented neutrophils. Antibodies to intrinsic factor prevent binding and absorption of B_{12}.
- Resection of distal ileum
- Tropical sprue
- Crohn's disease

Result of Deficiency
- Neuropathy typically involving dorsal columns (position and vibration sense)

Folic Acid

- Required for synthesis of nitrogen bases in DNA/RNA
- Deficiency causes macrocytic anemia without neurologic symptoms.

Vitamin C

- Required for hydroxylation of proline and lysine (cross-linking) in collagen synthesis
- Deficiency causes scurvy (bleeding gums, poor wound healing, hyperkeratosis).

FAT-SOLUBLE VITAMINS

Vitamin A

- Deficiency causes night blindness and dry skin.
- Excess causes neurologic symptoms, osteolysis, yellow skin, and alopecia.

Vitamin D

- Absorbed by GI (D_2) or synthesized in skin (D_3)

- Converted by liver/kidney to active form 1,25 (OH) D$_3$
- Deficiency causes rickets (children), osteomalacia (adults), symptoms of hypocalcemia.
- Excess causes symptoms of hypercalcemia.

Vitamin K

- Synthesized by intestinal flora, cofactor in synthesis of clotting factors
- Deficiency leads to disorders of bleeding and hemostasis.
- Excess can cause hemolytic anemia and hepatotoxicity.

Vitamin E

- Provides defense against lipid peroxidation
- Protects membranes of intracellular organelles from damage
- Found in green leafy plants and seeds
- No consistent ill effects are noted with deficiency or excess states, which are uncommon to begin with.

ECGs

See cardiovascular emergencies chapter for a more complete discussion:
- Electrocardiograms provide a tremendous amount of information in both the acutely ill patient and for a long-term view of cardiac function.
- To become proficient, one must have a system so as not to miss anything, and one must practice, practice, practice.
- Don't believe the machine's reading.

Rate

- Normal
- Bradycardic (< 60 bpm)
- Tachycardic (> 100 bpm)

Rhythm

- Sinus: P waves before every QRS, P upright in I and aVF, all P waves are of same shape (see Figure 3-5 for ECG lead placement)
- Atrial fibrillation: No P waves, irregularly irregular rhythm
- Atrial flutter: No P waves, saw tooth–shaped waves
- Ventricular tachycardia: No P wave, no discernible QRS, regular undulating smooth waves
- Ventricular fibrillation: Grossly irregular waves of varying amplitude, no discernible P or QRS

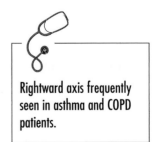

ECG paper runs at 25 mm/s.
One small box = .040 sec
One large box = 200 ms

Axis

- Normal: 0 to +90
- Rightward: +90 to +270
- Leftward: 0 to −90

See Figure 3-6 for ECG axes.

Rightward axis frequently seen in asthma and COPD patients.

Precordial Leads

V_1	R parasternal in ICS 4
V_2	L parasternal in ICS 4
V_3	midpoint between V_2 & V_4
V_{3R}	R-sided V_3 (pediatric lead)
V_4	L midclavicular line in ICS 5
V_5	L anterior axillary line in ICS 5
V_6	L midaxillary line in ICS 5

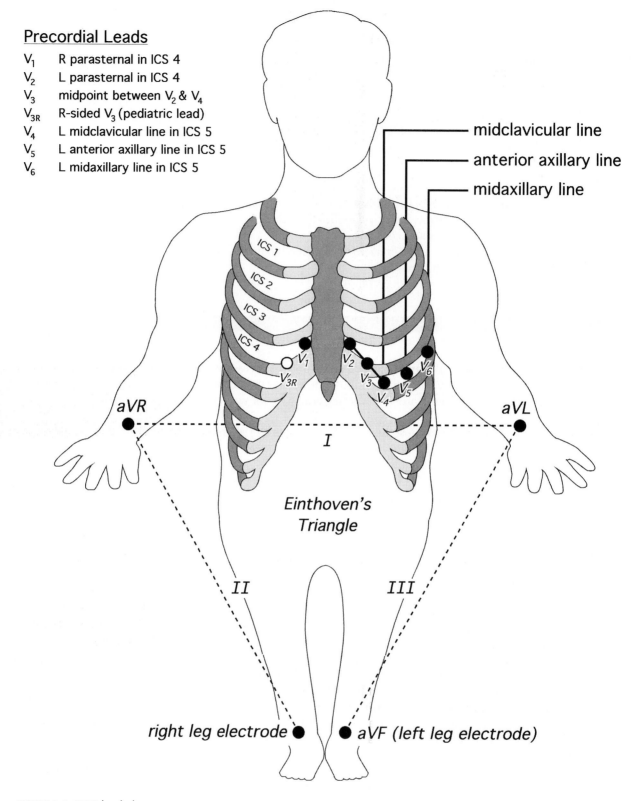

FIGURE 3-5. ECG lead placement.

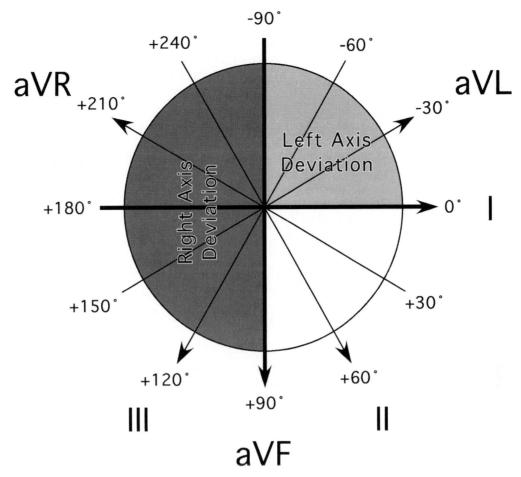

FIGURE 3-6. ECG axes.

Intervals

Intervals are important to determine if there is an atrioventricular (AV) nodal block, intraventricular conduction delay, or prolonged Q:

- PR interval—normal = 200 ms:
  - Consistently > 200 ms is first-degree AV block.
  - Progressively longer and eventually dropping a beat with a repeated pattern is Mobitz type I.
  - Consistent PR with dropped beats in a repeating pattern is Mobitz type II.
  - No association between P wave and QRS is third-degree AV block.
- QRS duration—normal < 120 ms. Greater than 120 ms indicates an intraventricular conduction delay or a left or right bundle branch block.
- QT interval—normal varies with rate but corrected QT (QT/√RR) < 450 ms:
  - Must take patient's age and sex into consideration
  - Prolonged by hypokalemia, hypomagnesemia, hypocalcemia, and certain medications
  - Risk of Torsade de pointes with prolonged QT

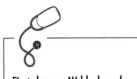

Beta blockers and Ca^{2+} channel blockers may cause first-degree block.

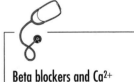

First-degree AV block and Mobitz type I are considered stable.

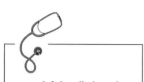

Mobitz type II and third-degree AV block are considered unstable. Treatment is pacemaker.

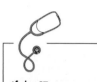

A new left bundle branch block is considered an acute myocardial infarction (MI) unless proven otherwise.

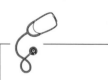

If the ST segment can hold water (concave up), usually not injury.

Diffuse (across all leads) ST elevations are seen in pericarditis.

Remember, have a system and practice, practice, practice. Even senior cardiologists don't agree with each other on some ECGs, so don't be discouraged.

Morphology

Morphology of the waves is important as well:
- P wave morphology may indicate right or left atrial enlargement (tall P waves) or ectopic atrial focus (different looking P waves).
- QRS complex morphology may indicate right ventricular or left ventricular hypertrophy (tall QRS), right bundle or left bundle branch block (M-shaped QRS complex), or paroxysmal supraventricular tachycardia (wide).
- T waves are helpful to determine ischemic changes or hyperkalemia:
  - In general, T waves should have the same deflection as the QRS. If they're flat or inverted, this may be a sign of ischemia or hypertrophic repolarization changes.
  - Peaked T waves are an early ECG change in hyperkalemia.

ST Segments

ST segments are helpful in determining injury or ischemia. In general:
- Elevation means injury.
- Depression means ischemia.

The concavity is also helpful:
- Concave up is usually not acute injury.
- Concave down: Think of acute injury.

Q Waves

Q waves are pathologic except in aVR, lead III and V1:
- Most commonly used criteria for significant Q waves is > 40 ms wide and at least one fourth of R wave in same lead.
- Usually form completely 2 days after transmural infarction
- May not be seen in subendocardial infarctions (non–Q wave MI)

U Waves

- U waves are sometimes seen after T waves.
- May indicate hypocalcemia or hypokalemia
- Contraindications to thrombolysis include recent surgery, active bleeding, recent stroke, suspected dissection, uncontrolled hypertension, or prolonged cardiopulmonary resuscitation.

Criteria for Thrombolysis

Criteria for thrombolysis in acute MI barring contraindications:
- Elevated ST segments > 1 mm in two consecutive leads
- Chest pain or original equivalent consistent with MI

Miscellaneous

- Look for pacemaker spike, may be very subtle.
- S in I, Q in III, inverted T in III—think pulmonary embolus.
- If injury is evolving, repeat ECGs are very helpful.

- X-rays have become a routine part of the evaluation of emergency patients.
- They are used to detect fractures, foreign bodies, pneumonias, CHF, pneumothoraces, and bowel obstruction.
- They are relatively inexpensive and readily available, making them an excellent adjunct when used properly.
- The emergency physician must be comfortable reading his or her own radiographs.

Chest X-Ray

- Use the ABCs for a systematic approach:
  - A —airway. Evaluate the trachea for deviation.
  - B—bones. Evaluate the ribs and other visible bones for evidence of fractures or bony pathology.
  - C—cardiac. Look at the cardiac silhouette. It is considered enlarged when greater than one half the thoracic diameter.
  - D—diaphragms. Look for free air beneath, flattening, or rising of one side as well as loss of the costophrenic angles.
  - E—everything else. Now look at the lung fields for pathology.
- Know the technique used. You may be fooled thinking of cardiomegaly, which shouldn't be read on a portable anteroposterior (AP) chest x-ray.
- Small pneumothoraces may be very subtle and require a hot lamp evaluation.

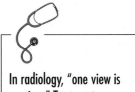

In radiology, "one view is no view." Try to get a lateral when possible.

Obstruction Series

- Consist of upright chest and abdominal x-rays, as well as a supine abdominal x-ray
- Look for free air, bowel gas patterns, air–fluid levels, and stool in the intestine.

Loss of costophrenic angle indicates approximately 250 cc of fluid accumulation.

Facial Films

- Useful for trauma and sinus evaluation
- Complicated fractures are usually followed up with computed tomography (CT) scan.
- Look for opacification of sinuses, air–fluid levels, and mucosal thickening, which are indicative of sinusitis.

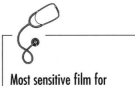

Most sensitive film for free air is an upright chest x-ray.

Neck Films

- Cervical spine series consists of lateral, AP, and open mouth views:
  - Must see from C1 to top of T1 for complete lateral film
  - May try shoulder pull or Swimmer's view for larger patients to expose bottom cervical vertebrae
  - Open mouth used to evaluate dens and lateral masses
- Soft tissue of neck useful if suspecting epiglottitis or foreign body

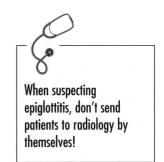

When suspecting epiglottitis, don't send patients to radiology by themselves!

HIGH-YIELD FACTS

Diagnostics

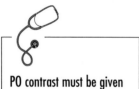

*Use **BLT RATS** when describing fractures:*
Bone
Location
Type of fracture

Rotation
Angulation
Transposition
Shortening

Acute ischemic strokes may initially present with a negative CT scan.

Chest CT will miss small, peripheral emboli.

PO contrast must be given time to reach the end of the GI tract (approximately 1 to 3 hours).

Extremity Films

- Ordered when suspecting fracture or foreign body
- Multiple views are better.
- Post-reduction views to check for proper positioning are necessary when extremity has been manipulated.
- Can also be used to evaluate for effusions and soft-tissue swelling

CT SCANS

CT scans have become widely available in the United States and have proven to be invaluable in the diagnosis and treatment of many emergency conditions. A good CT scan, when correlated with the history and patient's condition, can help save a life.

Head CTs

- Useful in atraumatic and traumatic patients
- Noncontrast CTs can help to see new-onset strokes, bleeds, masses, hydrocephalus, and edema.
- Can also be used to diagnose skull fractures, facial bone fractures, and sinus disease
- Usually done prior to lumbar puncture to rule out increased intracerebral pressure
- If HIV+ and infection is suspected, it is best to do without and with contrast to look for toxoplasmosis, cryptococcus, and lymphoma.
- C-spine/neck CTs are useful for penetrating trauma to the neck and to further delineate fractures and subluxations seen on plain C-spine films.

Chest CTs

- Newer-generation, high-resolution spiral CTs with IV contrast are useful for diagnosing large pulmonary emboli.
- Have high sensitivity for small pleural effusions and small pneumothoraces not picked up by plain films
- Useful in evaluating aorta and aortic root in suspected dissection or rupture

Abdominal/Pelvic CTs

- Very common ED test
- Useful to detect free fluid in the abdomen
- With PO and IV contrast administered appropriately, excellent test for infectious processes in the abdomen such as appendicitis, diverticulitis, and abscesses
- Also useful in evaluating intestinal pathology, although not good for penetrating intestinal trauma
- Sensitivity not great for pelvic organs. Ultrasound more useful for gynecologic pathology

IV Contrast

- Adds a tremendous amount of information
- Risk of allergy, renal impairment, or asthma exacerbation. Must weigh risks against benefits
- Exercise caution in patients with renal disease.

ULTRASOUND

- **Ultrasound** studies have gained an increasing role in Emergency Medicine.
- Portable machines have found their way to the bedside, and increased training of residents and attendings in ultrasonography has helped patients throughout the country.
- Future uses in the ED may include deep vein thrombosis evaluation, cardiac sonography, and use during procedures such as central lines.
- The two most common uses in the ED currently are pelvic sonography and Focused Abdominal Sonogram for Trauma (FAST) studies.

Pelvic Ultrasound

- Useful in evaluating the pregnant female with pain or bleeding, ruling out ectopic pregnancies, or evaluating the nonpregnant female with pelvic complaints
- Order of appearance of structures in pregnancy:
  - Double ring sign
  - Double gestational sac
  - Intrauterine fetal pole
  - Fetal heart activity
- Should be able to visualize uterus, ovaries, bladder, and Douglas' pouch for free fluid

Intrauterine pregnancy (IUP) on transvaginal sonogram is seen at beta-hCG of 1,800 IU/L. IUP on transabdominal seen at beta-hCG of 6,000 IU/L.

FAST

- Used to detect free peritoneal blood following blunt trauma to the abdomen
- Four sites of visualization:
  - Hepatorenal interface (Morison's pouch)
  - Splenic–renal interface
  - Pericardial sac
  - Bladder (Douglas' pouch)
- Sensitivity and specificity vary with experience of user and patient factors.
- Disadvantages:
  - Poor in obese patients or those with lots of bowel gas
  - Poor in evaluating solid-organ or bowel injury
  - May not pick up small amounts of fluid

HIGH-YIELD FACTS

Diagnostics

- Nuclear Medicine studies involve the use of hormones or cells that are labeled radioactively to evaluate the function of different organ systems.
- The two most common studies ordered in the ED are hepato-iminodiacetic acid (HIDA) scans and V/Q scans.

HIDA Scan

- IDA is labeled and taken up by hepatocytes and secreted into bile canaliculi.
- Failure to visualize the gallbladder despite seeing the hepatic and common ducts indicates cystic duct obstruction.
- Ninety-eight percent negative predictive value for cholecystitis
- Sensitivity as high as 97%

HIDA scan loses sensitivity as bilirubin levels rise above 5 mg.

V/Q Scan

- Indicated for patients when pulmonary embolism is suspected and other diagnoses can't be proven
- Perfusion scan done by labeling albumin
- Eight views need to be obtained for complete scan.
- Perfusion scans alone are not sensitive or specific.
- Ventilation scan performed with radioactive aerosols
- Four results are reported by radiology:
  - Normal scans have specificity of 96% and sensitivity of 98%.
  - Low-probability and intermediate-probability scans are considered nondiagnostic:
    - Correlate with clinical suspicion.
    - Intermediate probability—41% sensitive, positive predictive value (PPV) only 30%
    - Low probability—16% sensitive, 14% PPV
  - High-probability scans—41% sensitive, 87% PPV
- If your clinical suspicion is high enough, go further in workup than V/Q scan (lower extremity Doppler study, spiral chest CT, empiric treatment).

Famous PIOPED study: "Low-probability" V/Q studies miss 16% of pulmonary emboli.

Trauma

ADVANCED TRAUMA LIFE SUPPORT

"Golden Hour" of Trauma

Period immediately following trauma in which rapid assessment, diagnosis assessment, diagnosis, and stabilization must occur

Prehospital Phase

Control of airway and external hemorrhage, immobilization, and rapid transport of patient to nearest appropriate facility

Preparation

- Gown up, glove up, face shields on!
- Standard precautions!
- Set up: Airway equipment, monitor, O_2, urinary catheter (Foley), IV and blood tubes (complete blood count, chemistry, prothrombin time/partial thromboplastin time, type and cross, human chorionic gonadotropin, +/− toxicologies), chest tube tray, etc.

Trauma History

Whenever possible, take an **AMPLE** history:
- **A**llergies
- **M**edications/**M**echanism of injury
- **P**ast medical history/**P**regnant?
- **L**ast meal
- **E**vents surrounding the mechanism of injury

Primary Survey

- Initial assessment and resuscitation of vital functions
- Prioritization based on ABCs of trauma care

ABCs

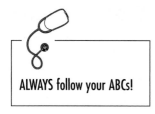

ALWAYS follow your ABCs!

- Airway (with cervical spine precautions)
- Breathing and ventilation
- Circulation (and Control of hemorrhage)
- Disability (neurologic status)
- Exposure/Environment control
- Foley

Airway and C-Spine

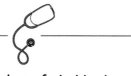

Assume C-spine injury in trauma patients until proven otherwise.

- Assess patency of airway.
- Use jaw thrust or chin lift initially to open airway.
- Clear foreign bodies.
- Insert oral or nasal airway when necessary. Obtunded/unconscious patients should be intubated. Surgical airway—cricothyroidotomy is used when unable to intubate airway.

Breathing and Ventilation

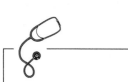

All trauma patients should receive supplemental O_2.

- Inspect, auscultate, and palpate the chest.
- Ensure adequate ventilation and identify and treat injuries that may immediately impair ventilation:
  - Tension pneumothorax
  - Flail chest and pulmonary contusion
  - Massive hemothorax
  - Open pneumothorax

Control of Hemorrhage

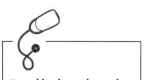

Draw blood samples at the time of intravenous catheter placement.

- Place *two* large-bore (14- or 16-gauge) IVs.
- Assess circulatory status (capillary refill, pulse, skin color) (see Shock section below).
- Control of life-threatening hemorrhage using **direct pressure;** do not "clamp" bleeding vessels with hemostats.

Disability

AVPU *scale:*
Alert
Verbal
Pain
Unresponsive

- Rapid neurologic exam
- Establish pupillary size and reactivity, and level of consciousness using the AVPU or Glasgow Coma Scale.

Exposure/Environment/Extras

- Completely undress the patient, most often with the help of your trauma shears.
- Hook up monitors (cardiac, pulse oximetry, blood pressure, etc.).

Foley Catheter

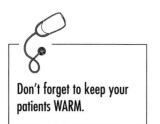

Don't forget to keep your patients WARM.

- Placement of a urinary catheter is considered part of the resuscitative phase, which takes place during the primary survey.

- Important for monitoring urinary output, which is a reflection of renal perfusion and volume status
- Adequate urinary output:
  - Adult: 0.5 cc/kg/hr
  - Child (> 1year of age): 1.0 cc/kg/hr
  - Child (< 1year of age): 2.0 cc/kg/hr
- Foley is contraindicated when urethral transection is suspected, such as in the case of a pelvic fracture. If transection is suspected, perform retrograde urethrogram before Foley.

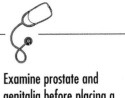

Examine prostate and genitalia before placing a Foley.

Signs of Urethral Transection
- Blood at the meatus
- A "high-riding" prostate
- Perineal or scrotal hematoma

Gastric Intubation

Placement of nasogastric (NG) or orogastric (OG) tube may reduce risk of aspiration by decompressing stomach, but does not assure full prevention.

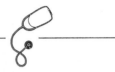

Place OG tube rather than NG tube when fracture of cribriform plate is suspected.

- Begins during the primary survey
- Life-threatening injuries are tended to as they are identified.

Intravenous Catheters

The rate of maximal fluid administration is directly related to the internal diameter of the IV catheter (to the fourth power of the radius according to Poiseuille's law) and inversely related to the length of the tubing.

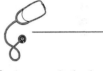

Trauma resuscitation is a team sport with many different activities overlapping in both time and space.

Intravenous Fluid

- Fluid therapy should be initiated with 1 to 2 L of an isotonic (either lactated Ringer's or normal saline) crystalloid solution (see below).
- Pediatric patients should receive an IV bolus of 20 cc/kg.

Crystalloid versus Colloid

- Crystalloids are sodium-based solutions that provide a transient increase in intravascular volume.
- Approximately one third of an isotonic solution will remain in the intravascular space. The remainder almost immediately distributes to the extravascular and interstitial spaces. This occurs because crystalloid solutions easily diffuse across membranes.
- Colloids have a harder time diffusing across membranes, thus remaining in the intravascular space for longer periods of time thereby requiring smaller volumes for resuscitation. However, it is costly and carries the risks of transfusion reactions and viral transmission.
- Neither crystalloids nor colloids have been shown to be superior for volume resuscitation. Therefore, volume resuscitation begins with crystalloids (see below).

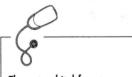

The antecubital fossae are a good place to find nice veins for which to place large-bore IVs.

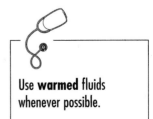

Use warmed fluids whenever possible.

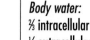

"3 to 1 Rule"

Used as a rough estimate for the total amount of crystalloid volume needed acutely to replace blood loss

Shock

- Inadequate delivery of oxygen on the cellular level secondary to tissue hypoperfusion
- In traumatic situations, shock is the result of hypovolemia until proven otherwise.

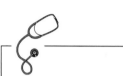

- Crystalloids include saline, Ringer's lactate, and glucose.
- Colloids include blood products such as red blood cells (RBCs) and albumin.

Hypovolemic Shock

Caused by the acute loss of blood in most cases. Blood volume estimate based on body weight in kilograms:
- Adults: 7% of weight
- Peds: 8 to 9% of weight

For example, 70-kg adult ($70 \times 7\% = 4.9$ L of blood)

Classes of Hemorrhagic Shock

Table 4-1 lists the types of hemorrhagic shock.

Treatment of Hemorrhagic Shock

- Response to the initial fluid bolus (e.g., change in vital signs, urinary output, and/or level of consciousness) should direct further resuscitative efforts.
- Early blood transfusion and surgical intervention should be a consideration in patients who fail to respond to initial fluid resuscitation.

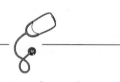

Hemorrhage is the most common cause of shock in the injured patient.

TABLE 4-1. Types of Hemorrhagic Shock

Class	Blood Loss (%)	Vol. Blood Loss (cc)	HR	Pulse Pressure	sBP	Urine Output	Altered Mental Status?	Treatment
I	Up to 15	Up to 750	< 100	N	N	N	No	Crystalloids (3 to 1 rule); no blood products necessary
II	15–30	750–1,500	↑	↓	↓	↓	No	Crystalloids initially, then monitor response; may or may not need blood products; can wait for type-specific blood.
III	30–40	1,500–2,000	↑↑	↓↓	↓↓	↓↓	Yes	Crystalloids followed by type-specific blood products
IV	> 40	> 2,000	↑↑↑	↓↓↓	↓↓↓	↓↓↓	Yes	2-L crystalloid bolus followed by uncrossed (O negative) blood; death is imminent.

N = normal; ↑ = increased; ↓ = decreased.

Nonhypovolemic Shock

- **Cardiogenic shock** occurring during trauma may occur secondary to blunt myocardial injury, cardiac tamponade, tension pneumothorax, air embolus, or an acute myocardial infarction.
- **Neurogenic shock** may occur secondary to sympathetic denervation in patients who have suffered a spinal injury.
- **Septic shock** is due to infection and may be seen when there is a significant delay in patients' arrival to the emergency department (ED) or in patients with penetrating abdominal injuries, for example.

Radiologic and Diagnostic Studies

- X-rays of the chest, pelvis, and lateral cervical spine usually occur concurrently with early resuscitative efforts; however, their procedure should never interrupt the resuscitative process.
- Diagnostic peritoneal lavage (DPL) and Focused Abdominal Sonogram for Trauma (FAST) are also tools used for the rapid detection of intra-abdominal bleeding that often occurs early in the resuscitative process (see section on abdominal trauma).

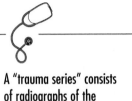

A "trauma series" consists of radiographs of the C-spine, chest, and pelvis.

Secondary Survey

- Begins once the primary survey is complete and resuscitative efforts are well under way
- Includes a **head-to-toe evaluation** of the trauma patient and **frequent reassessment** of status
- Neurologic examination, procedures, radiologic examination, and laboratory testing take place at this time if not already accomplished.

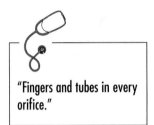

"Fingers and tubes in every orifice."

Tetanus Prophylaxis

Immunize as needed.

HEAD TRAUMA

Anatomy and Physiology

- Scalp:
  - The scalp consists of five layers.
  - Highly vascular structure
  - May be the source of major blood loss
  - The loose attachment between the galea and the pericranium allows for large collections of blood to form a subgaleal hematoma.
  - Disruption of the galea should be corrected and may be done so with single-layer, interrupted 3.0 nonabsorbable sutures through the skin, subcutaneous tissue, and galea.
  - Prophylactic antibiotics are not indicated in simple scalp lacerations.
- Skull:
  - Rigid and inflexible (fixed volume)
  - Composed of the cranial vault and base

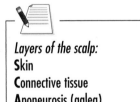

Layers of the scalp:
Skin
Connective tissue
Aponeurosis (galea)
Loose areolar tissue
Pericranium

45

- Brain:
  - Makes up 80% of intracranial volume
  - Partially compartmentalized by the reflections of dura (falx cerebri and tentorium cerebelli)
  - *Note:* CN III runs along the edge of the tentorium cerebelli.
- Cerebrospinal fluid (CSF):
  - Formed primarily by the choroid plexus at a rate of approximately 500 cc/day with 150 cc of CSF circulating at a given moment.
  - Cushions the brain
- Cerebral blood flow:
  - Brain receives approximately 15% of cardiac output.
  - Brain responsible for ~20% of total body O_2 consumption
- Cerebral perfusion pressure (CPP):
  - CPP = MAP − ICP
  - MAP = mean arterial blood pressure
  - ICP = intracranial pressure

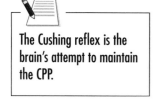

Concept of CPP is important in a hypertensive patient. Lowering the BP too fast will also decrease the CPP, creating a new problem.

Monro–Kellie Hypothesis

- The sum of the volume of the brain, blood, and CSF within the skull must remain constant. Therefore, an increase in one of the above must be offset by an decreased volume of the others. If not, the ICP will increase.
- Increased ICP can thus result in cerebral herniation, or when ICP = systolic blood pressure (BP), cerebral blood flow ceases and brain death occurs.

Assessment

History: Identify mechanism and time of injury, loss of consciousness, concurrent use of drugs or alcohol, medications that may affect pupillary size (e.g., glaucoma medications), past medical history (especially previous head trauma and stroke with their residual effects, and previous eye surgery, which can affect pupillary size and response), and the presence of a "lucid interval."

Vital Signs

Cushing reflex: Hypertension and bradycardia in the setting of increased ICP

The Cushing reflex is the brain's attempt to maintain the CPP.

Physical Exam

- Search for signs of external trauma such as lacerations, ecchymoses, and avulsions, as these may be clues to underlying injuries such as depressed or open skull fractures.
- Anisocoria (inequality of pupils) is found in a small percentage of normal people; however, unequal pupils in the patient with head trauma is pathologic until proven otherwise.

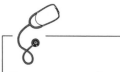

Hypotension is usually not caused by isolated head injury. Look for other injuries in this setting.

Glasgow Coma Scale (GCS)

GCS (Figure 4-1) may be used as a tool for classifying head injury:

Eyes	Open spontaneously	4
	Open to verbal command	3
	Open to pain	2
	No response	1
Best motor response	Obeys verbal command	6
	Localizes pain to painful stimulus	5
	Flexion withdrawal	4
	Decorticate rigidity	3
	Decerebrate rigidity	2
	No response	1
Best verbal response	Oriented and converses	5
	Disoriented and converses	4
	Inappropriate words	3
	Incomprehensible sounds	2
	No response	1
TOTAL		**15**

FIGURE 4-1. Glasgow Coma Scale.

An enlarging pupil with a concurrent decrease in level of consciousness is strongly suggestive of uncal (brain) herniation.

- Severe head injury: GCS 8 or less
- Moderate head injury: GCS 9 to 13
- Mild head injury: GCS 14 or 15

Diagnostic Studies

- Assume C-spine injury in head injury patients and immobilize until cleared.
- Skull films have largely been replaced by computed tomography (CT) scan.
- Indications for head/brain CT:
  - Neurologic deficit
  - Persisting depression or worsening of mental status
  - Moderate to severe mechanism of injury
  - Depressed skull fracture or linear fracture overlying a dural venous sinus or meningeal artery groove (as demonstrated with skull x-rays).

Skin staples interfere with CT scanning and should therefore not be used until after CT scanning is complete.

SKULL FRACTURES

Linear (Nondepressed)

Becomes clinically important if it occurs over the middle meningeal artery groove or major venous dural sinuses (formation of an epidural hematoma), air-filled sinuses, or if associated with underlying brain injury

Stellate

Suggestive of a more severe mechanism of injury than linear skull fractures

Depressed

- Carries a much greater risk of underlying brain injury and complications, such as meningitis and post-traumatic seizures
- Treatment involves surgical elevation for depressions deeper than the thickness of the adjacent skull.

Basilar

- Often a clinical diagnosis and sign of a significant mechanism of injury
- Signs include periorbital ecchymoses (raccoon's eyes), retroauricular ecchymoses (Battle's sign), otorrhea, rhinorrhea, hemotympanum, and cranial nerve palsies.

Open

- A laceration overlying a skull fracture
- Requires careful debridement and irrigation. Avoid blind digital probing of the wound.
- Obtain neurosurgical consultation.

Ring test for CSF rhinorrhea (in the presence of epistaxis):
Sample of blood from nose placed on filter paper to test for presence of CSF. If present, a large transparent ring will be seen encircling a clot of blood.

DIFFUSE INTRACRANIAL LESIONS

Cerebral Concussion

- Transient loss of consciousness that occurs immediately following blunt, nonpenetrating head trauma, caused by impairment of the reticular activating system
- Recovery is often complete; however, residual effects such as headache may last for some time.

Typical scenario:
A 20-year-old female sustains brief loss of consciousness following head injury. She presents to the ED awake but is amnestic for the event and keeps asking the same questions again and again. *Think: Concussion.*

Diffuse Axonal Injury (DAI)

- Caused by microscopic shearing of nerve fibers, scattered microscopic abnormalities
- Frequently requires intubation, hyperventilation, and admission to a neurosurgical intensive care unit
- Patients are often comatose for prolonged periods of time.
- Mortality is approximately 33%.

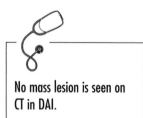

No mass lesion is seen on CT in DAI.

FOCAL INTRACRANIAL LESIONS

Cerebral Contusion

- Occurs when the brain impacts the skull; may occur directly under the site of impact (coup) or on the contralateral side (contrecoup)
- Patients may have focal deficits; mental status ranges from confusion to coma.

Intracerebral Hemorrhage

Caused by traumatic tearing of intracerebral blood vessels. Difficult to differentiate from a contusion.

Epidural Hematoma

- Collection of blood located between the dura and the skull
- Majority are associated with tearing of the middle meningeal artery from an overlying temporal bone fracture.
- Typically biconvex or lenticular in shape (see Figure 4-2)
- Patients may have the classic "lucid interval," wherein they "talk and die." Requires early neurosurgical involvement

Subdural Hematoma

- Collection of blood below the dura and over the brain (see Figure 4-3). Results from tearing of the bridging veins, usually secondary to an acceleration–deceleration mechanism
- Classified as acute (< 24 hours), subacute (24 hours to 2 weeks), and chronic (> 2 weeks)
- Acute and subacute subdurals require early neurosurgical involvement.
- Alcoholics and the elderly (patients likely to have brain atrophy) have increased susceptibility.

Typical scenario:
A 19-year-old male with head injury has loss of consciousness followed by a brief lucid interval. He presents to the ED in a coma, with an ipsilateral fixed and dilated pupil and contralateral hemiparesis. *Think: Epidural hematoma.*

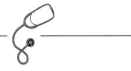

Acute subdural hematomas have a high mortality: Approximately one third to two thirds.

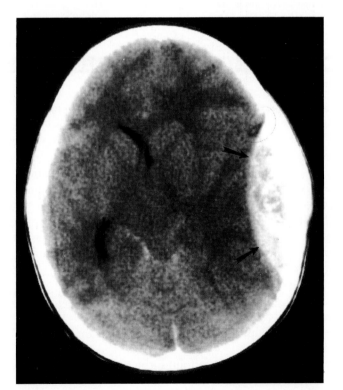

FIGURE 4-2. Epidural hematoma. Arrows indicate the characteristic lens-shaped lesion.
(Reproduced, with permission, from Schwartz SI, Spencer SC, Galloway AC, et al. *Principles of Surgery*, 7th ed. New York: McGraw-Hill, 1999: 1882.)

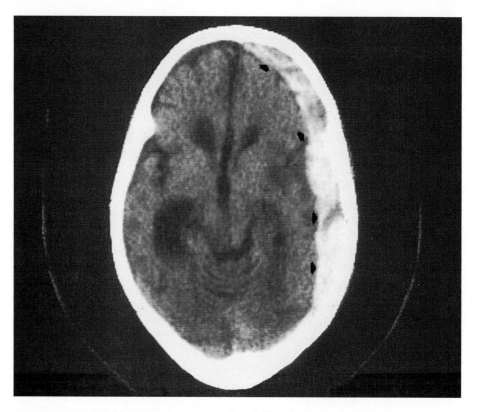

FIGURE 4-3. Subdural hematoma. CT scan of a child with shaken baby syndrome. Arrows indicate the hematoma. Note the characteristic inward concavity of the lesion.
(Reproduced, with permission, from Knoop K, Stack LB, and Storrow AB. *Atlas of Emergency Medicine.* New York: McGraw-Hill, 1997: 436.)

MANAGEMENT OF MILD TO MODERATE HEAD TRAUMA

When in doubt, admit the patient for observation.

- Safe disposition of the patient depends on multiple factors.
- Any patient with a persisting or worsening decrease in mental status, focal deficits, severe mechanism of injury, penetrating trauma, open or depressed skull fracture, or seizures or who is unreliable or cannot be safely observed at home should be admitted for observation.
- Patients with mild and sometimes moderate head trauma, brief or no loss of consciousness, no focal deficits, an intact mental status, and reliable family members who can adequately observe the patient at home can often be discharged home with proper discharge instructions.
- Discharge instructions should include signs and symptoms for family members to watch for such as:
  - Persisting or worsening headache
  - Dizziness
  - Vomiting
  - Inequality of pupils
  - Confusion
- If any of the above signs are found, the patient should be brought to the ED immediately.

- Patients must be treated aggressively starting with the ABCs.
- Secure the airway via endotracheal intubation using topical anesthesia, intravenous lidocaine, and paralytics when necessary to prevent any further increase in the ICP.
- Maintain an adequate BP with isotonic fluids.
- Treatment of increased ICP:
  - Hyperventilation to an arterial P_{CO_2} of 28 to 32 will decrease the ICP by approximately 25% acutely.
  - Mannitol (1 g/kg in a 20% solution) is an osmotic diuretic and lowers ICP by drawing water out of the brain. Contraindicated in the hypotensive patient
- Corticosteroids (used in penetrating spinal trauma) have not been shown to be useful in the patient with head trauma.
- Consider prophylactic anticonvulsant therapy with phenytoin 18 mg/kg IV at no faster than 50 mg/min (usually at the discretion of the neurosurgeon).
- Acute seizures should be managed with diazepam or lorazepam and phenytoin.
- Early ICP measurement via ventriculostomy should begin in the ED and is also at the discretion of the neurosurgeon.
- Treat the pathology whenever possible (e.g., surgical drainage of a hematoma).

> *Measures to lower ICP:*
> **HIVED**
> - **H**yperventilation
> - **I**ntubation with pretreatment and sedation
> - **V**entriculostomy (burr hole)
> - **E**levate the head of the bed
> - **D**iuretics (mannitol, furosemide)

General

Described in broad terms as penetrating versus blunt injuries even though considerable overlap exists between the management of the two

Anatomy

The neck is divided into triangles (anterior and posterior) as well as zones (I, II, and III).

Anterior Triangle
- Bordered by the midline, posterior border of the sternocleidomastoid muscle (SCM) and the mandible

Posterior Triangle
- Bordered by the trapezius, posterior border of the SCM, and the clavicle. There is a paucity of vital structures in its upper zone (above the spinal accessory nerve). In the lower zone lies the subclavian vessels and brachial plexus. The apices of the lungs are in close proximity.

Zones (Figure 4-4)
- Further division of the anterior triangle:
  - Zone I lies below the cricoid cartilage.
  - Zone II lies between I and III.

> Within the anterior triangle lie the majority of the vital structures of the neck.

HIGH-YIELD FACTS

Trauma

51

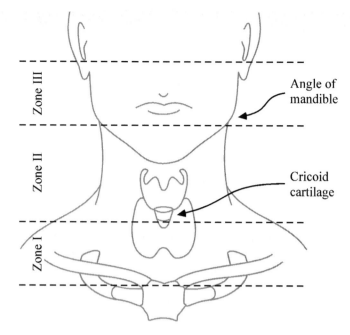

FIGURE 4-4. Zones of the neck.

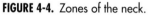

- Zone III lies above the angle of the mandible.
- These divisions help to drive the diagnostic and therapeutic management decisions for penetrating neck injuries.

Penetrating Injuries

Any injury to the neck in which the platysma is violated

Vascular Injuries
- Very common and often life threatening.
- Can lead to exsanguination, hematoma formation with compromise of the airway, and cerebrovascular accidents (from transection of the carotid artery or air embolus, for example)

Nonvascular Injuries
- Injury to the larynx and trachea including fracture of the thyroid cartilage and dislocation of the tracheal cartilages and arytenoids, for example, leading to airway compromise and often a difficult intubation
- Esophageal injury does occur and, as with penetrating neck injury, is not often manifest initially.

Resuscitation

AIRWAY

- Special attention should be paid to airway management of the patient with neck trauma.
- Anatomy may be distorted and an apparently patent airway can rapidly evolve into a compromised, difficult airway.
- Initial attempts at securing the airway should be via endotracheal intubation; however, alternative methods of airway management, such as

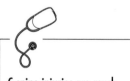

Fracture of the hyoid bone is suggestive of a significant mechanism of injury.

C-spine injuries are much more common with blunt neck injury.

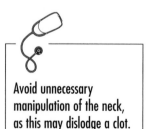

Avoid unnecessary manipulation of the neck, as this may dislodge a clot.

percutaneous transtracheal ventilation and surgical airway, should be readily available.

BREATHING

- Inability to ventilate the patient after an apparently successful intubation should prompt rapid reassessment of that airway.
- Creation and/or intubation of a "false lumen" in the patient with laryngotracheal or tracheal transection may be a fatal error if not identified immediately.
- Look for pneumohemothorax, as the apices of the lungs lie in close proximity to the base of the neck.

CIRCULATION

- If the patient remains unstable after appropriate volume resuscitation, he or she should be taken rapidly to the operating room (OR) for operative control of the bleeding.
- If injury to the subclavian vessels is suspected, IV access should be obtained in the opposite extremity, or more appropriately in the lower extremities.
- If a hemopneumothorax is suspected and central venous access is necessary, a femoral line is the first option, followed by placement of the access on the side ipsilateral to the "dropped lung" (because the patient doesn't like it when both lungs are down!).

Secondary Survey

- After stabilization, the wound should be carefully examined.
- Obtain soft-tissue films of the neck for clues to the presence of a soft-tissue hematoma and subcutaneous emphysema, and a chest x-ray (CXR) for possible hemopneumothorax.
- Surgical exploration is indicated for:
  - Expanding hematoma
  - Subcutaneous emphysema
  - Tracheal deviation
  - Change in voice quality
  - Air bubbling through the wound
- Pulses should be palpated to identify deficits and thrills and auscultated for bruits.
- A neurologic exam should be performed to identify brachial plexus and/or central nervous system deficits as well as Horner's syndrome.

Management

- Zone II injuries are taken to the OR for exploration.
- Injuries to zones I and III may be taken to the OR or managed conservatively using a combination of angiography, bronchoscopy, esophagoscopy, gastrografin or barium studies, and CT scanning.

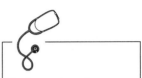

Keep cervical in-line stabilization until C-spine fracture has been ruled out.

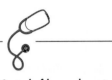

Tracheostomy is the procedure of choice in the patient with laryngotracheal separation.

Control of hemorrhage in the ED is via direct pressure (no blind clamping).

Never blindly probe a neck wound, as this may lead to bleeding in a previously tamponaded wound.

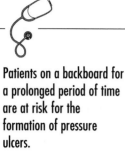

Patients on a backboard for a prolonged period of time are at risk for the formation of pressure ulcers.

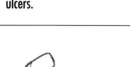

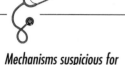

Mechanisms suspicious for spinal injury:
- Diving
- Fall from > 10 feet
- Injury above level of shoulders (C-spine)
- Electrocution
- High-speed motor vehicle crash
- Rugby or football injury (tackling)

General

- Spinal trauma may involve injury to the spinal column, spinal cord, or both.
- Over 50% of spinal injuries occur in the cervical spine, with the remainder being divided between the thoracic spine, the thoracolumbar junction, and the lumbosacral region.
- As long as the spine is appropriately immobilized, evaluation for spinal injury may be deferred until the patient is stabilized.

Anatomy

- There are 7 cervical, 12 thoracic, 5 lumbar, 5 sacral, and 4 coccygeal vertebrae.
- The cervical spine is the region that is most vulnerable to injury.
- The thoracic spine is relatively protected due to limited mobility from support of the rib cage (T1–T10); however, the spinal canal through which the spinal cord traverses is relatively narrow in this region. Therefore, when injuries to this region do occur, they usually have devastating results.
- The thoracolumbar junction (T11–L1) is a fairly vulnerable region, as it is the area between the relatively inflexible thoracic region and the flexible lumbar region.
- The lumbosacral region (L2 and below) contains the region of the spinal canal below which the spinal cord proper ends and the cauda equina begins.

Pathology and Pathophysiology

Spinal injuries can generally be classified based on:
- Fracture/dislocation type (mechanism, stable versus unstable)
- Level of neurologic (sensory and motor) and bony involvement
- Severity (complete versus incomplete spinal cord disability)

Neurogenic Shock

- A state of vasomotor instability resulting from impairment of the descending sympathetic pathways in the spinal cord, or simply a loss of sympathetic tone
- Signs and symptoms include flaccid paralysis, hypotension, bradycardia, cutaneous vasodilation, and a normal to wide pulse pressure.

Spinal Shock

- State of flaccidity and loss of reflexes occurring immediately after spinal cord injury
- Loss of visceral and peripheral autonomic control with uninhibited parasympathetic impulses
- May last from seconds to weeks, and does not signify permanent spinal cord damage

- Long-term prognosis cannot be postulated until spinal shock has resolved.

Spinal Cord Injuries

COMPLETE VERSUS INCOMPLETE

- Complete spinal cord injuries demonstrate no preservation of neurologic function distal to the level of injury. Therefore, any sensorimotor function below the level of injury constitutes an incomplete injury.
- Sacral sparing refers to perianal sensation, voluntary anal sphincter contraction, or voluntary toe flexion and is a sign of an incomplete spinal cord injury.

> Deep tendon reflexes and sacral reflexes may be preserved in complete injuries.

Physical Exam

- Classification of spinal cord injuries as complete or incomplete requires a proper neurologic exam.
- The exam should include testing of the three readily assessable long spinal tracts (see Figure 4-5):
  - Corticospinal tract (CST):
    - Located in the posterolateral aspect of the spinal cord
    - Responsible for ipsilateral motor function
    - Tested via voluntary muscle contraction
  - Spinothalamic tract (STT):
    - Located in the anterolateral aspect of the spinal cord
    - Responsible for contralateral pain and temperature sensation and is tested as such
  - Posterior (dorsal) columns:
    - Located in the posterior aspect of the spinal cord

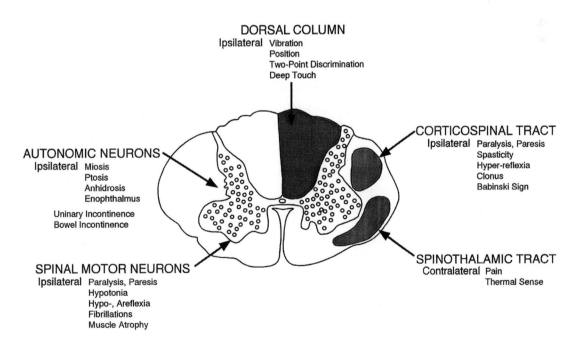

FIGURE 4-5. Effects of lesions in major spinal cord tracts.

(Reproduced, with permission, from Afifi AA, Bergman RA. *Functional Neuroanatomy: Text and Atlas.* New York: McGraw-Hill, 1998: 92.)

- Responsible for ipsilateral position and vibratory sense and some light touch sensation
- Test using a tuning fork and position sense of the fingers and toes.

Spinal Cord Syndromes

ANTERIOR CORD SYNDROME

- Pattern seen with injury to the anterior portion of the spinal cord or with compression of the anterior spinal arteries
- Involves full or partial loss of bilateral pain and temperature sensation (STT) and paraplegia (CST), with preservation of posterior column function
- Often seen with flexion injuries
- Carries a poor prognosis

BROWN–SÉQUARD SYNDROME

- Pattern seen with hemisection of the spinal cord usually secondary to a penetrating injury, but may also be seen with disc protrusion, hematoma, or tumor
- Consists of ipsilateral loss of motor function (CST) and posterior column function, with contralateral loss of pain and temperature sensation

CENTRAL CORD SYNDROME

- Pattern seen with injury to the central area of the spinal cord often in patients with a preexisting narrowing of the spinal canal
- Usually seen with hyperextension injuries: Its cause is usually attributed to buckling of the ligamentum flavum into the cord and/or an ischemic etiology in the distribution of branches of the anterior spinal artery.
- Characterized by weakness greater in the upper extremities than the lower extremities, and distal worse than proximal
- Has a better prognosis than the other partial cord syndromes with a characteristic pattern of recovery (lower extremity recovery progressing upwards to upper extremity recovery, then the hands recover strength)

Typical scenario:
A 70-year-old male presents to the ED after a whiplash injury. He is ambulating well but has an extremely weak handshake. *Think: Central cord syndrome.*

Treatment of Spinal Cord Syndromes

- Always start with the ABCs of trauma resuscitation.
- Maintain spinal immobilization throughout the resuscitation.
- Estimate level of neurologic dysfunction during the secondary survey.
- Obtain appropriate diagnostic studies.
- Establish early neurosurgical consultation.
- If penetrating spinal cord injury is diagnosed, begin high-dose methylprednisolone:
  - Loading dose of 30 mg/kg over 15 minutes during hour 1, followed by a continuous infusion of 5.4 mg/kg/hr over the next 23 hours.
- Consider traction devices in consultation with the neurosurgeon.
- Consider early referral to a regional spinal injury center.

General

As mentioned above, usually classified on the basis of mechanism (flexion, extension, compression, rotation, or a combination of these), location, and/or stability

Imaging

- Three views of the cervical spine are obtained (lateral, anteroposterior [AP], and an odontoid view) for best accuracy.
- A lateral view alone will miss 10% of C-spine injuries.
- Adequate AP and lateral films will allow visualization of C1–T1.
- If C1–T1 can still not be adequately visualized, CT scanning is indicated.

Reading a C-Spine Film

Alignment
- Evaluate the alignment of the four lordotic curves (see Figure 4-6):
  - Anterior margin of the vertebral bodies
  - Posterior margin of the vertebral bodies
  - Spinolaminar line
  - Tips of the vertebral bodies:
    - In the adult, up to 3.5 mm of anterior subluxation is considered a normal finding.

Bones
- Assess the base of the skull and each vertebral body, pedicle, facet, laminae, and spinous and transverse process for fracture/dislocation.

Cartilage
- Assess the intervertebral spaces and posterolateral facet joints for symmetry.

Soft Tissue
- Assess the prevertebral soft tissue: Wider than 5 mm suggests hematoma accompanying a fracture.
- Assess the predental space: Wider than 3 mm in adults and 4 to 5 mm in children is suggestive of a torn transverse ligament and fracture of C1.
- Assess the spaces between the spinous processes: Any increase in distance between the spinous processes is likely associated with a torn interspinous ligament and a spinal fracture.

ATLANTO-OCCIPITAL DISLOCATION

- Results from severe traumatic flexion
- Survival to the hospital setting is rare.
- Traction is not recommended.

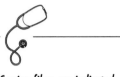

C-spine films are indicated for:
- Tenderness along C-spine
- Neurologic deficit
- Good mechanism of injury
- Presence of distracting injury patients with altered sensorium

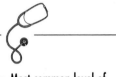

- Most common level of fracture is C5.
- Most common level of subluxation is C5 on C6.

HIGH-YIELD FACTS

Trauma

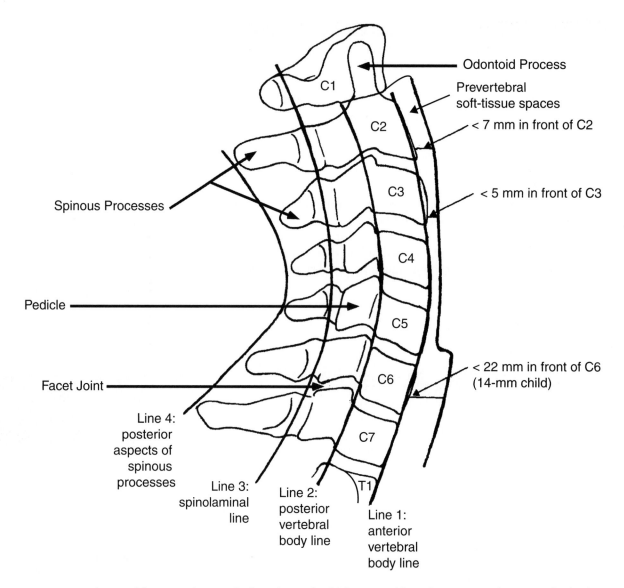

Odontoid Process

Prevertebral
soft-tissue spaces

< 7 mm in front of C2

< 5 mm in front of C3

< 22 mm in front of C6
(14-mm child)

Spinous Processes

Pedicle

Facet Joint

Line 4:
posterior
aspects of
spinous
processes

Line 3:
spinolaminal
line

Line 2:
posterior
vertebral
body line

Line 1:
anterior
vertebral
body line

FIGURE 4-6. *Lateral view of the cervical spine. The four "lines" should flow smoothly, without stepup. The prevertebral soft-tissue spaces should be within normal.*

JEFFERSON FRACTURE

- C1 (atlas) burst fracture
- Most common C1 fracture
- Consists of a fracture of both the anterior and posterior rings of C1
- Results from axial loading such as when the patient falls directly on his or her head or something falls on the patient's head
- Often associated with C2 fractures
- Consider all C1 fractures unstable even though most are not associated with spinal cord injury.
- Seen as an increase in the predental space on lateral x-ray and displacement of the lateral masses on the odontoid view

C1 Rotary Subluxation

- Seen most often in children or in patients with rheumatoid arthritis
- Seen as an asymmetry between the lateral masses and the dens on the odontoid view
- Patients will present with the head in rotation and should not be forced to place the head in the neutral position.

Odontoid Fractures

- Type 1: Involves only the tip of the dens
- Type 2: Involves only the base of the dens
- Type 3: Fracture through the base and body of C2
- Generally unstable

Hangman's Fracture

- Fracture of both pedicles ("posterior elements") of C2
- Usually due to a hyperextension mechanism
- Unstable fracture; however, often not associated with spinal cord injury because the spinal canal is at its widest through C2

Some type 1 fractures may be stable when the transverse ligament remains intact.

Burst Fracture of C3–7

- An axial loading mechanism causing compression of a vertebral body with resultant protrusion of the anterior portion of the vertebral body anteriorly and the posterior portion of the vertebral body posteriorly into the spinal canal often causing a spinal cord injury (usually the anterior cord syndrome)
- Stable fracture when ligamentous structure remains intact

Simple Wedge Fracture

- A flexion injury causing compression on the anterior portion of the vertebral body
- Appears as a wedge-shaped concavity, with loss of vertebral height on the anterior portion of the vertebral body
- Usually stable when not associated with ligamentous damage

Flexion Teardrop Fracture

- A flexion injury causing a fracture of the anteroinferior portion of the vertebral body
- Appears as a teardrop-shaped fragment
- Unstable fracture, as it is usually associated with a tearing of the posterior ligament and often neurologic damage

Extension Teardrop Fracture

- Also appears as a teardrop-shaped fragment on the anteroinferior portion of the vertebral body
- However, occurs as an extension injury with avulsion of the fragment, rather than a compression mechanism
- The posterior ligaments are left intact, making this a stable fracture.
- However, differentiation between a flexion versus extension teardrop fracture may be difficult and should be treated initially as if it were unstable.

59

CLAY SHOVELER'S FRACTURE

- Usually a flexion injury resulting in an avulsion of the tip of the spinous process (C7 > C6 > T1)
- May also result from a direct blow

UNILATERAL FACET DISLOCATION

- Occurs as a flexion–rotation injury
- Usually stable, but is potentially unstable as it often involves injury to the posterior ligamentous structures
- Often identified on the AP view of the C-spine films when the spinous processes do not line up

BILATERAL FACET DISLOCATION

- Occurs as a flexion injury and is extremely unstable
- Associated with a high incidence of spinal cord injury
- Appears on lateral C-spine films as a subluxation of the dislocated vertebra of greater than one half the AP diameter of the vertebral body below it

SUBLUXATION

- Occurs with disruption of the ligamentous structures without bony involvement
- Potentially unstable
- Findings on C-spine films may be subtle, and flexion–extension views may be needed.

Thoracic Spine Fractures

- As mentioned above, the majority of injuries take place at the junction between the relatively fixed upper thoracic spine and the mobile thoracolumbar region (T10–L5).
- When thoracic fractures do take place, they can be devastating because the spinal canal through this region is relatively narrow and the blood supply to this region of spinal cord is in a watershed area (the greater radicular artery of Adamkiewicz enters the spinal canal at L1 but provides blood flow as high as T4).
- Most thoracic spine fractures are caused by hyperflexion leading to a wedge or compression fracture of the vertebral body.
- The majority of fractures/dislocations in this area are considered stable because of the surrounding normal bony thorax.
- However, as mentioned, neurologic impairment resulting from injuries in this area is often complete.

THORACOLUMBAR JUNCTION AND LUMBAR SPINE FRACTURES AND DISLOCATIONS

Frequency: L1 > L2 > T1

Compression (Wedge) Fracture

- Results from axial loading and flexion
- Potentially unstable

- Neurologic injury is uncommon.
- Treatment is symptomatic (patients usually experience pain and are at increased risk for the formation of an ileus).

Burst Fracture

- Fracture of the vertebral end plates with forceful extrusion of the nucleus pulposus into the vertebral body causing comminution of the vertebral body
- Results from axial loading
- See loss of vertebral height on lateral spine film.

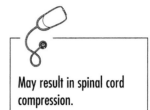

May result in spinal cord compression.

Distraction or Seat Belt Injury

- Frequently referred to as a "chance fracture"
- Horizontal fracture through the vertebral body, spinous processes, laminae, and pedicles and tearing of the posterior spinous ligament
- Caused by an acceleration–deceleration injury of a mobile person moving forward into a fixed seat belt

Fracture–Dislocations

- Result from flexion with rotation
- Unstable and often associated with spinal cord damage

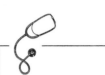

Abdominal injuries frequently coexist with fracture–dislocations.

SACRAL AND COCCYGEAL SPINE FRACTURES AND DISLOCATIONS

- Fractures in this area are relatively uncommon.
- Sacral injuries must often be diagnosed via CT scan.
- Neurologic impairment is rare; however, damage to the sacral nerve roots results in bowel/bladder and sexual dysfunction as well as loss of sensory and motor function to the posterior lower extremities.
- Fractures of the coccyx are usually caused by direct trauma.
- Diagnosis is made upon palpation of a "step-off" on rectal examination, and rectal bleeding must also be ruled out (severe fractures may lead to a rectal tear).
- Treatment of uncomplicated coccygeal fracture is symptomatic and includes pain management and a doughnut pillow.

THORACIC TRAUMA

Cardiac Tamponade

- Life-threatening emergency usually seen with penetrating thoracic trauma, but may be seen with blunt thoracic trauma as well
- Signs include tachycardia, muffled heart sounds, jugular venous distention (JVD), hypotension, and electrical alternans on electrocardiogram (ECG) (see Figure 4-7).

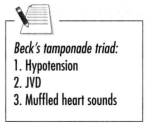

Beck's tamponade triad:
1. Hypotension
2. JVD
3. Muffled heart sounds

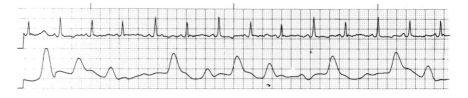

FIGURE 4-7. Simultaneous ECG (top) and plethysmograph (bottom) tracings in a patient with clinical signs of cardiac tamponade. Note the varying amplitude of the R wave on the ECG, known as electrical alternans.

(Reproduced, with permission, from Tintinalli JE, Kelen GD, Stapczynski JS. *Emergency Medicine: A Comprehensive Study Guide,* 5th ed. New York: McGraw-Hill, 2000.)

- Diagnosis may be confirmed with cardiac sonogram if immediately available.
- Requires immediate decompression via **needle pericardiocentesis,** pericardial window, or thoracotomy with manual decompression

Tension Pneumothorax

- Life-threatening emergency caused by air entering the pleural space (most often via a hole in the lung tissue) but being unable to escape
- Causes total ipsilateral lung collapse, mediastinal shift **(away from injured lung)** impairing venous return and thus decreased cardiac output, eventually resulting in shock
- Signs and symptoms include dyspnea, hypotension, tracheal deviation, absent breath sounds, and hyperresonance to percussion.
- Requires immediate needle decompression followed by tube thoracostomy

Hemothorax

- Defined as the presence of blood in the lungs
- > 200 cc of blood must be present before blunting of costophrenic angle will be seen on CXR.
- Treatment involves chest tube placement and drainage.

Indications for Thoracotomy
- 1,500 cc initial drainage from the chest tube
- 200 cc/hr continued drainage
- Patients who decompensate after initial stabilization
- > 50% hemothorax

Traumatic Aortic Rupture

- Most often seen with sudden deceleration injuries (high-speed motor vehicle crash, falls from > 25 feet)
- Most frequent site of rupture is ligamentum arteriosum.
- High-mortality injury: Almost 90% die at the scene, and another 50% die within 24 hours.
- Signs and symptoms:
  - Retrosternal chest pain
  - Dyspnea

A diagnosis of tension pneumothorax via x-ray is a missed diagnosis. Do not delay treatment of a suspected tension pneumothorax in order to confirm your suspicion (i.e., tension pneumothorax is a **clinical** diagnosis).

Needle decompression involves placing a needle or catheter over a needle into the second intercostal space, midclavicular line, over the rib on the side of the tension pneumothorax, followed by a tube thoracostomy (chest tube).

- New systolic murmur
- Pseudocoarctation syndrome: Increased BP in upper extremities with absent or decreased femoral pulses
- Pulse deficits between upper and lower extremities
- Findings on CXR:
  - Widened mediastinum
  - Tracheal or NG tube deviation to the right
  - Depression of left main stem bronchus
  - Widening of paratracheal stripe to the right
  - Indistinct aortic knob
  - Indistinct space between pulmonary artery and aorta
  - Presence of left apical cap
  - Multiple rib fractures
- Diagnosis is via angiography.

Sucking Chest Wound

- Also known as a communicating pneumothorax
- Caused by an open defect in the chest wall, often due to gunshot injuries
- If the diameter of the defect is greater than two thirds the diameter of the trachea, air will preferentially enter through the defect.
- The affected lung will collapse on inspiration as air enters through the defect and expand slightly on expiration. This mechanism seriously impairs ventilation.
- Initial treatment involves covering wound with an occlusive dressing sealed on three sides. This will convert it to a closed pneumothorax while the unsealed side will allow air to escape, preventing conversion into a tension pneumothorax.

Pulmonary Contusion

- Damage to the lung parenchyma without pulmonary laceration
- Most common mechanism is direct chest trauma in a rapid deceleration injury.
- Signs and symptoms:
  - Dyspnea
  - Tachypnea
  - Local ecchymosis
- Arterial blood gas (ABG) findings:
  - Hypoxemia
  - Widened A-a gradient
- Findings on CXR:
  - Local irregular patchy infiltrate that corresponds to site of injury. This develops usually immediately, and always within 6 hours.
- Treatment involves supplemental oxygen and pulmonary toilet.
- Most frequent complication is pneumonia.

Typical scenario:
A 25-year-old female presents after a high-speed motor vehicle crash with dyspnea and tachycardia. There is local bruising over the right side of her chest. CXR shows a right upper lobe consolidation. *Think: Pulmonary contusion.*

The most frequently injured solid organ associated with penetrating trauma is the liver, followed by the small bowel.

The most frequently injured solid organ associated with blunt trauma is the spleen, followed by the liver.

General

Penetrating abdominal injuries (PAIs) resulting from a gunshot create damage via three mechanisms:

1. Direct injury by the bullet itself
2. Injury from fragmentation of the bullet
3. Indirect injury from the resultant "shock wave"

PAIs resulting from a stabbing mechanism are limited to the direct damage of the object of impalement.

Blunt abdominal injury also has three general mechanisms of injury:

1. Injury caused by the direct blow
2. Crush injury
3. Deceleration injury that occurs

Anatomy

- Anterior abdominal wall—bordered laterally by the midaxillary lines, superiorly by a horizontal line drawn through the nipples and inferiorly by the symphysis pubis and inguinal ligaments
- The "thoracoabdominal region" is that region below the nipples and above the costal margins and is the area within which the diaphragm travels. Penetrating injuries to this region are more likely to involve injury to the diaphragm.
- Flank—area between the anterior and posterior axillary lines
- Back—area posterior to the posterior axillary lines, bordered superiorly by a line drawn through the tips of the scapulae and inferiorly by the iliac crests
- Peritoneal viscera—liver, spleen, stomach, small bowel, sigmoid and transverse colon
- Retroperitoneal viscera—majority of the duodenum (fourth part is intraperitoneal), pancreas, kidneys and ureters, ascending and descending colon, and major vessels such as the abdominal aorta, inferior vena cava, renal and splenic vessels
- Pelvic viscera—bladder, urethra, ovaries and uterus in women, prostate in men, rectum, and iliac vessels

Physical Examination

- **Seat belt sign**—ecchymotic area found in the distribution of the lower anterior abdominal wall and can be associated with perforation of the bladder or bowel as well as a lumbar distraction fracture (chance fracture)
- **Cullen's sign** (periumbilical ecchymosis) is indicative of intraperitoneal hemorrhage.
- **Grey Turner's sign** (flank ecchymoses) is indicative of retroperitoneal hemorrhage.
- Inspect the abdomen for evisceration, entry/exit wounds, impaled objects, and a gravid uterus.

Diagnosis

- Perforation: Abdominal x-ray and CXR to look for free air
- Diaphragmatic injury: CXR to look for blurring of the diaphragm, hemothorax, or bowel gas patterns above the diaphragm (at times with a gastric tube seen in the left chest)

FAST

- Used as a rapid bedside screening study
- Noninvasive and not time consuming
- Positive if free fluid is demonstrated in the abdomen

Three abdominal views are utilized to search for free intraperitoneal fluid (presumed to be blood in the trauma victim), which collects in dependent areas and appears as hypoechoic areas on ultrasound:

- Morison's pouch in the right upper quadrant: Free fluid can be visualized between the interface of the liver and kidney.
- Splenorenal recess in the left upper quadrant: Free fluid can be visualized between the interface of the spleen and kidney.
- Pouch of Douglas, which lies above the rectum (probe is placed in the suprapubic region)
- Subxiphoid and parasternal views to look for hemopericardium

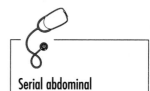

Serial abdominal examinations can and should be performed.

DPL

Advantages	Disadvantages
- Performed bedside	- Invasive
- Widely available	- Risk for iatrogenic injury
- Highly sensitive for hemoperitoneum	- Relatively low specificity (many false positives)
- Rapidly performed	- Does not evaluate the retroperitoneum

DPL Technique: Open

Make vertical incision carefully from the skin to the fascia. Grasp the fascial edges with clamps, elevate, then incise through to the peritoneum. Insert the peritoneal catheter and advance toward the pelvis.

DPL Technique: Closed

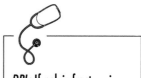

DPL: If pelvic fracture is suspected, a supra-umbilical approach should be used.

- Using skin clamps or an assistant's sterile gloved hands, elevate the skin on either side of the site of needle placement and make a "nick" with a #11 blade.
- Insert the needle (usually an 18-gauge needle comes with the kit) angled slightly toward the pelvis, through the skin and subcutaneous tissue, and into the peritoneum. Most often three areas of resistance are met (felt as "pops") as the needle is passed through: Linea alba, transversalis fascia, and peritoneum.
- Using the Seldinger technique, a guidewire is placed through the needle and advanced into the peritoneum.
- The needle is removed, leaving the guidewire in place.
- The peritoneal catheter is then threaded over the wire, and the wire is removed.

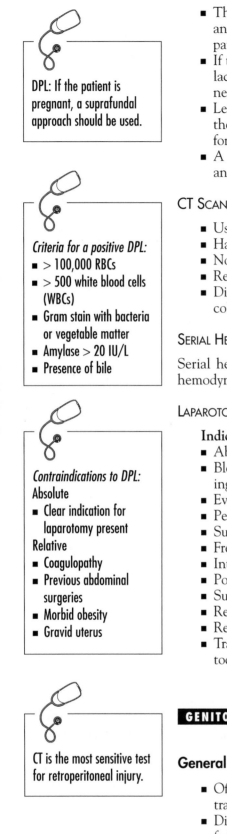

DPL: If the patient is pregnant, a suprafundal approach should be used.

Criteria for a positive DPL:
- > 100,000 RBCs
- > 500 white blood cells (WBCs)
- Gram stain with bacteria or vegetable matter
- Amylase > 20 IU/L
- Presence of bile

Contraindications to DPL:
Absolute
- Clear indication for laparotomy present
Relative
- Coagulopathy
- Previous abdominal surgeries
- Morbid obesity
- Gravid uterus

CT is the most sensitive test for retroperitoneal injury.

- The peritoneal catheter is in a syringe and is connected to the catheter and aspiration is performed. If gross blood appears (> 5 to 10 cc), the patient should be taken to the OR for exploratory laparotomy.
- If the aspiration is negative, instill 15 cc/kg of warmed normal saline or lactated Ringer's solution into the peritoneum through IV tubing connected to the catheter.
- Let the solution stand for up to 10 minutes (if the patient is stable), then place the IV bag from which the solution came from on the floor for drainage via gravity.
- A sample of the returned solution should be sent to the lab for STAT analysis.

CT SCANNING

- Useful for the hemodynamically stable patient
- Has a greater specificity than DPL and ultrasonography (US)
- Noninvasive
- Relatively time consuming when compared with DPL and US
- Diagnostic for specific organ injury; however, may miss diaphragmatic, colonic, and pancreatic injury

SERIAL HEMATOCRITS

Serial hematocrits should be obtained during the observation period of the hemodynamically stable patient.

LAPAROTOMY

Indications for Exploratory Laparotomy
- Abdominal trauma and hemodynamic instability
- Bleeding from stomach (not to be confused with nasopharyngeal bleeding)
- Evisceration
- Peritoneal irritation
- Suspected/known diaphragmatic injury
- Free intraperitoneal or retroperitoneal air
- Intraperitoneal bladder rupture (diagnosed by cystography)
- Positive DPL
- Surgically correctable injury diagnosed on CT scan
- Removal of impaled instrument
- Rectal perforation (diagnosed by sigmoidoscopy)
- Transabdominal missile (bullet) path (e.g., a gunshot wound to the buttock with the bullet being found in the abdomen or thorax)

GENITOURINARY (GU) TRAUMA

General

- Often overlooked in the initial evaluation of the multiply injured trauma victim
- Diagnostic evaluation of the GU tract is performed in a "retrograde" fashion (i.e., work your way back from the urethra to the kidneys and renal vasculature).

Anatomy

The GU tract injury is divided into upper (kidney and ureters) and lower tract (bladder, urethra, and genitalia) injury.

Signs and Symptoms

- Flank or groin pain
- Blood at the urethral meatus
- Ecchymoses on perineum and/or genitalia
- Evidence of pelvic fracture
- Rectal bleeding
- A "high-riding" or superiorly displaced prostate

Placement of Urethral Catheter

- A Foley or coudé catheter should be placed in any trauma patient with a significant mechanism of injury in the **absence** of any sign of urethral injury.
- Partial urethral tears warrant one careful attempt of a urinary catheter. If any resistance is met or a complete urethral tear is diagnosed, suprapubic catheter placement will be needed to establish urinary drainage.

Urinalysis

- The presence of gross hematuria indicates GU injury and often concomitant pelvic fracture.
- Urinalysis should be done to document presence or absence of microscopic hematuria.

Retrograde Urethrogram

- Should be performed in any patient with suspected urethral disruption (before Foley placement)
- A preinjection KUB (kidneys, ureter, and bladder) film should be taken.
- A 60-cc Toomey syringe (versus a Luer-lok syringe) should be filled with the appropriate contrast solution and placed in the urethral meatus.
- With the patient in the supine position, inject 20 to 60 cc contrast over 30 to 60 seconds.
- A repeat KUB is taken during the last 10 cc of contrast injection.
- Retrograde flow of contrast from the meatus to the bladder without extravasation connotes urethral integrity and Foley may then be placed.
- May be performed in the OR in patients requiring emergency surgery for other injuries

Bladder Rupture

Intraperitoneal
- Usually occurs due to blunt trauma to a full bladder
- Treatment is surgical repair.

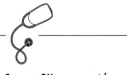

Suspect GU trauma with:
- Straddle injury
- Penetrating injury to lower abdomen
- Falls from height

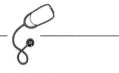

Blood at the urethral meatus is virtually diagnostic for urethral injury and demands early retrograde urethrogram before Foley placement.

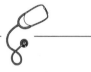

Do not probe perineal lacerations, as they are often a sign of an underlying pelvic fracture, and disruption of a hematoma may occur.

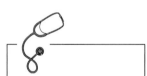

History of enlarged prostate, prostate cancer, urethral stricture, self-catheterization, or previous urologic surgery may make Foley placement difficult or can be confused with urethral disruption.

Extraperitoneal
- Usually occurs due to pelvic fracture
- Treatment is nonsurgical management by Foley drainage.

Retrograde Cystogram

- Should be performed on patients with gross hematuria or a pelvic fracture
- Obtain preinjection KUB.
- Fill the bladder with 400 cc of the appropriate contrast material using gravity at a height of 2 feet.
- Obtain another KUB.
- Empty the bladder (unclamp the Foley), then irrigate with saline and take another KUB ("washout" film).
- Extravasation of contrast into the pouch of Douglas, paracolic gutters, or between loops of intestine is diagnostic for intraperitoneal rupture and requires operative repair of the bladder.
- Extravasation of contrast into the paravesicular tissue or behind the bladder as seen on the "washout" film is indicative of extraperitoneal bladder rupture.

Ureteral Injury

- Least common GU injury
- Must be surgically repaired
- Diagnosed at the time of intravenous pyelogram (IVP) or CT scan during the search for renal injury

Renal Contusion

- Most common renal injury
- Renal capsule remains intact.
- IVP is usually normal and CT scan may show evidence of edema or microextravasation of contrast into the renal parenchyma.
- Often associated with a subcapsular hematoma
- Management is conservative and requires admission to the hospital.
- Recovery is usually complete unless there is underlying renal pathology.

Renal Laceration

- Classified as either minor (involving only the renal cortex) or major (extending into the renal medulla and/or collecting system)
- Diagnosed by CT scan or IVP
- Minor renal lacerations are managed expectantly.
- Management of major renal lacerations varies and depends on the surgeon, hemodynamic stability of the patient, and the extent of injury and its coincident complications (ongoing bleeding and urinary extravasation).

Renal Fracture ("Shattered Kidney")

- Involves complete separation of the renal parenchyma from the collecting system
- Usually leads to uncontrolled hemorrhage and requires surgical intervention

EXTREMITY TRAUMA

Signs and Symptoms

- Tenderness to palpation
- Decreased range of motion
- Deformity or shortening of extremity
- Swelling
- Crepitus
- Laceration or open wound over extremity (open fracture)
- Temperature or pulse difference in one extremity compared to the other
- Loss of sensation in extremity
- Abnormal capillary refill

Treatment

- Reduction of fracture or dislocation under sedation
- Splint extremity
- Irrigation, antibiotics, and tetanus prophylaxis for open fractures

Complications

- Compartment syndrome
- Neurovascular compromise
- Fat embolism
- Osteomyelitis
- Rhabdomyolysis (with prolonged crush injuries)
- Avascular necrosis
- Malunion
- Nonunion

Signs of compartment syndrome: **The 6 Ps**
Pain
Pallor
Paresthesias
Pulse deficit
Poikilothermia
Paralysis

Rhabdomyolysis causes myoglobin release, which can cause renal failure. Maintaining a high urine output together with alkalinization of the urine can help prevent the renal failure by reducing precipitation of myoglobin in the kidney.

HIGH-YIELD FACTS

Trauma

Neurologic Emergencies

Definition

Change in mental status is a term used to describe a spectrum of altered mentation including dementia, delirium, psychosis, and coma.

Causes

- Infection:
    - Meningitis
    - Encephalitis
    - Urosepsis
    - Pneumonia
- Metabolic:
    - Uremia
    - Hepatic encephalopathy
    - Electrolyte imbalance
    - Hyper/hypoglycemia
    - Thyroid disease
    - Adrenal disease
- Neurological:
    - Cerebrovascular accident (CVA)
    - Central nervous system (CNS) space-occupying lesions (neoplasm)
    - Seizures/postictal state
    - CNS trauma
- Vascular:
    - Hypertensive encephalopathy
    - Vasculitis
- Cardiopulmonary:
    - Hypoxic encephalopathy
    - Congestive heart failure (CHF)
    - Chronic obstructive pulmonary disease
    - Pulmonary embolism
- Toxic:
    - Drug overdose
    - Alcohol withdrawal

- Environmental:
  - Carbon monoxide exposure
  - Hypo/hyperthermia

DELIRIUM

Definition

- Impairment of brain function secondary to another disease state
- Delirium is usually transient in nature, reversing with removal or treatment of underlying cause.
- Patients with structural brain damage as cause of delirium may progress to chronic dementia.

Clinical Presentation

- Patients usually have difficulty in focusing or sustaining attention.
- Clinical course is usually fluctuating, waxing and waning.
- Onset is usually rapid, from days to weeks.
- Symptoms usually worsen at night.
- Some patients may experience hallucinations, usually visual in nature.
- Patients usually have clinical signs and symptoms suggestive of underlying cause.

Diagnosis

- Coma cocktail: Thiamine, glucose, naloxone
- Head CT and labs to identify underlying cause

Treatment

- Sedation as needed for patient comfort
- Treat underlying cause.

DEMENTIA

Definition

- A chronic, progressive decline in mental capacity that interferes with a patient's normal psychosocial activity
- The identification of *reversible dementia* is key because progression can be halted.

Nonreversible Causes

- Degenerative:
  - Alzheimer's disease
  - Parkinson's disease
- Vascular:
  - Multiple infarcts
  - Subarachnoid hemorrhage (SAH)
  - Anoxic brain damage

Treatment of delirium: **CAST**
Cocktail
Admission
Sedation
Tomography (CT)

Reversible causes of dementia: **DEMENTIA**
Drugs
Electrolyte disturbances, eye and ear problems
Metabolic abnormalities (uremia, thyroid)
Emotional problems (psych)
Neoplasm, nutritional (vitamin deficiency)
Trauma
Infection, inflammation (lupus)
Alcohol

Clinical Presentation

- Impairment is gradual and progressive.
- Attention is usually normal, without waxing or waning of consciousness.
- Distant memory is usually preserved.

Diagnosis

Identify *reversible* causes of dementia.

Treatment

- Address *reversible* causes of dementia.
- Supportive environmental, psychosocial interventions

DIFFERENTIATING DELIRIUM, DEMENTIA, AND PSYCHOSIS

See Table 5-1.

TABLE 5-1. Differentiating Delirium, Dementia, and Psychosis

Manifestations	Delirium	Dementia	Psychosis
Onset	Sudden	Insidious	Sudden
Duration	Days to weeks	Permanent	Years (history)
Arousal level	Fluctuating	Normal	Normal
Attention	Poorly maintained	Maintained	Varies
Memory	Usually not intact	Distant memory intact	Varies
Hallucinations	Usually visual	Usually absent	Usually auditory
Delusions	Transient	Absent	Sustained
Thought process	Poorly organized	Varies with degree	Varies

COMA

Definition

Diffuse brain failure leading to impaired consciousness

Management

- ABCs:
  - Airway—intubate if necessary to protect airway.
  - Breathing—oxygen, oral airway

Causes of coma:
AEIOU TIPS
Alcohol
Encephalopathy, endocrine (thyroid disease, etc.), electrolyte abnormality
Insulin-dependent diabetes
Opiates, oxygen deprivation
Uremia

Trauma, temperature
Infection
Psychosis, porphyria
Space-occupying lesion, stroke, SAH, shock

- Circulation—intravenous (IV) access, blood pressure
- **C-spine**—cervical collar unless absolutely sure no history of trauma
- **Vitals**—temperature, oxygen saturation (fifth vital sign) frequent reassessment
- **Electrocardiogram (ECG)/cardiac monitor**—arrhythmias, myocardial infarction (MI)
- **History:**
  - From patient, family member, bystander, or old chart
  - Past medical history
  - Past psychiatric history
  - Medications
  - Social history (drug or alcohol use)
- **Physical exam:**
  - General exam:
    - Check for signs of trauma.
    - Glasgow Coma Scale
    - Respiratory pattern:
      - Cheyne–Stokes: Periodic fluctuations of respiratory rate and depth suggest CNS pathology.
  - Ocular exam:
    - Pupillary function: If pupils are **reactive** to light bilaterally, brain stem is intact:
      - **Pinpoint pupils** suggest opioid toxicity or pontine dysfunction.
      - **Fixed and dilated pupils** suggest increased intracranial pressure (ICP) with possible herniation.
  - Ocular motions:
    - **Doll's eyes reflex:** Turn patient's head quickly to one side and observe eye movement. In a normal response, the eyes move in the opposite direction. Absence of motion suggests dysfunction in hemisphere or brain stem function.
  - Neurological exam: Refer to section on neurological examination.

Do not perform doll's eye maneuver in the presence of head or neck trauma.

Diagnosis

- Arterial blood gas: Acid–base disorders can help point to etiology (remember MUDPILES).
- Routine labs: Look for infection or electrolyte abnormalities.
- Toxicology screen: Look for drugs and alcohol.
- X-rays: C-spine in suspected cases of trauma
- Head CT: Look for intracranial pathology.
- Lumbar puncture (LP): Look for SAH or infection.

Treatment

Coma cocktail: **DON'T**
Dextrose (1 amp)
Oxygen
Naloxone
' (To remind you to give thiamine before dextrose)
Thiamine

- Coma cocktail
- Supportive care
- Monitoring (cardiac, oxygen saturation)
- Identify specific cause and apply appropriate treatment.
- Appropriate specialty consult as deemed necessary

Definitions

- **CVAs:** Neurologic deficit caused by a disruption of blood flow to the brain
- **Transient ischemic attacks (TIAs):** Neurological deficits that resolve within 24 hours
- **Stroke in evolution:** Neurological deficits that fluctuate or worsen over time
- **Completed stroke:** Neurological deficits that have remained stable for over 24 hours

Anatomy

Anterior Circulation
- Originates from the carotid system, then leads to anterior and middle cerebral artery
- Supplies blood to the eye, the frontal and parietal lobes, and majority of the temporal area

Posterior Circulation
- Originates from the vertebral arteries, then forms the basilar artery, cerebellar arteries, then the posterior cerebral artery (PCA)
- Supplies the brain stem, ears, cerebellum, occipital cortex, and parts of the temporal lobe

General Classification

Ischemic Stroke (Figures 5-1 and 5-2)
- 80% of all strokes
- Thrombotic stroke
- Embolic stroke
- Lacunar stroke
- Systemic hypoperfusion

Hemorrhagic Stroke (Figure 5-3)
- 20% of all strokes
- Intracerebral hemorrhage
- SAH

Specific Classification

See Table 5-2.

Thrombotic Stroke
- Risk factors:
  - Atherosclerosis (most common cause)
  - Vasculitis
  - Often preceded by TIA
- Pathophysiology:
  - Vessel narrowing and occlusion secondary to plaque formation

HIGH-YIELD FACTS

Neurologic Emergencies

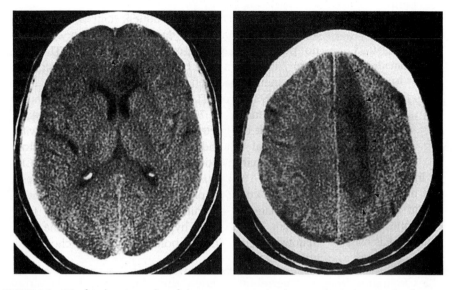

FIGURE 5-1. CT of ischemic stroke of the anterior cerebral artery (ACA). Note the lesion is hypodense.
(Reprinted, with permission, from Johnson MH. CT evaluation of the earliest signs of stroke. *The Radiologist* 1(4): 189–199, 1994.)

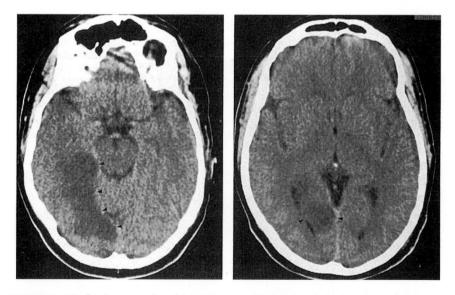

FIGURE 5-2. CT of ischemic stroke of the PCA. Note the lesion is hypodense.
(Reprinted, with permission, from Johnson MH. CT evaluation of the earliest signs of stroke. *The Radiologist* 1(4): 189–199, 1994.)

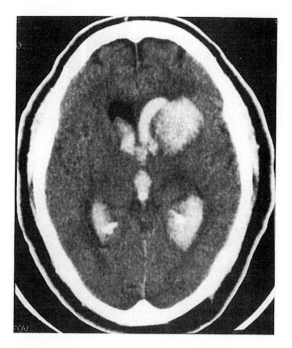

FIGURE 5-3. Hemorrhagic stroke due to hypertension. Note the lesion is hyperdense. Note bleeding into the ventricles. Effacement of sulci suggests edema. Mild mass effect is also present.

(Reprinted, with permission, from Lee SH, Zimmerman RA, Rao KC. *Cranial MRI and CT,* 4th ed. New York: McGraw-Hill, 1999.)

Embolic Stroke
- Risk factors:
  - Atrial fibrillation
  - Dilated cardiomyopathy
  - Recent MI
  - Endocarditis
  - IV drug abuse
- Pathophysiology:
  - Occlusion from intravascular material (clot, air bubble, fat, etc.) from distal sites
  - Sources of emboli:

TABLE 5-2. Differentiating Stroke Types

	Thrombotic	Embolic	Hemorrhagic
Timing	Upon awaking	Any time	Any time
Onset	Gradual, evolves	Sudden	Sudden
Associated symptoms	Prior TIA	Palpitations	Severe, sudden headache Nausea, vomiting Stiff neck Coma Seizure

- Most common sources of emboli are from heart or ruptured plaque from major vessels.
- Dislodged vegetation from cardiac valves (fibrin clots, septic vegetations, etc.)
- Dislodged mural thrombi from atrial fibrillation, dilated cardiomyopathy, or recent MI

Lacunar Stroke
- Risk factor: Chronic hypertension
- Pathophysiology: Occlusion of small penetrating arteries

Intracerebral Hemorrhage
- Risk factors:
  - Age
  - History of prior stroke
  - Smoking
  - Hypertension
  - Anticoagulation (e.g., warfarin therapy)
  - Amyloidosis
  - Cocaine use
- Pathophysiology:
  - Vessel rupture with bleeding into brain parenchyma, causing increased ICP

SAH
- Risk factors:
  - Ruptured berry aneurysms
  - Arteriovenous malformations
- Pathophysiology:
  - Vessel rupture with blood leaking into subarachnoid space
  - Usually occurs at bifurcation of vessels

Physical Exam

- Vitals:
  - Cushing reflex: Hypertension, bradycardia, and abnormal breathing could represent an increase in ICP.
- Eyes:
  - Do funduscopic exam.
  - Papilledema is a sign of increased ICP.
  - Subhyaloid hemorrhage is pathognomonic for SAH.
  - Note papillary function and extraocular movements.
- Neurological exam: Localize lesion and differentiate between ischemic and hemorrhagic CVA.

Localization

- Middle cerebral artery:
  - Most common
  - Contralateral weakness and numbness of arms greater than legs
  - Aphasia
  - Homonymous hemianopsia: Loss of vision on right or left side of both eyes
- ACA: Contralateral weakness of legs greater than arms

Signs of lacunar strokes:
DAMS
- **D**ysarthria — clumsy hand: Slurred speech with weak, clumsy hands
- **A**taxic hemiparesis: Ataxia with leg weakness
- Pure **M**otor hemiplegia: Motor hemiplegia without sensory changes
- Pure **S**ensory stroke: Sensory deficits of face, arms, legs without motor deficits

- PCA:
    - Vision changes
    - Sensory changes
    - Usually have subtle presentations
- Small penetrating arteries: Lacunar strokes present as "DAMS"
- Vertebrobasilar artery:
    - Syncope
    - Weakness
    - Cranial nerve changes
    - **Crossed findings** (ipsilateral cranial nerve changes with contralateral motor weakness)
    - Ataxia
- Cerebellar arteries:
    - **Central vertigo**
    - Headache
    - Nausea and vomiting
    - Loss of posture (inability to sit or stand without support)

Diagnosis

- Routine labs
- ECG
- CT scan of head:
    - Helps differentiate ischemic from hemorrhagic CVA
    - Helpful up to 12 hours; before that, CT can be negative in ischemic strokes.
    - Area of cerebellum could be distorted by bony artifact.
    - Detects 1-cm and larger intracerebral hemorrhage (acute bleed looks white on CT scan)
    - Detects SAH 90% of time
    - Magnetic resonance imaging (MRI)
    - Can detect subtle ischemic infarcts
    - Good study for brain stem or cerebellar lesions
    - Availability of MRI is a limiting factor.

Emergency Department Management of Ischemic Stroke

- ABCs: Give supplemental O_2.
- Blood pressure (BP) control:
    - Since autoregulation is lost in ishemic brain, perfusion is directly dependent on the cerebral perfusion pressure (CPP), which in turn is dependent on the mean arterial pressure (MAP).
    - CPP = MAP – ICP
    - MAP = ⅓ SBP + ⅔ DBP. Ideally want MAP ≥ 60
    - Use pressors for MAP < 60 or sBP < 90.
- Serum glucose control:
    - Hyperglycemia provides more substrate for anaerobic metabolism, worsening acidosis.
    - It is recommended to keep serum glucose < 150 mg/dL
    - Use sliding scale regular insulin for glucose > 300 mg/dL
- Temperature control:
    - Hyperthermia increases oxygen demand when the ischemic brain is already hypoxic.
    - Administer acetaminophen for fever.

Vertebrobasilar strokes present with **3 Ds:**
Dizziness (vertigo)
Diplopia
Dysphasia

Identification of strokes involving the cerebellum is important due to risk of edema and increased pressure to brain stem.

Optimization for ischemic stroke:
- Supplemental O_2
- BP: MAP ≥ 60, sBP ≥ 90
- Serum glucose: < 150
- Normal temperature
- Screen for thrombolytics

- Thrombolytic therapy:
  - Only approved specific therapy (Class I within 3 hours of symptom onset)
  - Very specific inclusion criteria: Need a clinical diagnosis of stroke with National Institute of Health stroke scale score < 22. Stroke needs to be moderate; massive strokes and very mild strokes are not eligible.
  - Same contraindications as for thrombolytic therapy in MI

Emergency Department Management of Hemorrhage Stroke

Up to 25% of patients with a hemorrhagic stroke will seize in the first 72 hours.

- ABCs: Consider early intubation.
- BP control:
  - Keep MAP < 130 and sBP < 220.
  - Agents of choice: Labetalol, nitroprusside
- Control seizures with lorazepam acutely, followed by phenytoin.
- Control cerebral edema with dexamethasone.
- Control elevated ICP with mannitol, hyperventilation, and by elevating the head of the bed.
- Nimodipine (Ca^{2+} channel blocker) to decrease vasospasm in SAH
- Prompt neurosurgical evaluation

Prevention

Antiplatelet agents: **CAT**
Clopidogrel
Aspirin
Ticlopidine

- Antiplatelet therapy for ischemic strokes
- Anticoagulation with warfarin for embolic strokes
- Smoking cessation
- Strict hypertension control
- Control of hyperlipidemia

NEUROLOGICAL EXAMINATION

Mental Status

- Orientation: Person (×1), place (×2), time (×3)
- Level of consciousness: Awake, lethargic, comatose
- Affect: Appropriate, alert, confused
- Speech: Presence of dysphasia or dysarthria, appropriateness of speech, and language content

Definitions of Expression

- *Dysarthria:* Difficulty in speech secondary to muscle weakness or paralysis
- *Dysphasia:* Disorder in the comprehension or expression of speech
- *Expressive dysphasia:* Difficulty in finding words or expression of speech without a defect in comprehension
- *Receptive dysphasia:* Problems in understanding words or written speech

80

CN I: Olfactory

Distinguishing two odors (e.g., coffee and garlic powder)

CN II: Optic

Test visual fields of each eye.

CN III: Oculomotor

Check pupillary function and extraocular motions. Don't forget to do a funduscopic exam.

CN IV: Trochlear

Controls Superior Oblique (SO4)

CN V: Trigeminal

- Sensation to face (V1, V2, and V3)
- Check motor function of muscles of mastication (masseter, pterygoids, temporalis).

CN VI: Abducens

Controls Lateral Rectus (LR6)

CN VII: Facial

- Check motor function of face—ask patients to puff out cheeks (buccinator muscle) and smile.
- Check for facial symmetry.

Peripheral versus Central CN VII Palsy

In patients with a seventh nerve palsy, ask patient to raise eyebrows and examine forehead for symmetry:
- Peripheral lesion: Asymmetrical or absent wrinkles on the side of the lesion
- Central lesion: Symmetrical wrinkles due to crossed fibers (innervation from both sides of the cerebral hemispheres)

CN VIII: Vestibulocochlear

- Check auditory acuity.
- Look for nystagmus (onset, direction, fatigability).

CN IX: Glossopharyngeal

- Check gag reflex (shared with CN X).
- Check taste on posterior one third of tongue.

Fracture of cribriform plate can disrupt odor sensation.

Corneal reflex: Touch side of cornea with cotton wisp. A blink is a normal response indicating normal reflex arc. This reflex requires V1 division of trigeminal nerve (V) for sensory input and motor response from intact facial nerve (VII).

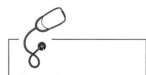

If vertical nystagmus is found in a patient, a central lesion within the brain stem or cerebellum must be ruled out.

HIGH-YIELD FACTS

Neurologic Emergencies

CN X: Vagus

Check for uvula deviation.

CN XI: Accessory

Check trapezius and sternocleidomastoid muscles. Ask patient to shrug his shoulders.

CN XII: Hypoglossal

Check for tongue deviation. Deviation indicates ipsilateral lesion.

MOTOR SYSTEM

Decorticate posture: COR — visualized as covering of chest, and CORonaries

Posture

- **Decorticate posture:** Abnormal flexion of the arm and wrist, with extension of the leg
- **Decerebrate posture:** Abnormal extension of both the arms and legs

Strength

5 = Normal strength
4 = Able to move against resistance
3 = Movement against gravity
2 = Movement with gravity eliminated
1 = Flickers of motion
0 = No movement

Pronator Drift

- Have patient hold arms outstretched, palms upward, with eyes closed.
- Pronation of the hand with downward drift of the arms is considered an abnormal sign.
- Normal strength and proprioception is required to prevent arms from drifting.

SENSORY SYSTEM

Symmetry

- Right versus left
- Upper versus lower

Sensation

- Touch
- Pain
- Temperature
- Position
- Vibratory sensation

Level of Reactivity

- Hyperactive reflexes are associated with upper motor neuron lesions.
- Hypoactive reflexes are associated with lower motor neuron lesions.

Symmetry

Visualize spinal roots starting from feet up to arms.

Spinal Roots	Reflex
S1–2	Ankle
L3–4	Knee
C5–6	Biceps
C7–8	Triceps

Cerebellar Tests

- Finger to nose
- Heel to shin
- Check rapid repetitive motions (dysdiadokinesis).
- Gait

HEADACHE

Primary Headache Syndromes

- Migraine
- Tension headache
- Cluster headache

Secondary Causes

- CNS infection:
  - Meningitis
  - Encephalitis
  - Cerebral abscess
- Non-CNS infection:
  - Sinusitis
  - Upper respiratory infection
  - Fever
  - Herpes zoster
  - Ear infections
  - Dental infections
- Vascular:
  - SAH
  - Subdural hematoma
  - Epidural hematoma
  - Intracerebral hemorrhage
  - Temporal arteritis
  - Carotid or vertebral artery dissection
- Ophthalmologic:
  - Glaucoma

- Iritis
- Optic neuritis
- Toxic/metabolic:
  - Carbon monoxide (CO) poisoning
  - Nitrates and nitrides
  - Hypoglycemia
  - Hypoxia
  - Hypercapnia
  - Caffeine withdrawal
  - Withdrawal from chronic analgesics
  - Malignant hypertension
  - Preeclampsia
  - Pseudotumor cerebri
  - Post LP
  - Intracranial tumor

Diagnostic Approach

- Differentiate between primary headache syndromes and secondary causes of headache.
- Recognize critical life-threatening causes of headache.
- Treat primary causes of headache.

History

- Pattern:
  - First episode or chronic in nature
  - In chronic headache, assess duration, severity, or associated symptoms.
- Onset: Gradual versus sudden or severe
- Location:
  - Migraines typically unilateral
  - Tension headache usually bilateral
  - SAH headache usually occipital
- Associated symptoms:
  - Syncope
  - Changes in mental status
  - Fever
  - Vision changes
  - Seizures
  - Neck pain and stiffness
  - History of head trauma
- Past medical history:
  - Hypertension
  - CVA
  - Migraines
  - Human immunodeficiency virus (HIV)
- Medications:
  - Nitrates
  - Analgesics
  - Anticonvulsants
- Family history:
  - Migraines
  - SAH
- Age:
  - Look for secondary causes in elderly.
  - Migraines less likely in children

Consider CO poisoning if similar symptoms of headache, nausea, vomiting in other members of household.

HIGH-YIELD FACTS

Neurologic Emergencies

84

Physical Exam

- Vitals: Fever, BP, Cushing reflex
- Eyes: Funduscopic exam may reveal absence of venous pulsations or papilledema, suggesting increased ICP.
- Neurological exam: Refer to section on neurological exam.

Labs/Radiology

- Routine labs:
  - Check glucose.
  - Erythrocyte sedimentation rate (ESR): Positive if over 50 mm/hr
- CT scan of the brain:
  - Helps to identify:
    - Mass lesions
    - Midline shift of intracranial contents
    - CNS bleeds
    - Increased ICP (increased size of ventricles, enlargement of sulci)
  - Contrast is useful for:
    - Cerebral toxoplasmosis
    - Small brain mass
    - Intracranial abscess
- LP indications:
  - Meningitis
  - Encephalitis
  - SAH

MIGRAINE HEADACHE

Epidemiology

- Onset in adolescence
- Increased frequency in females

Pathophysiology

Theorized that brain responds to some trigger causing abnormal vascular changes

Signs and Symptoms

- Frequently associated with aura (should not last more than 1 hour)
- May have visual auras (scintillating scotoma, or flashing lights)
- Slow onset
- Last 4 to 72 hours
- Worsen with exertion
- Unilateral and pulsating
- Nausea, vomiting, photophobia
- Neurological deficits (history of similar deficits in prior episodes)

Treatment

- Whatever worked in the past
- Metoclopramide
- Compazine
- Dihydroergotamine
- Nonsteroidal anti-inflammatory drugs (NSAIDs) such as ketorolac
- Opioid analgesia

CLUSTER HEADACHE

Epidemiology

- More common in men
- Onset usually > 20 years old

Pathophysiology

Mechanism unknown

Signs and Symptoms

- Short lived
- Severe, unilateral, lasting up to 3 hours
- Appear in clusters, multiple attacks in same time of day or month
- Patients appear restless.
- Associated with ipsilateral conjunctival injection, lacrimation, nasal congestion, rhinorrhea, miosis, and ptosis

Treatment

- 100% oxygen
- NSAIDs

TENSION HEADACHE

Pathophysiology

Muscle tension has been theorized as the causative factor.

Signs and Symptoms

- Bilateral
- Nonpulsating
- Not worsened with exertion
- Usually no nausea or vomiting
- Associated neck or back pain

Treatment

NSAIDs

Causes

- Arteriovenous malformation
- Rupture of aneurysm
- Idiopathic

Signs and Symptoms

- Sudden, severe occipital headache
- Nausea, vomiting
- CT of head detects up to 90% (see Figure 5-4).
- If CT negative, perform LP to check cerebrospinal fluid (CSF) for blood or xanthochromia.

Head CT can miss up to 15% of SAH; therefore, an LP must be done to look for blood or xanthochromia if CT is negative.

Sudden, severe headache described as "worst headache of my life" should be considered SAH until proven otherwise (do CT + LP).

HIGH-YIELD FACTS

Neurologic Emergencies

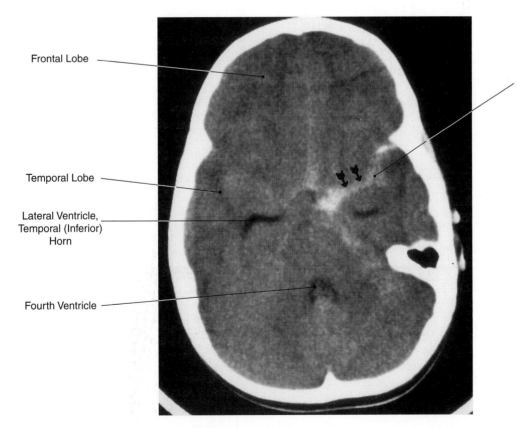

FIGURE 5-4. SAH. Arrows indicate fresh blood in the Sylvian fissure.

(Reproduced, with premission, from Afifi AK, Bergman RA. *Functional Neuroanatomy: Text and Atlas.* New York: McGraw-Hill, 1998: 554.)

Treatment

- To prevent vasospasm: Nimodipine 60 mg PO q 4 hours × 21 days, start within 96 hours of SAH
- For cerebral edema: Dexamethasone 10 mg IV × 1
- Prevent hypo- or hypertension.
- To lower ICP: Hyperventilation to a P_{CO_2} of 30 to 35 mm Hg
- To prevent seizures: Phenytoin 15 to 18 mg/kg loading dose
- Elevate head of the bed to 30° if C-spine is not a concern.
- Admit patients for observation.

TEMPORAL ARTERITIS

Epidemiology

More common in women age > 50

Pathophysiology

Systemic panarteritis affecting temporal artery

Signs and Symptoms

- Severe, throbbing in nature
- Frontal headache
- Tender temporal artery

Diagnosis

- ESR > 50 mm/hr
- Temporal artery biopsy showing giant cells is definitive—do not await biopsy results before initiating treatment.

Treatment

- Prednisone
- If left untreated, can lead to **vision loss**

SUBDURAL HEMATOMA

- History of head trauma (see chapter on trauma)
- Disruption of bridging vessels intracranially
- High-risk patients include alcoholics, elderly, and patients on anticoagulants.

CEREBRAL ISCHEMIA/INFARCT

Rarely produces headaches

INTRACEREBRAL HEMORRHAGE

- Commonly produces headache
- Neurological exam usually abnormal
- Refer to section on CVA for more detail.

BRAIN TUMOR

- Commonly presents with insidious headache
- Headache positional and worse in morning
- Neurological abnormalities usually present on physical exam

PSEUDOTUMOR CEREBRI (BENIGN INTRACRANIAL HYPERTENSION)

Epidemiology

- Occur in young, obese females
- History of headaches in past

Etiology

Unknown

Signs and Symptoms

- Papilledema
- Absent venous pulsations on funduscopic exam
- Headache, nausea, vomiting

Diagnosis

- Usually normal CT of head
- LP reveals elevated CSF opening pressures.

Treatment

- Steroids
- Acetazolamide
- LP to remove CSF
- CSF shunt

CAROTID OR VERTEBRAL ARTERY DISSECTION

- Idiopathic
- Secondary to trauma
- Unilateral neck pain with headache
- Diagnosed via angiography

POST LP HEADACHE

- Occurs within 24 to 48 hours post LP
- Headache secondary to persistent CSF leak
- Mild cases treated with analgesics
- Severe cases treated with blood patch (epidural injection of patient's blood to patch leak)

VERTIGO AND DIZZINESS

> The approach in the emergency department is to first distinguish between *true* vertigo and syncope, presyncope or weakness. Once *true* vertigo is differentiated, one must distinguish between *central* and *peripheral* vertigo. Consider all clinical information, including age and comorbidities.

Definitions

- **Dizziness** is a nonspecific term that should be clarified. It can be used to describe true vertigo or other conditions such as syncope, presyncope, light-headedness, or weakness.
- **Vertigo** is the perception of movement when there is no movement. The patient typically describes the room as spinning or the sensation of falling.
- **Nystagmus** is the rhythmic movement of eyes with two components (fast and slow). The direction of nystagmus is named by its fast component. Activation of the semicircular canals causes the slow component of the nystagmus to move away from the stimulus. The fast component of nystagmus is the reflex counter movement back to midline by the cortex.

Distinguishing Peripheral from Central Vertigo

See Table 5-3.

Peripheral Vertigo

Causes
- Benign paroxysmal positional vertigo
- Ménière's disease
- Vestibular neuronitis
- Labyrinthitis
- Ototoxicity (drugs)
- Eighth (vestibulocochlear) CN lesion
- Post-traumatic vertigo
- Middle ear disease
- Cerebellopontine angle tumors

TABLE 5-3. Peripheral versus Central Vertigo

	Peripheral Vertigo	**Central Vertigo**
Pathophysiology	Disorders affecting the vestibular apparatus or the eighth (vestibulocochlear) cranial nerve	Disorder affecting the brain or cerebellum
Severity	Intense	Less intense
Onset	Sudden	Slow, insidious
Pattern	Intermittent	Constant
Nausea/vomiting	Usually present	Usually absent
Positional (worsened by motion)	Usually	Usually not
Hearing changes or physical findings on ear exam	May be present	Usually absent
Focal neurologic findings	Absent	Usually present
Fatigability of symptoms	Yes	No
Nystagmus	Horizontal, vertical, rotary	Vertical

Benign Paroxysmal Positional Vertigo

EPIDEMIOLOGY

- Common
- Can occur at any age

PATHOPHYSIOLOGY

Transient vertigo precipitated by certain head motions

SIGNS AND SYMPTOMS

- Sudden onset
- Nausea
- Worse in morning, fatigable
- Normal ear exam, no hearing changes

DIAGNOSIS

Dix–Hallpike maneuver:
- Have patient with eyes open go from sitting to a supine position with head rotated to the side you want to test.
- Positive test entails reproduction of vertigo and nystagmus that resolves within 1 minute.
- Not to be performed on patients with carotid bruits

TREATMENT

- Antiemetics
- Antihistamines (meclizine)
- Benzodiazepines

Ménière's Disease

EPIDEMIOLOGY

Occurs between the ages of 30 and 60

PATHOPHYSIOLOGY

Etiology unknown; postulated that symptoms are due to extravasation of endolymph into the perilymphatic space

SIGNS AND SYMPTOMS

- Deafness, tinnitus, vertigo
- Nausea, vomiting, diaphoresis
- Recurrent attacks
- Deafness between attacks
- Attacks occur several times a week to months.

Ménière's triad: **DVT**
Deafness
Vertigo
Tinnitus

TREATMENT

Symptomatic treatment with antihistamines, antivertigo and antiemetic agents

Labyrinthitis

DEFINITION

Infection of labyrinth

SIGNS AND SYMPTOMS

- Hearing loss
- Peripheral vertigo
- Middle ear findings

DIAGNOSIS

Head CT or clinical

TREATMENT

Symptomatic treatment with antihistamines, antivertigo and antiemetic agents

Post-Traumatic Vertigo

PATHOPHYSIOLOGY

- Injury to labyrinth structures
- History of head trauma

SIGNS AND SYMPTOMS

- Peripheral vertigo
- Nausea, vomiting

DIAGNOSIS

CT of head to check for intracranial bleed or hematoma

TREATMENT

Symptomatic treatment with antihistamines, antivertigo and antiemetic agents

Vestibular Neuronitis

PATHOPHYSIOLOGY

Viral etiology

SIGNS AND SYMPTOMS

- Sudden onset, lasts several days
- Upper respiratory tract infection

TREATMENT

Symptomatic treatment with antihistamines, antivertigo and antiemetic agents

Other Causes of Central Vertigo

- Cerebellar hemorrhage or infarct
- Lateral medullary infarct **(Wallenberg syndrome)**
- Vertebrobasilar insufficiency
- Multiple sclerosis
- Neoplasm

OTOTOXICITY

Many drugs such as aminoglycosides, furosemide, and PCP cause ototoxicity.

HERPES ZOSTER OTICUS (RAMSAY HUNT SYNDROME)

Presents as deafness, facial nerve palsy, and vertigo with vesicles present in auditory canal

CEREBELLOPONTINE ANGLE TUMORS

Present with multiple findings (cerebellar signs, ataxia, vertigo, and loss of corneal reflex)

CEREBELLAR HEMORRHAGE OR INFARCTION

- Acute vertigo
- Profound ataxia or inability to stand or sit without support
- Cerebellar findings
- Headache

WALLENBERG SYNDROME

- Occlusion of posterior inferior cerebellar artery
- Acute onset
- Nausea, vomiting
- Nystagmus
- Ipsilateral facial pain, Horner's syndrome
- Contralateral pain and temperature loss

> Obtain neurology consult in all cases of central vertigo or cases in which you are unsure.

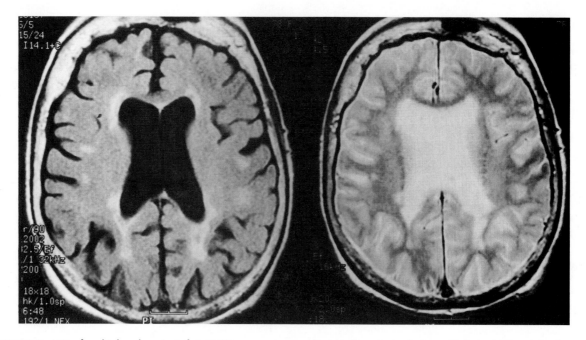

FIGURE 5-5. MRI of multiple sclerosis. Left is FLAIR sequence revealing periventricular lesions. Right is a T2-weighted image in which lesions are less obvious as they merge with the white ventricular CSF.

(Reproduced, with permission, from Gilman S. *Clinical Examination of the Nervous System.* New York: McGraw-Hill, 2000).

VERTEBROBASILAR VASCULAR DISEASE

- Vertebrobasilar vascular insufficiency can produce symptoms of vertigo.
- Other findings include diplopia, dysphagia, dysarthria, ataxia, **crossed findings** (refer to section on CVA—localizing the lesion).

MULTIPLE SCLEROSIS (SEE FIGURE 5-5)

- Demyelinating disease that can also affect the brain stem, causing vertigo
- May present with optic neuritis, ataxia, weakness, incontinence, or facial pain
- Best clue is inability to explain multiple neurologic symptoms and deficits by a single lesion.
- CSF may reveal oligoclonal banding.

CNS INFECTIONS

Meningitis

DEFINITION

Inflammation of the membrane surrounding the brain and spinal cord

CAUSES

- The majority of meningitides are caused by an infectious etiology, which varies according to age group (see Table 5-4).
- Noninfectious causes of meningitis include neoplasms, sarcoidosis, and CVA.

TABLE 5-4. Bugs in Meningitis by Age

	< 2 Months (Require Follow-up LP in 24–36 Hours)	2 Months to 50 Years	> 50 Years Debilitated or Immunocompromised
Organisms	■ Group B strep ■ *Listeria* ■ *Escherichia coli* ■ *Klebsiella* ■ *Enterobacter* ■ *Staphylococcus aureus* ■ *Haemophilus influenzae*	■ *Streptococcus pneumoniae* ■ *Neisseria meningitidis* ■ *H. influenzae*	■ *S. pneumoniae* ■ *Listeria* ■ Gram-negative bacteria
Treatment (IV)	■ Ampicillin 50 mg/kg q 8 h AND ■ Cefotaxime 50 mg/ kg q 8 h ■ ADD dexamethasone 0.4 mg/kg q 12 h × 2 d (for positive Gram stain or coma)	■ Cefotaxime 2 g q 4–6 h OR ■ Ceftriaxone 2 g q 12 h	■ Ampicillin 2 g q 4 h AND ■ Cefotaxime 2 g q 4–6 h OR ■ Ceftriaxone 2 g q 12 h
Penicillin-allergic Rx (IV)	■ TMP/SX 5mg/kg q 12 h AND ■ Vancomycin 15 mg/kg q 6 h	■ Vancomycin 15 mg/kg q 6 h AND ■ Gentamicin 2 mg/kg loading then 1.7 mg/kg q 8 h AND ■ Rifampin 10–20 mg/kg qd	

SIGNS AND SYMPTOMS

Altered mental status, photophobia, headache, fever, meningeal signs (nuchal rigidity, Kernig and Brudzinski's signs)

DIAGNOSIS

- Diagnosis made by LP: Obtain 5 tubes containing 1 to 2 mL of CSF.
- Make sure there is no risk of herniation prior to performing LP. (Head CT scan can support this.)
- CSF findings suggestive of bacterial meningitis include increased white blood cells with a high percentage of polymorphonuclear leukocytes, low glucose, and high protein.

TREATMENT

- Mainstay of treatment in adults is ceftriaxone, which has good CSF penetration.
- If resistance is an issue for *Streptococcus pneumoniae*, vancomycin or rifampin can be added to the regimen.
- Ampicillin should be added to any age group at risk for *Listeria monocytogenes*.

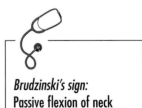

Kernig's sign:
Pain or resistance with passive extension of knee with hip flexed 90°.

Brudzinski's sign:
Passive flexion of neck causes flexion of the hips.

- Vancomycin and ceftazidime are used in post–head trauma patients, neurosurgical patients, or ventriculoperitoneal shunts.
- Antifungal agents should be considered in HIV+ and other immuno-compromised patients.

CNS Encephalitis

DEFINITION

Inflammation of the brain parenchyma secondary to infection

CAUSES

Usually viral in origin

SIGNS AND SYMPTOMS

- Abnormal behaviors and "personality changes"
- Seizures
- Headache
- Photophobia
- Focal neurological findings
- Signs of peripheral disease:
  - Herpes—skin vesicles, rash
  - Rabies—animal bite
  - Arboviruses—bug bite

DIAGNOSIS

Primarily diagnosed via CSF culture or serology: Blood in the CSF is a non-specific clue.

TREATMENT

- Mainly supportive
- Acyclovir for herpes

Brain Abscess

DEFINITION

A focal purulent cavity, covered by granulation tissue located in the brain

CAUSES

Brain abscesses develop secondary to:
- Hematogenous spread
- Contiguous infections
- Direct implantation via penetrating trauma or neurosurgery

SIGNS AND SYMPTOMS

- Headache
- Fever
- Focal neurological findings
- Signs of primary infection
- History of trauma

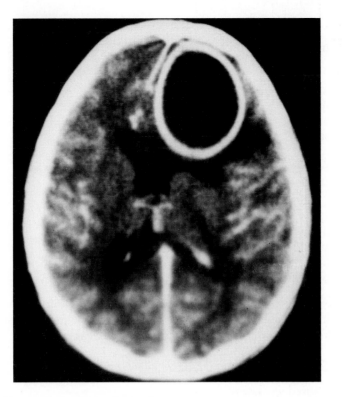

FIGURE 5-6. CT scan demonstrating brain abscess.
(Reproduced, with permission, from Schwartz SI, ed. *Principles of Surgery,* 7th ed. New York: McGraw-Hill, 1999: 1902.)

DIAGNOSIS

CT scan of head with contrast (see Figure 5-6)

TREATMENT

Antibiotics tailored to suspected source of primary infection

Guillain–Barré Syndrome

DEFINITION

- Ascending peripheral neuropathy
- Can affect all ages
- History of viral illness

CAUSES

Idiopathic

SIGNS AND SYMPTOMS

- Loss of deep tendon reflexes
- Distal weakness greater than proximal (legs greater than arms)
- Weakness is symmetrical.
- Numbness or tingling of the extremities
- Risk of respiratory failure

DIAGNOSIS

LP reveals increased CSF protein with a normal glucose and cell count.

TREATMENT

- Plasmapheresis
- IV immunoglobulin
- Intubate if there is respiratory compromise.

Myasthenia Gravis

DEFINITION

- Autoimmune disease of the neuromuscular junction
- Affects old males, and young females

PATHOPHYSIOLOGY

- Acetylcholine receptor antibodies bind acetylcholine receptors, preventing binding of acetylcholine and subsequent muscular stimulation.
- Failure of neuromuscular conduction causes weakness.

SIGNS AND SYMPTOMS

- Generalized weakness
- Usually proximal weakness affected more than distal weakness
- Weakness relieved with rest
- Ptosis and diplopia usually present
- Symptoms may fluctuate, but usually worsen as the day progresses.
- Overuse of specific muscle groups can cause specific weakness of those muscle groups.

DIAGNOSIS

- Edrophonium test: Edrophonium is an anticholinesterase that prevents the breakdown of acetylcholine. Increased level of acetylcholine overcomes the receptor blockage from autoantibodies. There is rapid return of muscle strength. Since the duration is short acting, this is only used as a diagnostic modality.
- Myasthenia gravis can be diagnosed by detection of acetylcholine receptor antibodies in the serum.

TREATMENT

- Anticholinesterase
- Plasma exchange
- Immunoglobulins
- Respiratory support (intubate as needed)

SEIZURES

Definition

Abnormal electrical discharge of neurons causing a clinical episode of neurological dysfunction

Neurologic Emergencies

Typical scenario:
A 37-year-old female presents with severe weakness of respiratory muscles, diplopia, ptosis, and proximal muscle weakness. *Think: Myasthenic crisis.*

TABLE 5-5. Classification of Seizures

Type	Description
Generalized	All generalized seizures involve loss of consciousness.
Tonic–clonic (grand mal)	Loss of consciousness immediately followed by tonic (rigid) contraction of muscles, then clonic (jerking) contraction Patients may be cyanotic or apneic. Urinary incontinence may occur. *Postictal period:* Confusion or disorientation following seizure
Absence (petit mal)	Loss of consciousness without loss of postural tone Patients do not respond to verbal stimuli, nor do they lose continence.
Myoclonic	Loss of consciousness with brief muscular contractions
Clonic	Loss of consciousness with repetitive clonic jerks
Tonic	Loss of consciousness with sustained, prolonged contraction of body
Atonic	Loss of consciousness with sudden loss of postural tone
Partial (focal)	Usually involve focal area of abnormal electrical discharge in cerebral cortex Partial seizures may progress to generalized seizure.
Simple partial	Abnormal focal neurological discharge in which consciousness remains intact
Complex partial	Otherwise known as *temporal lobe seizures* Consciousness may be impaired. Patient usually has an abrupt termination of ongoing motor activity.
Partial with secondary generalization	A partial seizure that has spread to both hemispheres

Classification

See Table 5-5.

Management

ABCs
- Airway: Maintain adequate airway with nasal trumpet.
- Breathing: Administer oxygen.
- Circulation: Obtain IV access.

History
- Important history can be obtained from bystanders or witnesses.
- Include **syncope** as part of your differential diagnosis.
- Seizures can cause loss of bladder control.
- Differentiate between partial and generalized seizure (ask patient if they can recall event).
- First seizure or known seizure history
- Baseline seizure history (frequency and last seizure episode)
- Recent history of trauma
- Consider factors that may lower seizure threshold.

> Patients having an actual seizure usually require only protection from injury.

Factors that lower seizure threshold: **I AM H⁴IP**
Infection

Alcohol withdrawal, drugs
Medication (changes in dosing or compliance)

Head injury, **H**ypoxia, **H**ypoglycemia, **H**yponatremia (and other electrolyte abnormalities)
Intracranial lesions
Pregnancy (eclampsia)

Seizures can cause posterior shoulder dislocations, as well as intraoral lacerations.

Todd's paralysis: Focal neurological deficit persisting from partial (focal) seizure, which usually resolves within 48 hours.

Signs and Symptoms

Physical Exam
- Check for injuries caused as a result of seizure activity.
- Look for signs of infection, especially CNS infections.
- Assess and reassess mental status for signs of deterioration.

Diagnosis

- Routine labs
- Magnesium, calcium, toxicology screen, alcohol level, liver function tests
- Consider LP.
- Consider CT scan of head.

Treatment

- Prevention of injury and adequate oxygenation in the actively seizing patient
- Benzodiazepines are the mainstay of treatment in the seizing patient.
- Correct subtherapeutic levels of anticonvulsants.
- Treat underlying causes (meningitis, hypoglycemia, etc.).
- Most often, treatment is mainly supportive.

ANTICONVULSANT THERAPY

Phenytoin

- Most commonly used anticonvulsant
- Requires loading dose
- Phenytoin cannot be mixed with glucose-containing solutions.
- Can act as a myocardial depressant, therefore contraindicated in CHF, heart block, or acute MI
- Requires cardiac monitoring when given IV
- Must be infused slowly because the diluent propylene glycol causes hypotension

Fosphenytoin

- Prodrug of phenytoin
- Same onset and effectiveness
- Myocardial depressant
- Can be infused faster due to lack of propylene glycol
- Expensive

PRIMARY SEIZURE DISORDER

- Idiopathic
- One to 2% of population has disease.

- *Epileptic:* Term used to describe an individual with recurrent seizures
- These patients are usually placed on lifelong anticonvulsants.

SECONDARY SEIZURE DISORDER

Definition

Seizures that occur as a result of another disease condition

Causes

- Metabolic:
  - Hyper/hypoglycemia
  - Hyper/hyponatremia
  - Uremia
  - Hypocalcemia
- Infection:
  - Meningitis
  - Encephalitis
  - Intracerebral abscess
- Trauma:
  - Subdural hematoma
  - Epidural hematoma
  - Intracerebral hemorrhage
  - SAH
- Toxic:
  - Theophylline
  - Amphetamines
  - Cocaine
  - Tricyclic antidepressants
  - Alcohol withdrawal
  - CO
  - Cyanide
- Neurological:
  - Cortical infarction
  - Intracranial hemorrhage
  - Hypoxia
  - Hypertensive encephalopathy
- Eclampsia

Causes of secondary seizures: **MITTEN**
Metabolic
Infection
Trauma
Toxins
Eclampsia
Neurological lesions

Neurologic Emergencies

STATUS EPILEPTICUS

Definition

Seizures occurring continuously for at least 30 minutes, or two or more seizures occurring without full recovery of consciousness between attacks

Treatment

- Treat with benzodiazepines and phenytoin.

Continuous seizures can cause significant CNS injury.

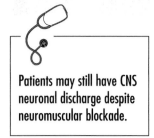

- Use phenobarbital as second-line drug.
- Consider isoniazid toxicity in refractory cases and treat with vitamin B$_6$.
- Neuromuscular blockage can be used as last resort.

Patients may still have CNS neuronal discharge despite neuromuscular blockade.

ECLAMPSIA

- Usually occurs in patients > 20 weeks' gestation
- Present with hypertension, edema, proteinuria, headache, vision changes, confusion, and seizure
- Magnesium sulfate can be used to treat eclampsia.

DELIRIUM TREMENS

- Seizures can occur in alcohol withdrawal.
- Occurs secondary to autonomic hyperactivity
- Seizures can occur within 6 hours after last drink.
- Treated with benzodiazepines and supportive care

Head and Neck Emergencies

PHARYNGITIS

DEFINITION

Infection of the pharynx and tonsils that rarely occurs in infants and is uncommon under 2 years of age

EPIDEMIOLOGY

- Peak incidence is between 4 and 7 years old but occurs throughout adult life.

ETIOLOGY

Viruses
- Most common cause of all pharyngeal infection
- Rhinoviruses and adenoviruses are the most common viral causes.
- Epstein–Barr virus, herpes simplex virus, influenza, parainfluenza, and coronaviruses also contribute.

Bacteria
- *Streptococcus pyogenes* (group A, beta-hemolytic strep) is the most common cause of bacterial pharyngitis.
- *Mycoplasma, Chlamydia,* and *Corynebacterium* also occur.

Fungal and Parasitic
- Can also occur in the immunocompromised host

SIGNS AND SYMPTOMS

Symptoms
- Incubation period is 2 to 5 days, after which patients develop sore throat, dysphagia, chills, and fever.
- Headache, nausea, vomiting, and abdominal pain can also occur.

Signs
- Erythematous tonsils
- Tonsillar exudates
- Enlarged and tender anterior cervical lymph nodes
- Palatal petechiae

Signs and symptoms are the same for viral and bacterial pharyngitis. One cannot differentiate between the two causes without microbiology testing.

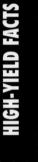

Treatment algorithm for strep pharyngitis:
- RADT (+): Treat
- RADT (−): Culture and treat until culture results are available.
- If culture is negative, discontinue antibiotics.
- No RADT available: Culture and treat until culture results are known. If negative, discontinue antibiotics.

Group-A, beta-hemolytic strep is associated with sequelae of RF and PSGN. Treating strep pharyngitis prevents RF, but not PSGN.

DIAGNOSIS

- Throat culture: Still the most effective means of diagnosis. There is a delay in obtaining results while the culture grows, and a good sample must be obtained.
- Rapid antigen detection tests (RADTs): Greater than 95% specific. A negative RADT should be confirmed with a throat culture.

TREATMENT

A one-time intramuscular injection of penicillin (benzathine penicillin 1.2 million units) or a 10-day course of oral penicillin is the treatment of choice. Erythromycin is an alternative for penicillin-allergic patients.

COMPLICATIONS

- Post-streptococcal glomerulonephritis (PSGN)
- Rheumatic fever (RF)
- Cervical lymphadenitis
- Peritonsillar abscess
- Retropharyngeal abscess
- Sinusitis
- Otitis media

EPIGLOTTITIS

DEFINITION

A life-threatening inflammatory condition (usually infectious) of the epiglottis and the aryepiglottic folds and periglottic folds.

ETIOLOGY

- *Haemophilus influenzae* type B (Hib) is the most common cause.
- *Streptococcus* is the next most common cause.
- Can also be caused by other bacteria and rarely viruses and fungi

EPIDEMIOLOGY

- The incidence in children has decreased dramatically after the introduction of the Hib vaccine.
- Most cases are now in adults and unimmunized children.

SIGNS AND SYMPTOMS

- Prodromal period of 1 to 2 days
- High fever
- Dysphagia
- Stridor
- Drooling
- Secretion pooling
- Dyspnea
- Erect or tripod position
- Pain on movement of the thyroid cartilage is an indicator of supraglottic inflammation.

DIAGNOSIS

- High clinical suspicion is necessary.
- Radiographs of the neck soft tissue can aid in diagnosis, as can fiberoptic laryngoscopy.
- Direct laryngoscopy is contraindicated because it may induce fatal laryngospasm.
- Do not examine the oropharynx unless surgical airway capability is available at the bedside.

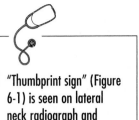

"Thumbprint sign" (Figure 6-1) is seen on lateral neck radiograph and demonstrates a swollen epiglottis obliterating the vallecula.

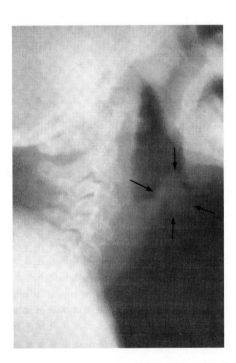

FIGURE 6-1. Epiglottitis. Arrows indicate classic thumbprint sign of enlarged, inflamed epiglottis.

(Reproduced, with permission, from Knoop K, Stack LB, and Storrow AB. Atlas of Emergency Medicine. New York: McGraw-Hill, 1997: 412.)

HIGH-YIELD FACTS

Head and Neck Emergencies

TREATMENT

- Intubation as needed to protect airway
- Ceftriaxone
- Intensive care unit admission

COMPLICATIONS

Airway obstruction and resultant respiratory arrest

DIFFERENTIAL DIAGNOSIS: CROUP

- Croup caused by parainfluenza virus also presents with sore throat and stridor.
- Anteroposterior soft-tissue neck radiograph may show the "steeple sign," which is indicative of subglottic narrowing.
- Treat with humidified oxygen, bronchodilators, and racemic epinephrine.

ACUTE SINUSITIS

Inflammation of the paranasal sinuses of less than 3 weeks' duration: There are one sphenoidal, two maxillary, and two frontal sinuses, along with the ethmoid air cells, which compose the paranasal sinuses. Sinusitis can occur when there is drainage obstruction of the sinuses.

PATHOPHYSIOLOGY AND ETIOLOGY

- Edema causes obstruction of the drainage pathways followed by reabsorption of the air in the sinuses.
- The resultant negative pressure causes transudate collection within the sinuses.
- When bacteria is present, a suppurative infection can occur.

RISK FACTORS

- Viral upper respiratory infection (URI)
- Allergic rhinitis

ETIOLOGY

Streptococcus pneumoniae causes 37% of bacterial sinusitis, with *H. influenza* causing 38%. Other common URI bacteria are also implicated.

SIGNS AND SYMPTOMS

- Pain over the sinuses
- Decreased sense of smell
- Fever
- Purulent nasal discharge
- Headache (may be aggravated by coughing, sneezing, and leaning forward)
- Tenderness to palpation or percussion over the affected area
- Nasal canal may be inflamed, and purulent exudates may drain from the ostia.

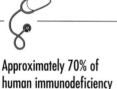

Approximately 70% of human immunodeficiency virus patients will develop sinusitis, which may be caused by opportunistic bacteria, viruses, or fungi.

DIAGNOSIS

- Usually clinical based on history and physical
- There is no defined role for sinus plain radiography in diagnosis.
- CT can be employed when the diagnosis is uncertain, or if the patient is immunocompromised or appears toxic.

TREATMENT

- Antibiotics improve symptoms, prevent complications, and decrease duration of illness if there is good clinical evidence that suppuration is present.
- Amoxicillin or amoxicillin with clavulanate is first-line therapy.
- If allergic to penicillin, erythromycin plus a sulfonamide can be used.
- Over-the-counter decongestant nasal sprays can provide symptomatic relief.

COMPLICATIONS

- The infection can extend beyond the sinuses and, in the case of ethmoidal involvement, may enter the central nervous system (CNS).
- Bony destruction can also occur and may result in facial deformity.
- Direct extension from sinuses to the venous or lymphatic system can cause cavernous sinus thrombosis.

ADMISSION CRITERIA

Presence of complications, toxicity, fever with neurological signs or orbital or periorbital cellulitis all warrant admission.

Only 38% of patients with sinusitis will have normal computed tomography (CT) scans. Sixteen percent of patients without sinusitis will have abnormal findings in the sinuses on CT scan.

CAVERNOUS SINUS THROMBOSIS

DEFINITION

Thrombosis (infectious or otherwise) in the dural sinus causing occlusion

ETIOLOGY

- Bacterial infection of the CNS, usually secondary to a staphylococcal infection of the face or sinuses
- Thrombosis may occur without antecedent infection.

PATHOGENESIS

- An infection in the face or sinuses spreads to the CNS causing inflammation of the linings of the dural sinuses.
- The inflammation predisposes to thrombosis with resultant occlusion of the cavernous sinus.

SIGNS AND SYMPTOMS

- Fever
- Headache
- Nausea
- Vomiting
- Occasionally seizures

The neurologic signs result from the third, fourth, and sixth cranial nerves passing through the cavernous sinus.

- Proptosis of the ipsilateral eye with chemosis and ophthalmoplegia
- Sensory loss in the first division of the trigeminal nerve
- Papilledema—late and ominous finding

DIAGNOSIS

Diagnosis can be made with magnetic resonance imaging or digital venous angiogram.

TREATMENT

- Infective sinus thrombosis is usually successfully treated with appropriate intravenous (IV) antibiotics (*Staphylococcus* should be covered).
- Sometimes, despite appropriate treatment, the clot propagates to cause cerebral infarction and death.
- Heparin/warfarin therapy may reduce mortality and prevent permanent neurological damage.

OTITIS EXTERNA

DEFINITION

Infection of the external ear or external canal: Can be localized (furuncle) or can affect the entire canal

ETIOLOGY

The most common causes are *Pseudomanas aeruginosa* and *Staphylococcus aureus*.

EPIDEMIOLOGY

It is more common in moist environments (summer, swimming pools, and the tropics).

SIGNS AND SYMPTOMS

- Sense of fullness in the ear
- White or green cheesy discharge
- Pain on retraction of pinna
- Itching
- Decreased hearing
- Fever
- A bulging or erythematous tympanic membrane

TREATMENT

- Cleanse ear canal thoroughly.
- Polymyxin–neomycin–hydrocortisone ear drops

COMPLICATIONS

Malignant external otitis media:
- Seen in diabetics and immunocompromised hosts
- Results in destruction of bone underlying the external ear canal
- Characterized by excruciating pain, fever, friable granulation tissue in external ear canal, and facial palsies
- Treated with anti-pseudomonal antibiotics

Otitis externa is also known as "swimmer's ear."

Typical scenario:
A 16-year-old swim team captain presents with a greenish discharge from his ear and complains that his ear feels "full." He withdraws as you tug on his ear to examine it. *Think: Otitis externa.*

Patients with otitis externa should avoid getting water into their ears for 2 to 3 weeks after treatment.

DEFINITION

A bacterial or viral infection of the middle ear, usually secondary to a viral URI

ETIOLOGY

- S. pneumoniae, nontypeable H. influenzae, and Moraxella catarrhalis are the most common causes.
- Newborns can also get suppurative otitis with Escherichia coli and S. aureus.

EPIDEMIOLOGY

- More common in colder months
- Most common age is ages 6 months to 3 years.

PATHOPHYSIOLOGY

- Dysfunction of the eustachian tube leads to retention of secretions, which leads to bacterial colonization.

SIGNS AND SYMPTOMS

- Ear pain and sense of fullness
- Perception of gurgling or rumbling sounds inside the ear
- Decreased hearing
- Dizziness
- Fever
- Purulent discharge
- A bulging or erythematous tympanic membrane
- Otorrhea
- Poor feeding and irritability in infants
- Decreased mobility of tympanic membrane on pneumatic otoscopy

TREATMENT

- Antibiotic therapy is controversial but has been shown to decrease the length of illness and decrease the incidence of complications.
- Amoxicillin for 10 to 14 days is the treatment of choice. In penicillin allergy, erythromycin can be substituted.
- Hospital admission

COMPLICATIONS

- Serous otitis media—an effusion of the middle ear resulting from incomplete resolution of otitis media
- Acute mastoiditis

Second-hand smoke is a risk factor for otitis media in children.

HIGH-YIELD FACTS

Head and Neck Emergencies

ACUTE MASTOIDITIS

DEFINITION

Bacterial infection of the mastoid process resulting in coalescence of the mastoid air cells: It is usually a complication of acute otitis media in which the infection has spread into the mastoid antrum.

SIGNS AND SYMPTOMS

- Swelling, erythema, tenderness, and fluctuance over the mastoid process
- Displacement of pinna laterally and inferiorly
- Fever
- Earache
- Otorrhea
- Decreased hearing

DIAGNOSIS

CT scan of the mastoid air cells reveals cell partitions that are destroyed, resulting in coalescence.

TREATMENT

- Antibiotics should cover the common acute otitis media pathogens and be resistant to beta-lactamase.
- Third-generation cephalosporins are preferred because they offer good penetration into the CNS at the proper doses.
- This therapy is usually effective in preventing neurological sequelae.

COMPLICATIONS

Subperiosteal abscess requires mastoidectomy.

LUDWIG'S ANGINA

DEFINITION

Cellulitis of bilateral submandibular spaces and the lingual space: This is a potentially life-threatening infection.

ETIOLOGY

- Usually a result of spread of a bacterial odontogenic infection into the facial tissue spaces
- Most common bug is mouth anaerobe *Bacteroides*.

RISK FACTORS

- Oral trauma
- Dental work
- Salivary gland infection

SIGNS AND SYMPTOMS

- Fever
- Drooling
- Trismus
- Odynophagia
- Dysphonia
- Elevated tongue
- Swollen neck
- Labored breathing

DIAGNOSIS

Soft-tissue radiographs of the neck can be obtained, but they should not delay treatment or place the patient in an area where emergent airway management is difficult.

TREATMENT

- Secure airway.
- IV antibiotics (penicillin and metronidazole or clindamycin)
- Definitive treatment is incision and drainage, then excision of fascial planes in the operating room (OR).
- Ear, nose, and throat (ENT) or oral and maxillofacial surgery consult

PERITONSILLAR ABSCESS

SIGNS AND SYMPTOMS

- Sore throat
- Muffled voice
- Decreased oral intake
- Tilting of head to affected side
- Trismus
- Deviation of uvula to affected side
- Swollen erythematous tonsils
- Fluctuant soft palate mass
- Cervical lymphadenopathy

DIAGNOSIS

By physical exam

TREATMENT

- Secure the airway; these abscesses are in a very precarious space and can cause complete upper airway obstruction.
- Antibiotics against gram-positive oral flora (including anaerobes)
- Consider steroids to decrease inflammation.
- ENT consult
- Incision and drainage of abscess may need to be done in the OR, depending on the size and degree of airway compromise.

Typical scenario:
A 29-year-old male who had been treated for strep throat the previous week presents with progressive difficulty swallowing. Physical exam reveals a fluctuant mass on the right side of the soft palate and deviation of the uvula to the right. *Think: Peritonsillar abscess.*

DEFINITION

Abscess in the pharyngeal spaces

SIGNS AND SYMPTOMS

- Difficulty breathing
- Fever, chills
- Severe throat pain
- Toxic appearance
- Hyperextension of neck
- Stridor
- Drooling
- Swollen, erythematous pharynx
- Tender cervical lymph nodes

Patients with epiglottitis prefer to sit leaning forward with the neck slightly flexed. Patients with retropharyngeal abscess prefer recumbency and hyperextension of the neck.

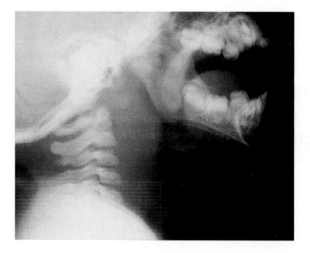

FIGURE 6-2. Retropharyngeal abscess. Note excess prevertebral swelling. Normal prevertebral space should be less than one half the distance between the vertebral bodies.
(Reproduced, with permission, from Knoop, Stack, and Storrow. *Atlas of Emergency Medicine.* New York: McGraw-Hill, 1997: 413.)

DIAGNOSIS

- Radiograph of the soft tissues of the neck (see Figure 6-2): Exaggerated swelling in the pharyngeal spaces is indicative of abscess.

TREATMENT

Same as for peritonsillar abscess, except that all parapharyngeal and retropharyngeal abscesses are drained in the OR

EPISTAXIS

DEFINITION

Nosebleed

EPIDEMIOLOGY

- Anterior epistaxis is more common in younger patients.
- Posterior epistaxis is more common in the elderly population.

ANATOMY

- The nose humidifies and warms air and has a rich blood supply.
- The internal and external carotid arteries supply blood to the nasal mucosa through a number of smaller branches.

Anterior Epistaxis

- Comprise 90% of nose bleeds
- Most commonly originates from Kiesselbach's plexus (a confluence of arteries on the posterior superior nasal septum)

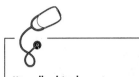

Kiesselbach's plexus is located in the "picking zone."

ETIOLOGY

- Trauma to the nasal mucosa (usually self-induced)
- Foreign body
- Allergic rhinitis
- Nasal irritants (such as cocaine, decongestants)
- Pregnancy (due to engorgement of blood vessels)
- Infection (sinusitis, rhinitis)
- Osler–Weber–Rendu syndrome (telangiectasias)

DIAGNOSIS

- Labs are not routinely required if there are no comorbidities.
- Facial or nasal films may be considered in the setting of nasal trauma.

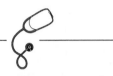

In anterior epistaxis, the bleeding is unilateral and the patient denies a sensation of blood in the back of the throat.

TREATMENT

- **Direct pressure:** Compress the elastic portions of the nose between the thumb and middle finger. Hold continuously for 10 to 15 minutes.
- **Vasoconstrictive agents:**
  - Phenylephrine or oxymetazoline can be instilled into the nasal cavity in conjunction with other treatment methods.
  - Cotton-tipped applicators can be used to apply vasoconstrictive agents if the bleed can be visualized.
- **Anterior nasal packing:**
  - Should be performed on any patient in which vasoconstrictive agents and direct pressure have failed
  - Patients should receive antistaphylococcal prophylaxis.
  - Nasal packs should be removed at ENT follow-up after 2 to 3 days.
- **Chemical cautery** with silver nitrate-tipped applicators
- **Electrocautery** performed by an otolaryngologist

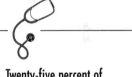

Twenty-five percent of properly placed nasal packs fail to control bleeding. In this case, an emergent ENT consult is indicated.

PROCEDURE FOR ANTERIOR NASAL PACKING

Nasal tampons can be inserted along the floor of the nasal canal. They expand to several times their original size when instilled with saline or blood:

1. Use one fourth–inch petroleum jelly–impregnated gauze. Grasp the gauze 3 cm from the end with bayonet forceps.
2. The first layer is placed on the floor of the nose through a nasal speculum. The forceps and the speculum are then withdrawn, and the gauze stays in place.
3. The nasal speculum is then reintroduced on top of the previous layer of gauze, and another layer of gauze is introduced using the forceps.

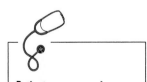

Patients may experience reflux of blood through the nasal puncta after packing and should be warned in advance. No specific therapy is recommended.

HIGH-YIELD FACTS

Head and Neck Emergencies

4. This process is repeated until several layers have been placed.
5. Remove the speculum and use the forceps to pack down the layers.

A successful anterior nasal pack is placed in an "accordion" fashion so that each layer lies anterior to the prior layer. This prevents the gauze from falling into the posterior nasal pharynx.

Posterior Epistaxis

DEFINITION

- Comprises approximately 10% of epistaxis in the emergency department
- More common in older patients and is thought to be secondary to atherosclerosis of the arteries supplying the posterior nasopharynx

ETIOLOGY

- Hypertension
- Anticoagulation therapy
- Liver disease
- Blood dyscrasias
- Neoplasm
- Atherosclerosis of nasal vessels

CLINICAL FEATURES

- Blood may be seen effluxing from both nares or down the posterior oropharynx.
- Visualization of the bleeding usually requires use of a fiber-optic laryngoscope.
- Bleeding is often more severe than with an anterior bleed.

DIAGNOSIS

Routine labs (including complete blood count, prothrombin time, and activated partial thromboplastin time are drawn to look for possible coagulopathies.

TREATMENT

- **Posterior nasal packing:** Commercial nasal packs and specialized hemostatic balloon devices are available and are more efficacious than the traditional methods of posterior nasal packing. The procedure for inserting a commercial nasal hemostatic balloon is described below:

  1. Prepare the nasal cavity with vasoconstrictors and anesthetic agents.
  2. Insufflate 25 cc of saline into the anterior balloon to test for leakage. The posterior balloon is tested with 8 cc of saline.
  3. Lubricate the device with 4% lidocaine jelly and insert it into the nasopharynx. Advance until the distal balloon tip is visible in the posterior oropharynx when the patient opens his mouth.
  4. Fill the posterior balloon tip with 4 to 8 cc of saline and pull the device anteriorly such that it wedges in the posterior nasopharynx.
  5. Fill the anterior balloon with 10 to 25 cc of saline while maintaining traction on the device.
  6. It may be necessary to pack both nares to obtain adequate hemostasis.
  7. Many patients require sedation following the procedure.

- **Embolization and ligation:** These treatments are indicated when the other treatments fail and should be performed by ENT specialists.
- All patients with posterior bleeds should have an emergent ENT consult and are usually admitted.

Approximately 50% of patients presenting with posterior epistaxis have a systolic blood pressure $\geq$ 180 mm Hg or a diastolic pressure > 110 mm Hg.

Respiratory Emergencies

PNEUMONIA

EPIDEMIOLOGY

- Most common cause of death from infectious disease in the United States
- Community-acquired pneumonia is an acute infection in patients not hospitalized or residing in a care facility for 14 days prior to onset of symptoms.

ETIOLOGY

Most common etiologies:
- Bacterial:
  - *Streptococcus pneumoniae*
  - *Haemophilus influenzae*
  - *Mycoplasma pneumoniae*
  - *Legionella pneumophila*
  - *Moraxella catarrhalis*
  - *Chlamydia pneumoniae*
  - *Staphylococcus aureus*
  - Gram-negative bacilli (*Pseudomonas*)
- Viral:
  - Influenza
  - Parainfluenza
  - Adenovirus
- *Mycobacterium tuberculosis* and endemic fungi are rare causes of community-acquired pneumonia.

SIGNS AND SYMPTOMS

- Physical findings associated with increased risk:
  - Respiratory rate > 30
  - Heart rate > 140
  - Blood pressure, systolic < 90 or diastolic < 60
  - Temperature > 101
  - Change in mental status
  - Extrapulmonary infection

Typical scenario:
A 27-year-old patient presents with pneumonia, bullous myringitis, and a chest film that looks worse than expected. *Think:* Mycoplasma pneumonia.

Typical scenario:
A patient with human immunodeficiency virus (HIV) has a CD4 count of 52, does not take antiretroviral medications or trimethoprim–sulfamethoxazole, is hypoxic on room air, has an elevated lactic dehydrogenase (LDH), and has diffuse bilateral infiltrates on chest x-ray (CXR). *Think:* Pneumocystis carinii *pneumonia*.

Typical scenario:
An elderly man presents with pneumonia, diarrhea, bradycardia, and hyponatremia. *Think:* Legionella.

If you see *currant jelly sputum* on physical exam or *bulging fissure* on CXR, think *Klebsiella*.

Pulmonary pathogens that can be found in the oropharynx:
- *S. pneumoniae*
- *M. pneumoniae*
- *H. influenzae*
- *Streptococcus pyogenes*
- *M. catarrhalis*

- Signs:
  - Tachypnea
  - Tachycardia
  - Rales
  - Diaphoresis
- Symptoms:
  - Dyspnea
  - Chest pain
  - Cough
  - Hemoptysis

DIAGNOSIS

Laboratory findings associated with increased risk:
- White blood count < 4 or $> 30 \times 10^3$/L
- Absolute neutrophil count $< 1 \times 10^3$/L
- $PaO_2 < 60$ mm Hg on room air
- $PaCO_2 > 50$ mm Hg on room air
- Abnormal renal function
- Blood urea nitrogen > 20 mg/dL, creatinine > 1.2 mg/dL
- Hemoglobin < 9 g/dL or hematocrit $< 30\%$

TREATMENT

- Treatment of viral pneumonia is supportive.
- Antibiotic selection for bacterial pneumonia depends on the organism involved. Empiric therapy and hospital admission are based on the patient's age, comorbidities, severity of symptoms, and particular risk factors.

ASPIRATION PNEUMONIA

DEFINITION

- Pathogens can enter the lung by inhalation of aerosols, by hematogenous spread, or by aspiration of oropharyngeal contents.
- Up to half of normal adults aspirate oropharyngeal contents during sleep. Individuals with swallowing disorders, impaired level of consciousness, or an impaired gag reflex are more likely to aspirate material into the lungs. The chances of developing a pneumonia depend on the volume aspirated and the virulence of the material.
- Different organisms can be present in the aspirate depending on the individual.

PATHOPHYSIOLOGY

- Anaerobic pulmonary pathogens colonize dental plaque and gingiva; aspiration can cause pneumonia or lung abscess.
- Common pulmonary pathogens can colonize the nasopharynx of normal individuals.
- Aerobic gram-negative bacilli can colonize the stomach and reach the oropharynx in vomit or by spreading colonization in debilitated individuals.
- Mucociliary dysfunction, common in smokers, and alveolar macrophage dysfunction will reduce the clearing of aspirate and increase the chances of infection.

- Presence of foreign bodies in the aspirate will also increase the chances of infection.

PULMONARY EDEMA

DEFINITION

Pulmonary edema is the accumulation of fluid in the interstitial space of the lung. The most common cause of pulmonary edema is cardiogenic in nature, which results from increased pulmonary capillary pressure.

CARDIOGENIC CAUSES

- Left ventricular failure (myocardial infarction [MI], ischemia, cardiomyopathy)
- Increased pulmonary venous pressure without failure (valvular disease)
- Increased pulmonary arterial pressure

NONCARDIOGENIC CAUSES

- Hypoalbuminemia (decreased oncotic pressure)
- Altered membrane permeability (adult respiratory distress syndrome)
- Lymphatic insufficiency
- High-altitude pulmonary edema
- Opiate overdose
- Neurogenic pulmonary edema

CONGESTIVE HEART FAILURE (CHF)

- Acute pulmonary edema (APE) secondary to left ventricular failure is commonly known as CHF.

TREATMENT

- Diuretics (furosemide)
- Oxygen
- Nitroglycerin to promote afterload reduction and vasodilation
- Aspirin: Antiplatelet agent, protective against MI
- Morphine to decrease preload and relieve anxiety

PULMONARY EMBOLUS (PE)

RISK FACTORS

- Genetic predisposition
- Age
- Obesity
- Cigarette smoking
- Hypertension
- Oral contraceptives
- Hormone replacement therapy
- Neoplasm

Typical scenario:
A 75-year-old male stroke victim is brought in by his home health aide, who states she has been having to shove food down his throat the past few days because he refuses to eat. Today, she noted he had trouble breathing and was making gurgling sounds. *Think: Aspiration pneumonia.*

Typical scenario:
An 81-year-old woman is brought in by EMS gasping for breath. Rales are noted almost all the way up her lungs bilaterally. She has pink frothy sputum and her skin is also wet. *Think: APE.*

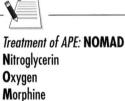

Treatment of APE: **NOMAD**
Nitroglycerin
Oxygen
Morphine
Aspirin
Diuretics

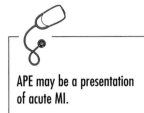

APE may be a presentation of acute MI.

There are no signs, symptoms, laboratory values, CXR, or electrocardiographic (ECG) findings that are diagnostic of PE or are consistently present. The absence of any of these should not be used to rule out PE. Diagnosis requires a high index of suspicion.

Typical scenario:
A 53-year-old female smoker who returned from a week-long road trip yesterday presents with dyspnea and tachycardia and appears extremely anxious. *Think: PE.*

- Immobilization
- Pregnancy and postpartum period
- Surgery and trauma
- Hypercoagulable state

SIGNS AND SYMPTOMS

Signs
- Tachypnea
- Tachycardia
- Hypoxia
- Rales
- Diaphoresis
- Lower extremity edema
- Thrombophlebitis
- Bulging neck veins
- Heart murmur

Symptoms
- Apprehension
- Dyspnea
- Chest pain
- Cough
- Hemoptysis

DIAGNOSIS

- ECG pattern of $S_1Q_3T_3$ (Figure 7-1) is seen in one fourth of patients. Most common rhythm is sinus tachycardia.
- Arterial blood oxygen levels are not useful in predicting the absence of PE.
- Venous studies are of value when positive but do not exclude PE when negative.
- Fifteen percent of patients with low-probability ventilation–perfusion scans have had angiographically proven PE.
- The gold standard for the diagnosis of PE is angiography. Spiral computed tomography is also excellant.

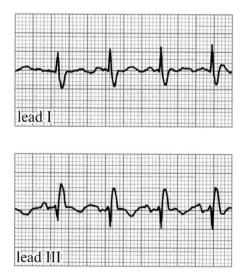

lead I

lead III

FIGURE 7-1. Classic $S_1Q_3T_3$ pattern of pulmonary embolism.

- Presently available d-dimer tests are not suitable for emergency department use.
- A-a gradient is also not suitable as a screening test.

TREATMENT

- All patients should get oxygen.
- Anticoagulation is the mainstay of therapy and may consists of heparin (inpatient) and coumadin or a low-molecular-weight heparin such as enoxaparin
- Thrombolytics should be considered for hemodynamically unstable patients.
- Surgical options include an inferior vena cava filter (good for patients with contraindications to anticoagulation) and embolectomy (poor prognosis).

Possible treatments of pulmonary embolism:
FATSO
Filter
Anticoagulation
Thrombolytics
Surgery
Oxygen

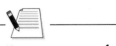

Most common causes of pleural effusion:
- CHF
- Bacterial pneumonia
- Malignancy

PLEURAL EFFUSION

DEFINITION

- The pleural space lies between the chest wall and the lung and is defined by the parietal and visceral pleuras. A very small amount of fluid is normally present, allowing the two pleural membranes to slide over each other during respiration. An abnormal amount of fluid (> 15 cc) in the pleural space is known as a pleural effusion.
- Pleural effusions are divided into transudates and exudates. Transudative effusions happen when there is either an increase in capillary hydrostatic pressure or a decrease in colloid osmotic pressure. Both of these conditions will cause a net movement of fluid out of capillaries into the pleural space.

CAUSES OF TRANSUDATIVE EFFUSIONS

- CHF
- Hypoalbuminemia
- Cirrhosis
- PE
- Myxedema
- Nephrotic syndrome
- Superior vena cava obstruction
- Peritoneal dialysis

CAUSES OF EXUDATIVE EFFUSIONS

- Infection (pneumonia, tuberculosis [TB], fungi, parasites)
- Connective tissue diseases
- Neoplasm
- PE
- Uremia
- Pancreatitis
- Esophageal rupture
- Intra-abdominal abscess
- Post surgery or trauma
- Drug induced

DIAGNOSIS

Pleural Fluid Analysis
- Transudate:
  - LDH < 200 U
  - Fluid-to-blood LDH ratio < 0.6
  - Fluid-to-blood protein ratio < 0.5
- Exudate:
  - Glucose < 60 mg/dL in infection, neoplasm, rheumatoid arthritis, pleuritis
  - Amylase: Elevated in esophageal rupture, pancreatitis, pancreatic pseudocyst, and some neoplasms
  - Cell count
  - Gram stain and culture
  - Cytology

TREATMENT

- Treat underlying cause.
- A thoracocentesis can be both diagnostic and therapeutic.

ASTHMA

DEFINITION

Asthma is a disease in which the tracheobronchial tree is hyperreactive to stimuli, resulting in variable, reversible airway obstruction.

EPIDEMIOLOGY

- Incidence greater in men than women
- Incidence greater in African Americans than whites
- Half of cases develop by age 17 and two thirds by age 40

EXTRINSIC ASTHMA

- Sensitivity to inhaled allergens
- Immunoglobulin E response
- Causally related in a third of asthma cases and a contributing factor in another third
- Frequently seasonal
- Early asthmatic response is mast cell dependent and results in acute bronchoconstriction.
- Late asthmatic response is an inflammatory reaction that leads to prolonged airway responsiveness.

NONIMMUNOLOGIC PRECIPITANTS OF ASTHMA

- Exercise
- Infections
- Pharmacologic stimuli
- Environmental pollution
- Occupational stimuli
- Emotional stress
- Diet

Steroids are given in asthma to decrease the late inflammatory response.

Drugs most commonly associated with acute asthma exacerbations are aspirin and beta blockers.

SIGNS AND SYMPTOMS

- Dyspnea
- Wheezing
- Cough

EMERGENCY TREATMENT

- The mainstay of therapy is oxygen and beta agonist nebulizers.
- Corticosteroids are added for moderate asthma.
- Severe asthma may require epinephrine or magnesium sulfate.

OUTPATIENT MANAGEMENT OPTIONS

- Leukotriene inhibitors (e.g., zafirlukast, montelukast)
- Mast cell stabilizing agents (e.g., cromolyn sodium)
- Methylxanthines (e.g., theophylline, aminophylline)

CHRONIC OBSTRUCTIVE PULMONARY DISEASE (COPD)

- Three separate disease entities are part of the classification of COPD. These are asthma, bronchitis, and emphysema. Asthma is discussed above.
- Chronic bronchitis is defined as a condition in which excessive mucus is produced. The mucus production is enough to cause productive cough for a minimum of 3 months out of the year in at least 2 consecutive years.
- Emphysema is a disease in which there is distention of the air spaces distal to the terminal bronchioles and destruction of alveolar septa. Alveolar septa are important for providing support of the bronchial walls. Their destruction leads to airway collapse especially during expiration.

RISK FACTORS

- Smoking
- Air pollution
- Occupational exposure
- Infection
- Genetic factors

SIGNS AND SYMPTOMS OF CHRONIC BRONCHITIS

- History of cough and sputum production
- History of smoking
- Commonly overweight
- Cyanosis
- Right ventricular failure
- Normal total lung capacity
- Increased residual volume
- Normal to slightly decreased vital capacity

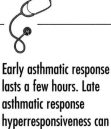

Early asthmatic response lasts a few hours. Late asthmatic response hyperresponsiveness can persist for weeks to months.

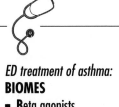

ED treatment of asthma:
BIOMES
- Beta agonists
- Ipratropium
- Oxygen
- Magnesium sulfate
- Epinephrine
- Steroids

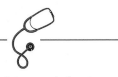

Patients with chronic bronchitis are sometimes referred to as "blue bloaters."

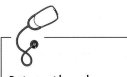

Patients with emphysema are sometimes referred to as "pink puffers."

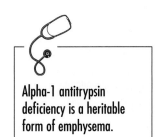

Alpha-1 antitrypsin deficiency is a heritable form of emphysema.

SIGNS AND SYMPTOMS OF EMPHYSEMA

- Exertional dyspnea
- Thin to cachectic
- Tachypnea
- Prolonged expiratory phase often with pursed lips
- Use of accessory muscles of respiration
- Increased total lung capacity and residual volume
- Decreased vital capacity

TREATMENT

- Smoking cessation
- Control of respiratory infections
- Nutrition
- Exercise
- Bronchodilators
- Corticosteroids
- Supplemental oxygen

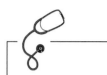

Smoking cessation is the most important treatment for COPD.

TB

DEFINITION

Mycobacterium tuberculosis is an intracellular, aerobic, acid-fast bacillus that infects humans. It is primarily spread through the respiratory route.

PATHOPHYSIOLOGY

- Bacillus normally enters through the lungs.
- Macrophage phagocytoses bacillus
- Bacillus multiplies intracellularly in the macrophage until it lyses the macrophage and repeats the process.
- Cell-mediated immunity, through T helper cells, activates macrophages, destroying infected cells.
- Epithelioid cell granulomas are produced that wall off the primary lesion; remaining bacilli can survive within granulomas for years.
- Months to years later, bacilli can reactivate.

SIGNS AND SYMPTOMS

- Primary TB is usually asymptomatic.
- Reactivation pulmonary TB is the syndrome most commonly seen:
  - Cough
  - Fever
  - Night sweats
  - Weight loss
  - Hemoptysis
  - Fatigue
  - Anorexia

SITES OF EXTRAPULMONARY TB

- Pleurisy with effusion
- Tuberculous pericarditis

Tuberculous adenitis is known as *scrofula*.

- Tuberculous adenitis
- Skeletal TB
- Genitourinary TB
- Gastrointestinal TB
- Tuberculous peritonitis
- Adrenal TB
- Cutaneous TB
- Miliary TB

Miliary TB results from hematogenous spread.

DIAGNOSIS

Purified Protein Derivative Testing
- > 5-mm induration considered positive in:
  - Persons with HIV or risk factors and unknown HIV status
  - Close household contacts of person with active TB
  - Persons with evidence of primary TB on x-ray
- > 10 mm positive in high-risk groups:
  - Intravenous drug users that are HIV⁻
  - Persons from high-prevalence areas
  - Persons with other medical conditions that render them debilitated or immunocompromised
- > 15 mm is considered positive in all other individuals.

HEMOPERICARDIUM

DEFINITION

Hemopericardium is the accumulation of blood in the pericardial sac, which is usually acute and can result in cardiac tamponade even when small volumes of blood accumulate.

CAUSES

- Penetrating trauma
- Blunt trauma
- Following invasive procedures in or around the heart
- Bleeding diathesis
- Aortic dissection
- Ventricular rupture

PERICARDIAL EFFUSION

DEFINITION

Pericardial effusions can accumulate slowly or quickly. The speed of fluid accumulation will in part determine how much fluid can accumulate before serious symptoms develop.

CAUSES

- Cancer
- Pericarditis

- Connective tissue diseases
- Cardiac disease
- Drugs
- Trauma
- Uremia
- Myxedema
- Bleeding diathesis
- Miscellaneous causes

TYPES OF VENTILATORS

- Pressure-cycled ventilation delivers volume until a preset peak inspiratory pressure is reached.
- Volume-cycled ventilation delivers a preset tidal volume.
- Time-cycled ventilation delivers volume until a preset time is reached.

VENTILATOR SETTINGS

- Ventilatory rate
- Tidal volume
- Inspired oxygen concentration
- Positive end-expiratory pressure (PEEP)
- Inspiratory–expiratory ratio

VENTILATOR MODES

- Controlled mechanical ventilation (CMV): The patient is ventilated at a preset rate; the patient cannot breathe between the delivered breaths.
- Assist–control ventilation: A minimum rate is set, but if the patient attempts to take additional breaths, the machine will deliver a breath with a preset tidal volume.
- Intermittent mandatory ventilation and synchronized intermittent mandatory ventilation (SIMV): The machine delivers a preset number of breaths at the preset tidal volume; additional breaths initiated by the patient will have a tidal volume dependent on the patient's effort. In SIMV, the machine breaths are synchronized so as not to interfere with spontaneous breaths.
- Pressure support: Patient determines respiratory rate, and tidal volume depends on both the patient's pulmonary compliance and the preset inspiratory pressure.

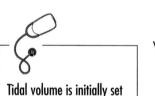

Ventilatory rate is initially set at 12 to 14 breaths per minute.

Tidal volume is initially set at 6 to 10 cc/kg.

PEEP improves oxygenation by keeping alveoli open during expiration.

CMV is useful in patients with no spontaneous respirations, heavily sedated patients, and paralyzed patients.

Cardiovascular Emergencies

CARDIOVASCULAR PHARMACOLOGY

Antiplatelet Agents

- Aspirin (acetylsalicylic acid [ASA]): Causes irreversible inhibition of platelet aggregation by prostaglandin inactivation and preventing thromboxane production
- Ticlopidine and clopidogrel: Irreversibly inhibits platelet aggregation by binding to adenosine diphosphate receptors on platelet. Used as ASA substitute in those who are allergic or in those in whom it's contraindicated
- Eptifibatide and tirofiban: Glycoprotein (GP) IIb-IIIa inhibitors irreversibly inhibit platelet aggregation by binding to GPIIb-IIIa (a common final pathway for platelet activation). Used in acute coronary syndromes (ACS)

Nitrates

- Preload and afterload reduction by vasodilatation of venules > arterioles, including coronaries
- Can rapidly lower blood pressure (BP) and cause headache
- Used in angina, congestive heart failure (CHF), pulmonary edema, and hypertensive crisis
- Comes as sublingual (SL) pill, transdermal paste, intravenous (IV) infusion, and long-acting oral tablet

Thrombolytics

- Also called clot-busters
- Given in acute myocardial infarction (AMI) within 6 to 12 hours of onset of symptoms with a history consistent with infarction and electrocardiogram (ECG) that has 1-mm ST segment elevation in two or more contiguous leads (see Figure 8-1)
- Streptokinase:
  - Protein obtained from beta-hemolytic *Streptococcus* bacteria
  - Given as 1.5 million units IV over 30 to 60 minutes
  - Antigenic response after first use—don't reuse.

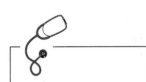

Absolute contraindications to thrombolytics:
- Systolic BP (SBP) > 180
- History of hemorrhagic stroke
- Any stroke within past year
- Suspected aortic dissection
- Active bleeding

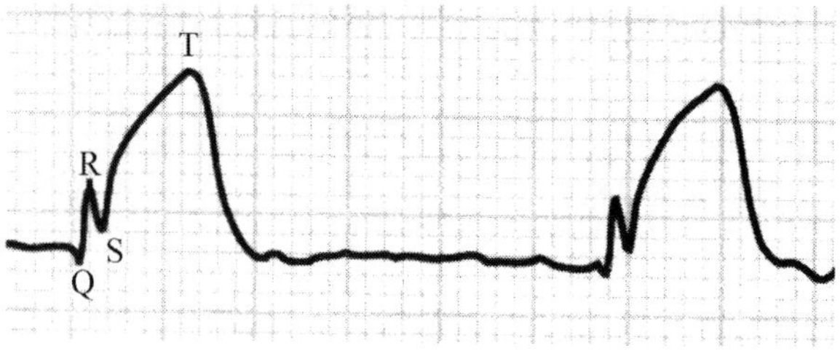

FIGURE 8-1. Large ST segment elevations "tombstones" indicative of MI. (Should be seen in at least two contiguous leads for diagnosis.) In the setting of chest pain, consider thrombolysis for this patient.

Antidysrhythmics are classified on their effect on the cardiac action potential and impulse conduction. All antidysrhythmic agents can be prodysrhythmic.

Absolute contraindications to beta blockers:
- HR < 60/min
- SBP < 100 mm Hg
- Second- or third-degree heart block
- Moderate to severe left ventricular (LV) dysfunction
- Severe chronic obstructive pulmonary disease (COPD) or asthma
- Signs of peripheral hypoperfusion

- Tissue plasminogen activator (tPA, alteplase):
  - Naturally occurring human protein produced by recombinant DNA technology
  - No antigenicity
  - Binds to plasminogen, which then binds to fibrin in clots, lysing them
  - Three megatrials showed no statistical difference between tPA and streptokinase (GISSI-2, GUSTO-1, ISIS-3).
  - Given as 15-mg IV bolus followed by 0.75 mg/kg over 30 minutes and 0.50 mg/kg over next 60 minutes (accelerated regimen)
- Altered recombinant plasminogen activator (reteplase):
  - Has longer half-life and greater fibrin specificity
  - Given as two separate boluses of 10 U 30 minutes apart

Antidysrhythmics

CLASS I

- Also called membrane stabilizers
- Slow phase 0 depolarization by blocking fast Na$^+$ channels
- Used mainly for ventricular ectopy and tachydysrhythmia

CLASS IA

- Quinidine, procainamide, disopyramide
- Moderate Na$^+$ channel–blocking activity
- *Prolong* repolarization and action potential duration

CLASS IB

- Lidocaine, mexiletine
- Mild Na$^+$ channel–blocking activity
- *Shorten* repolarization and action potential duration

CLASS IC

- Propafenone, flecainide, encainide
- Large Na$^+$ channel–blocking activity
- *Prolong* repolarization and action potential duration

CLASS II

- Beta blockers (esmolol, metoprolol, propranolol)
- Decrease heart rate (HR), ectopy, and contractility; increase ventricular fibrillation (V-fib) threshold.

126

- Used in AMI with increased HR, in supraventricular reentry tachycardias, to control ventricular response in rapid atrial fibrillation (A-fib), and in hypertrophic cardiomyopathy
- Shown to reduce cardiac mortality

CLASS III

- Amiodarone, bretylium, sotalol, ibutilide
- Na^+ channel activation
- K^+ channel blockage
- Prolong refractory period and action potential duration
- Increase V-fib threshold.
- Sotalol has beta-blocking effects.
- Ibutilide used to break new-onset A-fib to sinus rhythm
- Amiodarone used in new advanced cardiac life support (ACLS) protocols

CLASS IV

- Ca^{2+} channel blockers (verapamil, diltiazem, nifedipine, nicardipine, amlodipine)
- Blocks slow Ca^{2+} channels in vasculature and heart (phase 2 in action potential)
- Cause atrioventricular (AV) nodal conduction delay, negative inotropy, and decrease BP
- Verapamil affects mostly heart.
- Diltiazem affects heart and vessels.
- Nifedipine and others affect mostly vessels.
- Diltiazem and verapamil are used to control ventricular response in rapid A-fib and supraventricular tachycardia (SVT).

Adenosine

- Endogenous nucleoside with 10-second half-life that causes transient AV nodal conduction block
- Useful to decipher supraventricular reentry tachycardias.
- Monitor may show several seconds of asystole before natant rhythm returns.
- Patient typically describes an "uncomfortable feeling" during adenosine administration.

Digoxin

- Cardiac glycoside that disrupts Na^+-K^+ adenosine triphosphatase in cardiac muscle
- Negative chronotropy, positive inotropy
- Used to control rate in acute and chronic A-fib due to negative chronotropic effects
- Used for diminished LV function and failure (positive inotropy)
- Acute and chronic overdose possible (see toxicology section for diagnosis and treatment)

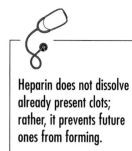

Heparin does not dissolve already present clots; rather, it prevents future ones from forming.

Heparin

- A mixture of different mucopolysaccharides that binds to antithrombin III and inactivates clotting factors X, IX, and XII
- Partial thromboplastin time (PTT) used to monitor adequate dosing (1.5 to 2 times normal)
- Protamine sulfate given to reverse its effects

Low-Molecular-Weight Heparin (LMWH)

- Fragments of normal heparin
- Binds more specifically to factor X and thrombin
- Better safety profile than heparin—don't have to monitor coagulation times
- Used for unstable angina, AMI, deep vein thrombosis (DVT), pulmonary embolism (PE)
- Protamine sulfate given to reverse its effects

Coumadin

- Prevents the formation of vitamin K–dependent coagulation factors (II, VII, IX, X) in the liver
- Prothrombin time (PT), international normalized ratio (INR) used for monitoring of dosage (INR: 2 to 3—tissue heart valves and A-fib; 2.5 to 3.5—postinfarct period and PE/DVT; 3.5 to 4.5—mechanical or multiple heart valves)
- Vitamin K given to reverse its effects

Angiotensin-Converting Enzyme (ACE) Inhibitor

- Prevents the conversion of angiotensin I to angiotensin II (which is a potent arteriolar vasoconstrictor and is involved in many other cellular and endocrine processes)
- Used in AMI, hypertension (HTN), and CHF (increases cardiac output, prolongs survival)
- Side effects include chronic dry cough.

Diuretics

LOOP

- Examples: Furosemide, bumetanide
- Act at the loop of Henle
- Used in acute and chronic CHF, chronic HTN, and acute pulmonary edema (APE) to decrease congestion and filling pressures
- Can cause Na^+ and K^+ depletion and hypotension

THIAZIDE

- Examples: Hydrochlorothiazide, metolazone
- Used primarily in chronic conditions (HTN, CHF) or in combination with other agents
- Giving metolazone 30 minutes before a loop diuretic can increase net diuretic effect.
- Can cause Na^+ and K^+ depletion

K+ SPARING

- Examples: Spironolactone, triamterene
- Only advantage is prevention of K+ depletion.
- Usually given in chronic conditions (CHF, cirrhosis, and ascites) and not with a second agent contributing to increased K+ (ACE inhibitors)

Morphine

- Decreases preload
- Alleviates pain and anxiety
- Reduces myocardial oxygen demand
- Used in MI and APE

Electricity

- Defibrillation—two indications:
  - V-fib
  - Pulseless ventricular tachycardia (V-tach)
- Cardioversion:
  - Synchronized electric shock coinciding with patient's natant beats
- Used for:
  - Unstable SVT
  - Recent (< 24 hours) unstable A-fib
  - V-tach with a pulse refractory to medication

AMI

DEFINITION

Damaged myocardial tissue secondary to ischemia

RISK FACTORS

- Male gender
- Age > 45
- MI in male relatives under age 50
- Cigarette smoking
- Cocaine use
- HTN
- Diabetes mellitus
- Hypercholesterolemia
- Postmenopausal

DIAGNOSIS

- World Health Organization criteria (two out of three):
  - Anginal pain > 20 minutes' duration
  - Ischemic change on ECG
  - Elevated cardiac enzyme levels

Inferior wall MI: ST elevation in II, III, and aVF (see Figure 8-2)
Anteroseptal MI: ST elevation in V_1, V_2, and V_3
Lateral wall MI: ST elevation in V_4, V_5, and V_6
Posterior wall MI: ST depression in V_1 and V_2

TABLE 8-1. Cardiac Enzymes

Enzyme	Rise (hrs post Chest Pain)	Peak	Return to Baseline
Myoglobin	1–2 hrs	4–6 hrs	24 hrs
Troponin	3–6 hrs	12–24 hrs	7–10 days
Creatine phosphokinase MB fraction	4–6 hrs	12–36 hrs	3–4 days
Lactic dehydrogenase	12 hrs	24–48 hrs	10–14 days

- Cardiac enzymes (see Table 8-1):
    - CPK-MB (creatine phosphokinase): An intracellular dimeric isoenzyme particular to brain cells (BB), skeletal muscle (MM), or cardiac muscle (MB), released into bloodstream upon cell death
    - Myoglobin: A heme-containing protein found in both skeletal and striated muscle released into the bloodstream when there is muscle cell death. It is released in a fixed ratio with carbonic anhydrase-III from skeletal muscle.
    - Troponin: Regulatory protein for cardiac muscle contraction; peaks earlier and remains elevated longer than other cardiac enzymes

SIGNS AND SYMPTOMS

- Chest pain:
    - Lasting 30 minutes to 3 hours

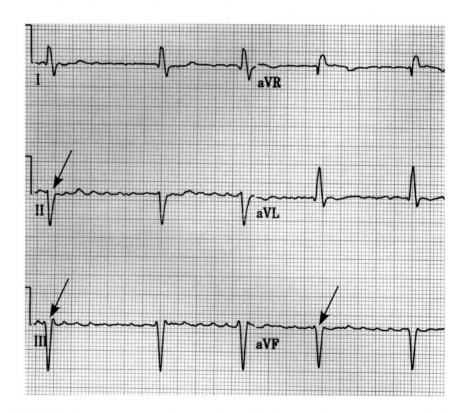

FIGURE 8-2. Q waves in II, III, and aVF indicate old inferior wall MI. Note, patient also has atrial flutter.

- Located over center of chest, typically demonstrated as a fist over the chest
- Typically radiates to left arm, left jaw, or shoulder
- May be associated with an impending sense of doom
- Typically described as a pressure or a heaviness
- Nausea
- Diaphoresis
- Dyspnea

TREATMENT

- O_2
- SL nitroglycerin
- Nitropaste 1 to 2″ to anterior chest wall
- ASA 160 mg, chewable
- Metoprolol 5 mg IV initially, titrate to HR of 60
- For > 0.1 mV ST elevation in at least two contiguous leads or new left bundle branch block (LBBB):
  - Intra-aortic balloon pump (IABP) if unstable, hypotensive, and cannot immediately go for coronary catheterization
  - Cardiac catheterization for percutaneous transluminal coronary angioplasty or coronary stenting if in a facility where available, otherwise tPA (if not contraindicated—see above)
  - If tPA is absolutely contraindicated or fails to improve condition, transfer patient to facility for "rescue cath."
- Heparin for nonthrombolysable MIs
- ACE inhibitor after patient stabilized, 6 to 24 hours into hospital course

CARDIAC CATHETERIZATION

- Arteriogram of coronaries allowing visualization of the anatomy and potential blockages of coronary arteries
- Access allows for balloon angioplasty or widening of narrowed, atherosclerotic coronary arteries and possible stent placement.

IABP

- Catheter with balloon at its tip that is inserted into femoral artery and tip placed by aorta
- Balloon is synchronized with ECG to inflate when aortic valve closes and deflate at onset of systole.
- Net effect:
  - Increased coronary perfusion
  - Decreased afterload
  - Increased cardiac output
  - Decreased diastolic BP (DBP)
  - Increased SBP
  - Decreased in myocardial O_2 consumption and ischemia
- Used in cases of refractory cardiac ischemia and hypotension as a temporizing measure prior to definitive treatment (catheterization/angioplasty/stenting, or coronary artery bypass graft
- Used in non–Q wave MI and unstable angina

COMPLICATIONS

- Heart failure
- Free wall rupture

Relative contraindications include arterial dissection and lesions that are technically difficult to lyse.

Anginal equivalents:
- Dyspnea at rest
- Nausea/vomiting
- Shoulder/arm pain
- Neck/jaw pain
- Diaphoresis
- Light-headedness
- Silent (up to one third of all MIs)

Typical scenario:
A 62-year-old smoker presents complaining of three episodes of severe heavy chest pain this morning. Each episode lasted 3 to 5 minutes, but he has no pain now. He has never had this type of pain before. He has *unstable angina.*

- New ventricular septal defect (VSD)
- Mitral regurgitation
- Ventricular dysrhythmias
- Supraventricular dysrhythmias
- Bradycardia
- AV block
- Pericarditis (Dressler's syndrome)
- Thromboembolism
- LV aneurysm

ACS

Emergency Department (ED) Differential Diagnosis of Chest Pain

- Heart: Peri-/myocarditis, ACS
- Lung: Pneumothorax, lobar pneumonia
- Vascular: Pulmonary embolus, aortic dissection
- Gastrointestinal (GI): Esophageal rupture, Mallory–Weiss tear

Stable Angina

- Established character, timing, and duration of chest pain
- Transient, reproducible, predictable
- Easily relieved by rest or SL nitrates
- Due to reduced coronary blood flow through fixed atherosclerotic plaques that narrow blood vessel lumina (see Atherosclerosis)

Unstable Angina

- Angina deviating from normal pattern
- Rest angina lasting longer than 20 minutes
- New-onset angina previously undiagnosed
- Increasing angina (severity, frequency, duration) or change in class
- Treated with O_2, ASA, LMWH

Variant Angina (Prinzmetal's)

- Same character as stable angina, but atherosclerosis is minimal and vasospasm is the etiology
- Canadian Cardiovascular Society Classification:
  - Class I—can perform normal activity pain free
  - Class II—slight limitation of normal activity (walking, climbing stairs, emotional stress)
  - Class III—severe limitation of normal activity (pain with walking one block or climbing one flight of stairs)
  - Class IV—pain with any activity, sometimes at rest
- Treated with nitrates and calcium channel blockers

DEFINITION

- Most pacers use a three-letter code:
    1. Pacing chamber: V (ventricular), A (atrial), or D (dual)
    2. Sensing chamber: V, A, or D
    3. I (inhibited), T (triggered), D (dual)
    4. P (programmable rate), C (communications stored), R (rate responsive)
    5. P (pacing), S (shock), D (dual), 0 (neither)

- Transcutaneous pacing: Indicated in refractory bradycardia with hypotension
- Transvenous pacing: Done when transcutaneous pacing is not tolerated or fails to capture. Pacemaker wire is passed through central venous access line into heart for pacing.

EMERGENT PACEMAKER PLACEMENT INDICATIONS

- New bi-/trifascicular block with acute ischemia:
    - Bi = RBBB + LAFB, RBBB + LPFB, LBBB
    - Tri = RBBB + LAFB + first-degree AV block, or RBBB + LPFB + first-degree AV block, or LBBB + first-degree AV block or alternating LBBB + RBBB
- Mobitz type II AV block
- Third-degree or complete AV block
- Symptomatic bradycardia

First-Degree AV Block

- First degree (prolonged PR interval—see Figure 8-3):
    - Prolonged conduction of atrial impulses without loss of any impulses
    - PR interval > 0.20 second
    - Benign and asymptomatic
    - Doesn't warrant further ED workup or treatment

Second-Degree AV Block, Type I

- Second degree, Mobitz type I (Wenckebach—see Figure 8-4):
    - Progressive prolongation of PR interval with each successive beat until there is a loss of AV conduction and hence a dropped beat or failure of ventricles to depolarize (P wave but no QRS)

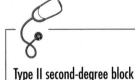

Type II second-degree block has a worse prognosis than type I.

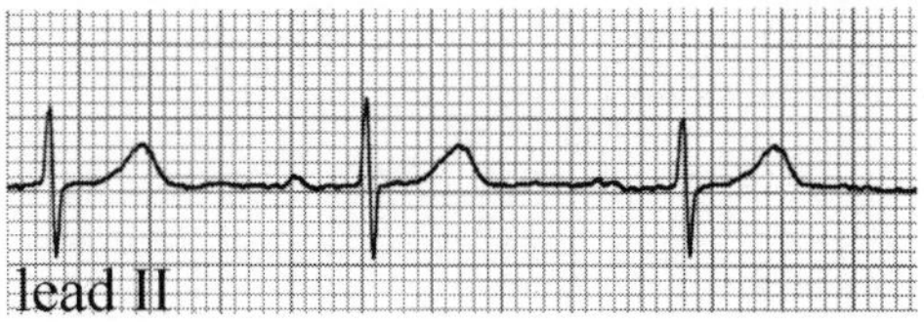

lead II

FIGURE 8-3. First-degree AV block.

HIGH-YIELD FACTS

Cardiovascular Emergencies

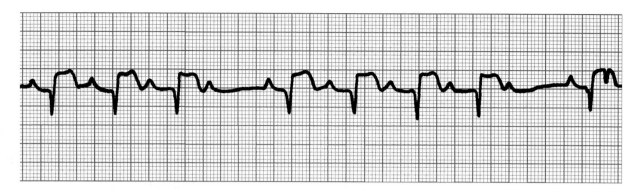

FIGURE 8-4. Mobitz I (Wenckebach) second-degree AV block.

Second-Degree AV Block, Type II

- Second degree, Mobitz type II (see Figure 8-5):
  - Random loss of conduction and beat below the AV node without change in PR interval (His–Purkinje system) (P, no QRS)
  - Potentially serious pathology present
  - Can be seen with anterior wall MI
  - Often progresses to complete AV block (third degree)

Third-Degree AV Block

- Third degree (complete AV dissociation [see Figure 8-6]):
  - No conduction of atrial signal and P wave through to the ventricle, and hence independent atrial and ventricular rhythms
  - Either congenital (with associated anatomic anomalies) or acquired (autoimmune connective tissue disease with scarring of normal electrical conduits)
  - Patients present with tachypnea, dyspnea on exertion, cyanosis, or syncope.
  - ECG shows no correlation between atrial (faster) and ventricular (slower) rhythms; P waves "march through" the rhythm strip ignoring the QRS complexes.

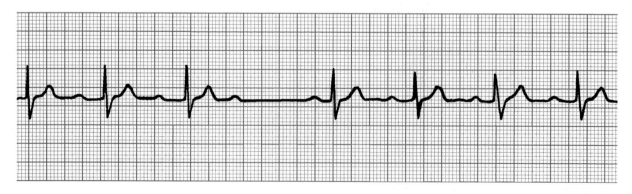

FIGURE 8-5. Mobitz II second-degree AV block.

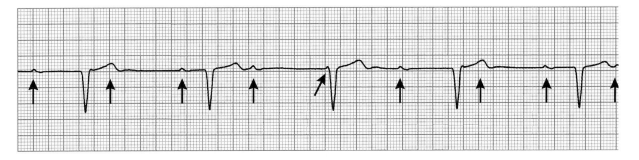

FIGURE 8-6. Third-degree (complete) AV block. Note the P waves (arrows) "marching through."

TREATMENT

- ABCs, IV access, O₂, monitor
- Immediate transcutaneous or transvenous pacemaker
- Eventual implantable pacemaker is warranted.
- Treat underlying cause if possible.

Left Anterior Fascicular Block (LAFB)

- Can reflect very focal lesions in conduction system
- Causes:
  - Ischemia
  - Cardiomyopathies
  - Myocarditis
  - Congenital
  - Surgery
  - Valvular disease
  - Age
  - Degenerative diseases
- ECG:
  - Left axis deviation (LAD)
  - QRS duration 0.10 to 0.12 second
  - Peak of terminal R in aVL precedes peak of terminal R in aVR
  - Deep S waves in II, III, and aVF
  - Lead I R wave > leads II or III

Left Posterior Fascicular Block (LPFB)

- Usually indicates widespread organic heart disease
- Causes are the same as LAFB.
- ECG:
  - R axis deviation
  - QRS duration 0.10 to 0.12 second
  - Small R and deep S in lead I
  - Lead III R wave > lead II
  - Small Q in II, III, and aVF

LBBB

- Conduction blocked before anterior and posterior fascicles split

Presence of new LBBB is indicative of AMI.

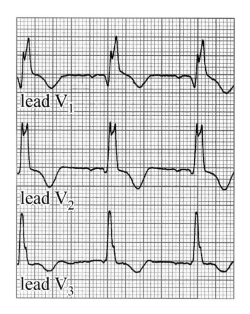

FIGURE 8-7. RBBB. Note the M-shaped QRS complex (R,R').

- Causes are the same as LAFB.
- Ischemia is masked with LBBB.
- Point system for determining acute ischemic change in the presence of LBBB (the more points, the more likely is ischemia):
    - ST segment elevation ≥ 1 mm concordant (in the same direction) with its QRS axis = 5 points
    - ST segment elevation ≥ 1 mm in V1–V3 = 3 points
    - ST segment elevation ≥ 5 mm, discordant with QRS = 2 points
- ECG:
    - LAD
    - QRS duration > 0.12 second
    - ST and T waves directed opposite to terminal 0.04-second QRS
    - No Q waves in I, aVF, V_5, V_6
    - Large wide R waves in I, aVL, V_5, V_6

Right Bundle Branch Block (RBBB)

- Ischemia is not masked with RBBB (see Figure 8-7).
- Causes are the same as LAFB.
- ECG:
    - QRS duration > 0.12 second
    - Triphasic QRS complexes
    - RSR´ described as "rabbit ears" in morphology in V_1, V_2
    - Wide S waves in I, aVL, V_5, V_6

DYSRHYTHMIAS

Prolonged QT Syndrome

DEFINITION

QT_c > 0.44 (see Diagnosis)

ETIOLOGY

- Congenital (Lange–Nielsen–Jervell and Romano–Ward syndromes)
- Electrolyte abnormalities (decreased Ca^{2+}, decreased Mg^{2+})
- Medications (quinidine, procainamide)

SIGNS AND SYMPTOMS

- Syncopal episodes
- Can predispose to paroxysmal episodes of V-tach and Torsade de pointes by "R-on-T phenomenon." This is when a premature ventricular complex–QRS fires at the same time as the peak of the T wave or "vulnerable period" in ventricular repolarization (when some but not all myocardial tissue is ready for the signal) inducing V-tach or V-fib via a ventricular reentry pathway.

DIAGNOSIS

- QT_I (QT interval) = 0.34 to 0.42 second or 40% of RR interval
- QT_c = HR corrected QT = $QT_I \div \sqrt{RR}$

See Figure 3-1 for ECG of prolonged QT.

TREATMENT

- ABCs, monitor
- Correct electrolytes.
- Discontinue medications.
- If inherited, beta blockers to decrease sympathetic stimulus and implantable overdrive pacemaker/defibrillator
- Magnesium sulfate IV for Torsade de pointes

Sinus Bradycardia

DEFINITION

- HR < 60 and regular:
  - P wave prior to every QRS complex
  - Upright Ps in I and aVF
  - Narrow (< 0.12 second) QRS complexes

ETIOLOGY

- Hypoxemia
- Hypothyroidism
- Excessive vagal tone
- Hypothermia
- Medication side effects: Beta blockers, digoxin, Ca^{2+} channel blockers, cholinergic toxins

TREATMENT

- Correct underlying problem.
- In code situation, give atropine 0.5 to 1.0 mg IV followed by epinephrine and transcutaneous pacing.
- May eventually require transvenous pacemaker

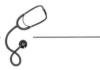

Causes of prolonged QT:
QT WIDTH
QT: Prolonged QT syndrome

Wolff–Parkinson–White (WPW) syndrome
Infarction
Drugs
Torsades
Heart disease (ischemic)

Prolonged QT and hypertrophic cardiomyopathy are causes of sudden death in young people.

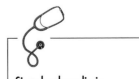

If the RR distance is at least one inch, consider:
One INCH
Overmedication

Inferior wall MI, increased intracranial pressure
Normal variant
Carotid sinus hypersensitivity
Hypothyroidism

Sinus bradycardia is commonly seen in inferior wall MI.

Sinus Tachycardia

DEFINITION

- HR > 100 and regular:
  - Usually < 150 bpm
  - P wave prior to every QRS complex
  - Upright Ps in I and aVF
  - Narrow QRS complexes

ETIOLOGY

- Anemia
- Dehydration/hypovolemia
- Fever
- Sepsis
- Drug overdose
- Anxiety
- Hypermetabolic state

TREATMENT

Correct underlying problem.

Atrial Ectopy

- **Premature atrial complexes (PACs):** Abnormal electrical focus triggers an atrial contraction before the sinus node fires, thus triggering a QRS and ventricular contraction. There is a compensatory pause (longer RR interval) before the next sinus beat. Benign and asymptomatic, they may reveal predisposition toward developing A-fib, atrial flutter, multifocal atrial tachycardia (MAT), or SVT.
- **Wandering atrial pacemaker:** ≥ 3 different P wave morphologies/foci in a normal 12-lead ECG rhythm strip with an HR between 60 and 100 bpm. QRS follows each P wave. Usually asymptomatic, may complain of palpitations or anxiety
- **MAT:** Wandering atrial pacemaker with a rate > 100 bpm. Patient is usually symptomatic (dyspnea, diaphoresis, ± angina).

Atrial Flutter

- Rapid atrial depolarization (240 to 350 bpm) from an abnormal focus within the atria and variable ventricular conduction described as block (i.e., 2:1–4:1 flutter [see Figure 8-8])
- Can be considered a transitional dysrhythmia between normal sinus and A-fib
- Causes are same as for A-fib.

A-fib

DEFINITION

Very rapid atrial depolarization (350 to 600 bpm) from many ectopic atrial foci, usually with ineffective conduction to ventricles

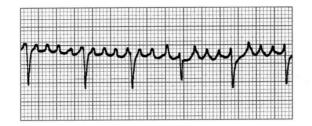

FIGURE 8-8. Atrial flutter.

ETIOLOGY

- Chronic lung disease
- HTN
- Thyrotoxicosis
- Ischemic heart disease
- Atrial septal defect (ASD)
- Pericarditis
- Acute alcohol intoxication (holiday heart)
- Rheumatic fever

PATHOPHYSIOLOGY

- Ventricular depolarization triggered by escape beats and occasional successful atrial depolarization giving rate of 150 to 180 bpm
- Rapid ventricular response gives ineffective systole (from poor filling) and subsequent heart failure/pulmonary edema/ACS.
- Presence of A-fib predisposes to atrial blood stasis and subsequent clotting, which can embolize and cause further disease.
- Ineffective atrial contraction results in complete loss of atrial kick and its contribution to cardiac output, especially those with heart failure.

DIAGNOSIS

- Chest x-ray (CXR) may show:
  - Cardiomegaly
  - Pulmonary edema
- ECG (see Figure 8-9):
  - Irregularly irregular ventricular rhythm
  - Wide or narrow QRS complexes

Causes of A-fib:
PIRATES
Pulmonary disease
Ischemia
Rheumatic heart disease
Anemia, atrial myxoma
Thyrotoxicosis
Ethanol
Sepsis

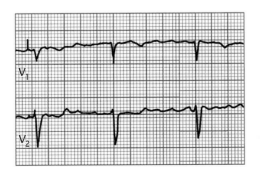

FIGURE 8-9. A-fib. Note lack of distinct P waves.

- P waves either too small to see or nonexistent
- Ventricular rate can be rapid (uncontrolled) or controlled (with medications).
- Echocardiography should be done to rule out atrial thrombi prior to electrical cardioversion.
- Labs:
  - Check complete blood count (CBC), cardiac enzymes, thyroid function tests (TFTs), and ethanol level to look for underlying cause.

TREATMENT

Treatment of A-fib:
1. Control ventricular response
2. Systemic anticoagulation
3. Chemical or electrical cardioversion

- ABCs, IV, O_2, monitor
- Control ventricular response rate (between 60 and 100) with IV diltiazem and digitalis.
- Synchronized electrical cardioversion for the hemodynamically unstable patient with A-fib for < 2 days (A-fib for ≥ 2 days is too great a risk for atrial thrombi); chemical cardioversion may be attempted with IV ibutilide or procainamide.
- Anticoagulation in new-onset A-fib is mandatory because of the significant risk for embolization, barring any contraindication (blue-toe, transient ischemic attack (TIA)/cerebrovascular accident (CVA), ischemic bowel, etc.).
- Treat for ACS as appropriate.

SVT

DEFINITION

Narrow QRS complex tachycardia with regular RR intervals at a rate of 150 to 250 bpm

SVT is the most common pediatric dysrhythmia.

ETIOLOGY

- Due to either increased atrial automaticity or reentry phenomenon
- Etiologies similar to A-fib

SIGNS AND SYMPTOMS

- Dyspnea
- Palpitations
- Angina
- Diaphoresis
- Varying degrees of hemodynamic stability
- Weak or nonpalpable pulses
- CHF
- Shock

DIAGNOSIS

- CXR: Most often normal
- ECG:
  - Narrow QRS complex
  - Tachycardia at a rate > 150 bpm
  - Typically regular, P waves may or may not be visible.

TREATMENT

- ABCs, IV, O$_2$, monitor
- Immediate synchronized cardioversion (50 J) if hemodynamically unstable, in CHF or ACS
- Vagal maneuvers or adenosine (6-mg rapid IV push followed by 20-cc flush, repeat as needed × 2 with 12 mg each time) to block AV nodal conduction
- Diltiazem (0.25 mg/kg IV over 2 minutes) or verapamil (0.15 mg/kg IV over 1 minute) to control rate: Watch out for hypotension.

WPW Syndrome

DEFINITION

- A syndrome in which there is an accessory electrical pathway that causes SVT in older children and adults
- Heart beats too fast for adequate filling, leading to shock.

ETIOLOGY

- Congenital

SIGNS AND SYMPTOMS

- < 24 hour pallor
- Diaphoresis
- Tachypnea
- Chest pain and palpitations
- Variable degrees of hemodynamic stability
- Weak to no pulses
- CHF
- Shock

Diagnosis

- ECG (see Figure 8-10):
  - Narrow QRS complex
  - HR > 200
  - P waves present
  - Slurred upstroke of QRS (delta wave)

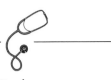

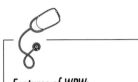

Vagal maneuvers:
- Carotid massage (check carotids for bruits prior to massage; never massage both sides simultaneously)
- Diving reflex (cold water immersion of head)
- Valsalva maneuver

Features of WPW:
- Short PR interval
- Widened QRS interval
- Delta wave slurring QRS upswing

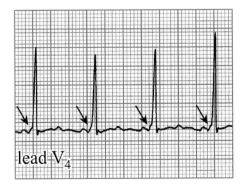

FIGURE 8-10. WPW syndrome. Arrows indicate pathognomonic delta waves.

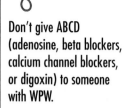

Don't give ABCD (adenosine, beta blockers, calcium channel blockers, or digoxin) to someone with WPW.

TREATMENT

- ABCs, monitor, IV access, O_2
- Patients with WPW, rapid A-fib, and rapid ventricular response require emergent cardioversion.
- Stable patients with WPW and A-fib are treated with amiodarone, flecainide, procainamide, propafenone, or sotalol.
- Adenosine, beta blockers, calcium channel blockers, and digoxin are *contraindicated* because they preferentially block conduction at the AV node, allowing unopposed conduction down the accessory bypass tract.

Sick Sinus Syndrome (SSS)

DEFINITION

- Sinus arrest: Also known as "pause" of sinoatrial node signal that usually results in "ectopic" or "escape" beats and rhythms that take over as source for ventricular impulse
- Also called tachy–brady syndrome: Any combination of intermittent fast and slow rhythms with associated AV block and inadequate escape rhythm:
  - Fast: A-fib, atrial flutter, SVT, junctional tachycardia
  - Slow: Sinus brady, varying sinus pauses, escapes

SIGNS AND SYMPTOMS

- Reflect fast or slow HR:
  - Palpitations
  - Syncope
  - Dyspnea
  - Angina
  - Embolic events

DIAGNOSIS

ECG: Any of above rhythms (see definition)

TREATMENT

- ABCs, IV, O_2, monitor
- Follow ACLS protocols
- Pacemaker

ESCAPE RHYTHMS

Junctional Ectopy

- Ectopic beats that originate from the junction of atria and ventricle
- Normal ventricular depolarization and repolarization
- Narrow QRS complexes
- Absent or late, retrograde P waves coming on or after the QRS
- Usually a sign of sinus node and/or atrial disease

Ventricular Ectopy

DEFINITION

- Ectopic beats that originate from below the AV node
- Usually slower than 60 bpm

ETIOLOGY

- Ischemia
- Increased K+
- Increased vagal tone
- Medications (digoxin, beta blockers, Ca^{2+} channel blockers)

DIAGNOSIS

- ECG (see Figure 8-11):
  - Wide QRS
  - No preceding P wave
  - Sign of sinus nodal or atrial disease, especially when "escape rhythm" or beats take over as the dominant rhythm.

TREATMENT

- If symptomatic: Immediate IV atropine or external pacemaker
- Definitive treatment is permanent pacemaker.

Torsade de Pointes

- French: "Twisting of the points"
- Refers to a V-tach variation in which QRS axis swings from positive to a negative in a single lead (see Figure 8-12)
- Can be caused by R-on-T phenomenon

V-tach

- ≥ 3 ectopic ventricular beats in a row
- See Chapter 2, Resuscitation.

V-fib

See Chapter 2, Resuscitation.

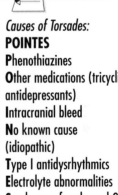

Causes of Torsades:
POINTES
Phenothiazines
Other medications (tricyclic antidepressants)
Intracranial bleed
No known cause (idiopathic)
Type I antidysrhythmics
Electrolyte abnormalities
Syndrome of prolonged QT

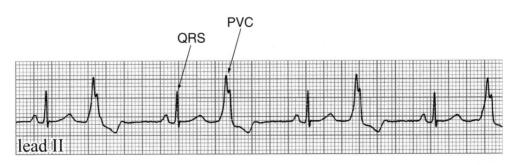

FIGURE 8-11. Ventricular bigeminy. Note the premature ventricular complex (PVC) that regularly follows the QRS complex.

143

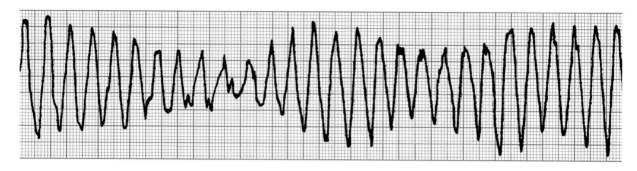

FIGURE 8-12. Torsade de pointes.

Dilated Cardiomyopathy

DEFINITION

Enlargement of all four chambers of the heart, resulting in impaired contractility (L > R ventricle), systolic dysfunction (ejection fraction < 45%), and thrombus formation

ETIOLOGY

Reversible
- Alcohol
- Pregnancy
- Thyroid disease
- Metabolic disturbances (hypocalcemia, hypophosphatemia, thiamine, selenium, vitamin C, or vitamin B_6 deficiency)

Irreversible
- Viral myocarditis
- Idiopathic
- Drugs (adriamycin, cocaine, lithium)
- Heavy metals (lead, mercury, cobalt)
- Familial predisposition
- Neuromuscular disease

SIGNS AND SYMPTOMS

- Symptoms of heart failure
- Angina due to increased O_2 demands of enlarged ventricles
- Neurological deficits, severe flank pain, or a cold pulseless extremity can be seen with peripheral embolization.
- Bilateral rales, jugular venous distention (JVD), hepatomegaly
- Presence of S_3 and S_4 gallop
- Mitral and tricuspid regurgitation

DIAGNOSIS

- ECG—atrial hypertrophy:
  - Notched P wave in lead II (P mitrale)
  - Peaked P wave in lead II (P pulmonale)
  - Negative terminal deflection of P wave in lead V1

Most common complaints in dilated cardiomyopathy are dyspnea on exertion and fatigue.

A-fib is the most common dysrhythmia in dilated cardiomyopathy.

HIGH-YIELD FACTS

Cardiovascular Emergencies

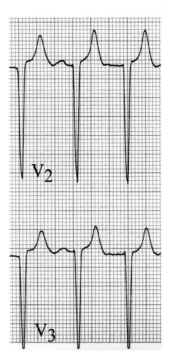

FIGURE 8-13. Left ventricular hypertrophy (LVH).

- Ventricular hypertrophy (see Figure 8-13):
    - Tall QRS complexes in precordial leads
- CXR—enlarged cardiac silhouette, pulmonary venous congestion
- Echocardiography—enlarged ventricles/atria, regurgitant valves, low ejection fractions

TREATMENT

- Correct any reversible causes (e.g., discontinue toxic agent).
- Anticoagulation for A-fib or signs of peripheral embolization
- Diuretics and nitrates as needed for management of CHF and APE
- Implanted automatic defibrillator for patients with life-threatening dysrhythmias

Restrictive Cardiomyopathy

DEFINITION

Deposition of protein or fibrous tissue leading to eventual scarring of myocardium causing decreased ventricular filling

PATHOPHYSIOLOGY

- Ventricular stiffness
- Diastolic dysfunction (decreased compliance and filling)
- Ventricular cavity obliteration (end stage)

- Endomyocardial fibroelastosis
- Eosinophilic endomyocardial disease (hypereosinophilic syndrome)
- Primary amyloidosis
- Hemochromatosis
- Sarcoidosis
- Carcinoid syndrome
- Scleroderma
- Glycogen storage disease type II

SIGNS AND SYMPTOMS

- Signs of right heart failure usually predominate.
- Bilateral rales, JVD, hepatomegaly
- Exercise intolerance is a common presenting symptom.
- Presence of S_3 and S_4 gallop
- Mitral or tricuspid regurgitation

DIAGNOSIS

- Auscultation—S_3/S_4 gallop murmurs, mitral/tricuspid regurgitation
- ECG—atrial and ventricular hypertrophy and nonspecific ST-T wave changes
- CXR—normal cardiac silhouette or enlarged atria, pulmonary venous congestion
- Echocardiography—normal-sized ventricles, large atria, thickened ventricular walls, normal or slightly decreased ejection fraction, tricuspid or mitral regurgitation

TREATMENT

- Treatment is generally ineffective.
- Phlebotomy and deferoxamine may be helpful for hemochromatosis.

Hypertrophic Cardiomyopathy

DEFINITION

- Hypertrophied, nondilated, asymmetric left ventricle (septum > free wall) with 2° atrial dilation
- Also known as idiopathic hypertrophic subaortic stenosis, or IHSS

PATHOPHYSIOLOGY

Results in:
- Systolic dysfunction (end-stage dilation)
- Diastolic dysfunction (poor filling and relaxation)
- Myocardial ischemia (increased O_2 demand because of increased myocardial mass, compression of small intramural coronaries during systole = decreased O_2 supply)

ETIOLOGY

- Idiopathic or inherited (50%)
- HTN
- Aortic or pulmonic stenosis

Remember **right** heart failure in **restrictive** cardiomyopathy.

In dilated cardiomyopathy, ventricular enlargement and left heart failure predominate; in restrictive cardiomyopathy, atrial enlargement and right heart failure predominate.

HIGH-YIELD FACTS

Cardiovascular Emergencies

SIGNS AND SYMPTOMS

- Angina:
    - Not well understood in terms of known pathophysiology
    - Occurs at rest and during exercise
    - Frequently unresponsive to nitroglycerin
    - May respond to recumbent position (pathognomonic but rare)
- Syncope:
    - Most often occurs following exercise—*decreased afterload* due to peripheral vasodilation resulting in peripheral pooling since muscular contractions no longer enhance return to heart causing *decreased preload*
    - Arrhythmias: A-fib, V-tach
- Palpitations due to arrhythmias
- Signs of CHF
- Pulsus bisferiens (rapid biphasic carotid pulse)
- S$_4$ gallop
- Systolic ejection murmur heard best along the left sternal border, decreases with increased LV blood volume (squatting), increases with increased blood velocities (exercise), and decreased LV end-diastolic volume (Valsalva)
- Paradoxical splitting of S$_2$
- Sudden death, the least useful sign, is usually due to an arrhythmia rather than obstruction.

DIAGNOSIS

- ECG: LVH, PVCs, A-fib, septal Q waves, nonspecific ST segment and T wave abnormalities
- Echocardiography: Septal hypertrophy, LVH but small LV size, atrial dilatation, mitral wall thickening

TREATMENT

- Amiodarone may reduce the incidence of life-threatening dysrhythmias.
- Beta blockers to reduce heart rate, increasing LV filling time and decreasing inotropy are first line; calcium channel blockers considered second line.
- Anticoagulation for A-fib or signs of peripheral embolization
- Septal myomectomy for severely symptomatic patients
- Mitral valve replacement can reduce obstruction.
- Permanent pacemaker to change pattern of ventricular contraction, reducing obstruction
- Implanted automatic defibrillator should be considered.
- Bacterial endocarditis prophylaxis for dental, GI, and genitourinary procedures
- Vigorous exercise should be discouraged.

ACUTE BACTERIAL ENDOCARDITIS (ABE)

DEFINITION

Bacterial infection of endocardium

Typical scenario:
A 25-year-old man becomes severely dyspneic and collapses while running laps. His father had died suddenly at an early age. *Think: Hypertrophic cardiomyopathy.*

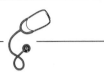

Hypertrophic cardiomyopathy: Symptoms prior to 30 years correlates with increased risk of sudden death, but severity of symptoms (whenever they occur) does not.

Very few murmurs *decrease* with squatting (this one does).

Causes of paradoxical splitting of S$_2$:
- Hypertrophic cardiomyopathy
- Aortic stenosis
- LBBB

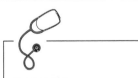

Hypertrophic cardiomyopathy: Digitalis and other positive inotropic agents are contraindicated even if presenting symptoms are those of CHF (because they increase outflow obstruction).

ETIOLOGY

Common pathogens:

- *Streptococcus viridans:* Declining in frequency, most common cause in normal population
- *Streptococcus* sp. (non-viridans)
- *Staphylococcus aureus:* 75% in IV drug users
- Coagulase-negative *Staphylococcus* sp. (prosthetic valves and neonates)
- Enterococci: 2 to 8% all groups
- HACEK group (*Haemophilus* species, *Actinobacillus actinomycetemcomitans*, *Cardiobacterium hominis*, *Eikenella corrodens*, *Kingella* species): 2 to 4% of all groups

RISK FACTORS

- Prosthetic valve
- Valvular heart disease
- IV drug abuse
- Indwelling venous catheters
- Dialysis
- Human immunodeficiency virus (HIV)
- Previous history of ABE

PATHOPHYSIOLOGY

- Valves and sometimes other areas of endocardium (walls, septa, papillary muscles) house bacteria in a platelet–fibrin matrix attached to damaged tissue.
- Bacteria is protected from host defenses by matrix and therefore proliferates, causing abscess and showering septic emboli distally.

SIGNS AND SYMPTOMS

- Fever, chills, malaise
- Arthralgias
- Pleuritic chest pain
- Back pain
- CHF
- Confusion
- Pneumonia
- Splinter hemorrhages under fingernails, petechiae
- Heart murmur (new)
- Hepatosplenomegaly
- Clubbing
- *Janeway lesions* (nontender palmar plaques)
- *Roth spots* (retinal hemorrhages)
- *Osler's nodes* (tender fingertip nodules)

DIAGNOSIS

- Labs: Normocytic anemia, increased white blood cell (WBC) count, increased erythrocyte sedimentation rate (ESR), positive rheumatoid factor
- Three separate blood cultures from different sites (the more cultures, the higher the yield) are used to make the diagnosis.
- Urinalysis demonstrates pyuria and hematuria.
- CXR: CHF, pneumonia, septic emboli
- ECG: Tachycardia, nonspecific changes
- Echocardiography: Transesophageal echocardiography (TEE) is more

Frequency of valves affected in ABE: aortic > mitral >> tricuspid

Typical scenario:
A 28-year-old female with a prosthetic valve presents with fever. Physical exam reveals a systolic ejection murmur and retinal hemorrhages. *Think: Bacterial endocarditis.*

148

sensitive than transthoracic (TTE) at picking up valvular vegetations and thickening, endocardial abscess, and wall motion abnormalities.

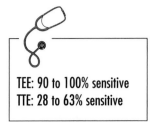

TEE: 90 to 100% sensitive
TTE: 28 to 63% sensitive

TREATMENT

- ABCs, IV access
- Treat for CHF if present.
- IV oxacillin or nafcillin 2 g q 4 hours with an aminoglycoside (e.g., gentamicin 1 mg/kg IV q 8 hours) to start empiric therapy
- If on antibiotics already, in an area with increased methicillin-resistant *S. aureus*, or patient has a prosthetic valve, add vancomycin IV 1 g.

HEART FAILURE

DEFINITION

- "Failure" of cardiac muscle to pump blood efficiently enough to meet metabolic demands of the body
- Causes are many and multifactorial and beyond the scope of this book.

Cor Pulmonale

Heart failure primarily of the right ventricle and atrium caused by lung disease (pulmonary HTN)

High-Output Heart Failure

- A hyperdynamic/hypermetabolic state will fatigue the heart (like any muscle) and cause it to fail from overuse.
- Caused by:
  - Decreased systemic vascular resistance (severe anemia or nutritional deficiency, thyrotoxicosis, medications, AV fistula, pregnancy)
  - Increased preload (mineralocorticoid-mediated renal retention of salt and water)
  - Increased sympathetic tone

Low-Output Heart Failure (CHF)

DEFINITION

Also called CHF

PATHOPHYSIOLOGY

Decreased systolic function and cardiac output with increased diastolic pressures is the clinical state of low-output failure regardless of cause. As blood cannot be pumped by a failing heart, hydrostatic pressures force fluid through capillary membranes "behind" the involved ventricle (usually both).

SIGNS AND SYMPTOMS

- Shortness of breath
- Dyspnea on exertion

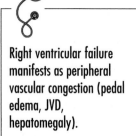

Right ventricular failure manifests as peripheral vascular congestion (pedal edema, JVD, hepatomegaly).

LV failure manifests as pulmonary edema or shock (dyspnea, orthopnea, hypotension).

- Orthopnea
- Paroxysmal nocturnal dyspnea
- Exercise intolerance ± angina
- Cough
- Leg swelling
- Abdominal girth
- Palpitations
- Tachycardia
- Tachypnea
- Decreased O_2 saturation
- Increased or decreased BP
- Rales
- Wheeze
- Peripheral edema
- JVD, hepatojugular reflex

DIAGNOSIS

- Labs: Check CBC, renal function (blood urea nitrogen/creatinine [BUN/Cr]), cardiac enzymes (troponin, creatine kinase [CK]-MB), urinalysis, pregnancy test (if applicable), coagulation factors (prothrombin time/partial thromboplastin time [PT/PTT]), arterial blood gas (ABG) to check CO_2 retention in COPD patients or A-a gradient.
- CXR: Cardiomegaly and pulmonary vascular congestion/edema, ± effusions, Kerley A and B lines, prominent major fissure
- ECG: Variable, tachycardia, look for ischemia/infarct
- Echocardiography: Global or segmental hypokinesis with or without valvular regurgitation/stenosis, chamber enlargement

TREATMENT

- ABCs, IV, O_2, monitor
- If normal pressure or hypertensive: Loop diuretics, nitrates, morphine, positive-pressure O_2 (biphasic positive airway pressure/continuous positive airway pressure), Foley catheter to evaluate fluid losses/diuresis
- If hypotensive or unstable: Arterial line for BP monitoring and ABG tests, inotropic agents (dobutamine, amrinone, digoxin), pressors (dopamine, norepinephrine, phenylephrine), IABP, Foley catheter, Swan–Ganz catheter for accurate measurement of intravascular pressures, antidysrhythmics as needed

MYOCARDITIS

DEFINITION

Inflammatory damage of myocardium

PATHOPHYSIOLOGY

- Myocyte necrosis/degeneration and correlating inflammatory infiltrate due to infectious and inflammatory etiologies
- Some infectious agents cause an autoimmune response to cardiac myocytes by molecular mimicry.

- Some cases spontaneously resolve.
- Some cases progress to end-stage dilated cardiomyopathy.

ETIOLOGIES

- Viral (coxsackie B4, adenovirus, influenza A and B, varicella-zoster virus, HIV, cytomegalovirus, hepatitis A and B, Epstein–Barr virus)
- Vaccine related
- Bacterial (*Mycoplasma, Streptococcus, Chlamydia*)
- Lyme disease (*Borrelia burgdorferi*)
- Chagas' disease (*Trypanosoma cruzi*)
- Kawasaki disease
- Steroid abuse

Typical scenario:
A 29-year-old male presents with fever and retrosternal chest pain. He had "the flu bug" 2 weeks ago. He is tachycardic. *Think: Myocarditis.*

CLINICAL FINDINGS

- Fever
- Chest pain
- Tachycardia out of proportion to fever
- Syncope
- Dyspnea
- Fatigue
- Palpitations
- Soft S_1
- S_3 or S_4 gallop
- Mitral or tricuspid regurgitation murmur

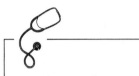

In new diagnosis of refractory asthma in a young adult, consider myocarditis.

DIAGNOSIS

- CXR: ± Cardiomegaly/pulmonary edema
- ECG: Sinus tachycardia, low voltage, long QT/PR/QRS, AV blocks, increased or decreased STs, decreased Ts
- Labs: Increased ESR, increased WBC count, increased CK-MB, increased troponin
- Echocardiography: Multichamber dysfunction, decreased left ventricular ejection fraction, global hypokinesis, focal wall motion abnormality

TREATMENT

- Intensive care unit admission
- Bed rest, supportive care, vital signs
- Antibiotics for bacterial and parasitic causes
- ASA and gamma globulin for Kawasaki disease
- ACE inhibitors for CHF associated with myocarditis

PERICARDITIS

Constrictive

- Fibrous reparative thickening of pericardial layers (sometimes calcified) that restricts diastolic ventricular filling
- Caused by trauma, uremia, tuberculosis (TB), radiation

Acute Inflammatory

- Inflammation of pericardial tissue resulting in pain and effusion
- Causes:
  - Trauma
  - Uremia
  - Infectious (viral > bacterial > parasitic > fungal)
  - Post irradiation
  - Post MI
  - Aortic dissection
  - Tumors

CLINICAL FINDINGS

- Fever
- Pleuritic and positional chest pain
- Tachycardia
- Myalgias
- Shallow breathing
- Anxiety
- Pericardial friction rub
- Distant heart sounds

DIAGNOSIS

- CXR: May see cardiomegaly if effusion present
- ECG (see Figure 8-14):
  - Stage 1 (first few hours/days): Diffuse ST elevations with PR depression
  - Stage 2: Normalization of STs and PRs
  - Stage 3: Diffuse T wave inversions
  - Stage 4: Normalization of T waves
- Labs: Increased ESR and WBC counts, + CK and troponin if concomitant myocarditis or endocarditis; check BUN/Cr, blood cultures
- Echocardiography: Normal global cardiac function unless an effusion is present

TREATMENT

- NSAIDs for viral, post MI, and idiopathic causes
- Antimicrobials for bacterial, fungal, TB, and parasitic causes
- Surgical pericardiectomy for purulent pericarditis
- Dialysis for uremic pericarditis

PERICARDIAL EFFUSIONS

DEFINITIONS

- Pericardial effusion: Excessive fluid in pericardial space
- Cardiac tamponade: Large pericardial effusion that restricts ventricular filling and eventually stroke volume, leading to systemic hypotension, shock, PEA, and death

---

Typical scenario:
A 31-year-old female presents with pleuritic chest pain that improves with leaning forward. Cardiac auscultation reveals a pericardial friction rub. ECG demonstrates diffuse PR depression. *Think: Pericarditis.*

Cardiac tamponade is one of the causes of pulseless electrical activity (PEA).

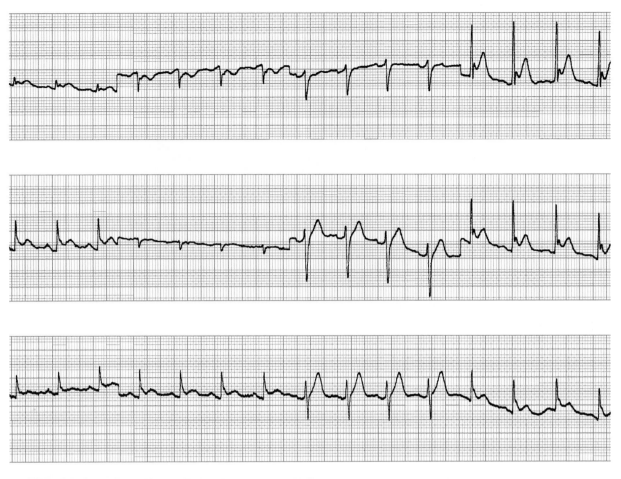

FIGURE 8-14. ECG in pericarditis. Note diffuse ST elevations with PR depression, early stage of pericarditis. ECG will change and normalize as disease progresses and resolves.

ETIOLOGIES

Same as pericarditis

CLINICAL FINDINGS

- Same as pericarditis, but alterations in vital signs may be more pronounced and shock state may exist
- Often asymptomatic when small
- Beck's triad for cardiac tamponade

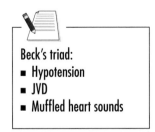

Beck's triad:
- Hypotension
- JVD
- Muffled heart sounds

DIAGNOSIS

- CXR: Cardiomegaly (see Figure 8-15)
- ECG: Differing QRS amplitudes ("alternans") and axes caused by ventricle swaying within fluid-filled pericardial sac with each beat
- Echocardiography: Effusion, decreased systolic and diastolic function

TREATMENT

- ABCs, IV, O$_2$, monitor
- Pericardiocentesis immediately if hemodynamically unstable or pulseless

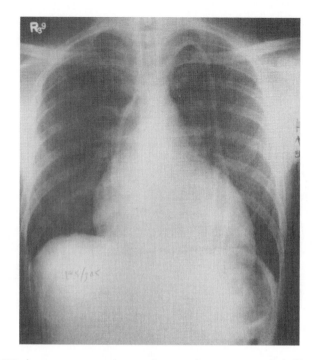

FIGURE 8-15. CXR demonstrating cardiomegaly secondary to pericardial effusion.

- If more stable, a pericardial window can be created in the operating room (OR) to prevent reaccumulation of effusion.

VALVULAR LESIONS

Aortic Stenosis (AS)

DEFINITION

Valve hardening obstructs blood flow from left ventricle. Results in progressive LVH, decreased cardiac output, decreased coronary blood flow, hypertrophic and later dilated cardiomyopathy. Predisposes to endocarditis.

ETIOLOGY

- Congenital
- Rheumatic fever
- Degenerative calcification

SIGNS AND SYMPTOMS

Dyspnea on exertion, angina, syncope on exertion, sudden death, low-pitched crescendo–decrescendo murmur at the base radiating to carotids, carotid pulse weak (parvus) and slow-rising (tardus), S_3, S_4

DIAGNOSIS

- CXR: Cardiomegaly ± pulmonary edema
- ECG: LVH ± ischemic change

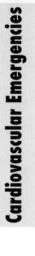

Prognosis: *Mean survival for patients with AS and:*
Angina = 5 years
Syncope = 2 to 3 years
Heart failure = 1 to 2 years

- Echocardiography: Will diagnose by measuring decreased ventricular outflow, diastolic dysfunction from wall stiffness, and diminished calculated aortic cross-sectional area

TREATMENT

- Definitive treatment is valve replacement.
- Acute presentation warrants ruling out ACS, CHF, and other etiologies.
- ABCs, IV, O_2, monitor
- Gentle hydration if hypotensive

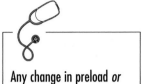

Any change in preload *or* afterload can cause acute decompensation in AS.

Aortic Insufficiency

DEFINITION

Regurgitation of blood flow back into the ventricle, with decreased stroke volume leading to dilated cardiomyopathy and failure

ETIOLOGY

Acute Causes
- Infective endocarditis
- Aortic root dissection

Chronic Causes
- Rheumatic fever
- Congenital
- Ankylosing spondylitis
- Syphilis
- Carcinoid
- Reiter's syndrome
- Fen-Phen use (fenfluramine and phentermine)

SIGNS AND SYMPTOMS

- Dyspnea
- Angina
- Presence of S_3 heart sound
- High-pitched blowing diastolic murmur at base, ± systolic flow murmur
- "Water-hammer" pulse: Peripheral pulse with quick upstroke and then collapse
- Wide pulse pressure
- Bounding "Corrigan" pulse, "pistol shot" femorals, pulsus bisferiens (dicrotic pulse with two palpable waves in systole)
- Duroziez sign: Presence of diastolic femoral bruit when femoral artery is compressed enough to hear a systolic bruit
- Hill's sign: Systolic pressure in the legs 20 mm Hg higher than in the arms
- Quincke's sign: Visible capillary pulse in nails
- De Musset's sign: Bobbing of head with heartbeat

Typical scenario:
A 70-year-old male presents with angina. Physical exam reveals bounding pulses and there is an SBP difference of 25 mm Hg between the upper and lower extremities. *Think: Aortic insufficiency.*

DIAGNOSIS

- CXR:
  - Chronic—cardiomegaly ± pulmonary edema
  - Acute—pulmonary edema without cardiomegaly

- ECG:
  - Chronic—LVH ± strain pattern
  - Acute—± ischemic change (especially inferior leads), low voltage, if dissection—tachycardia
- Echocardiography: Will diagnose disease by visualizing regurgitant flow ± valvular vegetations

TREATMENT

- ABCs, IV, O_2, monitor
- In acute and chronic cases of pulmonary edema, reduce afterload with nitrates and diuretics.
- Digoxin to increase inotropy
- Treat endocarditis as indicated.
- Dissection treated with surgical repair
- Valve replacement is indicated once CHF occurs.

Mitral Stenosis

DEFINITION

Decrease in cross-sectional area for blood flow from left atrium to left ventricle, resulting in atrial dilatation, A-fib, left heart failure, progressive pulmonary HTN, pulmonic and tricuspid valve regurgitation, and right heart failure

ETIOLOGY

- Rheumatic fever
- Atrial myxomas
- Congenital
- Degenerative calcification

SIGNS AND SYMPTOMS

- Dyspnea on exertion
- Orthopnea
- Early diastolic opening snap followed by diastolic rumble at the apex

DIAGNOSIS

- CXR: Can be normal; severe disease can show a straightening of the LV border ± pulmonary edema.
- ECG: Left atrial enlargement ± A-fib, right axis deviation
- Echocardiography: Will diagnose disease by showing thickened valve leaflets, decreased valve movement, and commissural fusion

TREATMENT

- ABCs, IV, O_2, monitor
- Acute A-fib: See above.
- Pulmonary edema: Nitrates, diuretics, oxygen, and morphine
- Surgical valvulotomy or valve replacement is indicated when there is pulmonary edema with good HR control.

Mitral Regurgitation

DEFINITION

Regurgitation of flow from ventricle to atrium during systole and hence an ineffective heart leading to hypertrophic and later dilated cardiomyopathy, with eventual failure

ETIOLOGY

Acute Causes
- MI with ischemic necrosis and subsequent rupture of papillary muscle or chordae tendineae usually from right coronary infarct
- Infective endocarditis
- Trauma

Chronic Causes
- Rheumatic fever heart damage
- Appetite suppressant drugs (Fen-Phen)
- Mitral valve prolapse
- Carcinoid tumor syndrome
- Marfan's syndrome

SIGNS AND SYMPTOMS

- Dyspnea
- Tachycardia and tachypnea
- Angina
- Presence of S_3 and S_4 heart sounds
- Loud crescendo–decrescendo murmur between S_1 and S_2 at the apex radiating to axilla
- Rales
- Rapidly rising and poorly sustained carotid pulse

DIAGNOSIS

- CXR:
  - Chronic: Cardiomegaly ± pulmonary edema
  - Acute: Pulmonary edema without cardiomegaly
- ECG:
  - Chronic: LVH, atrial enlargement, A-fib
  - Acute: ± Ischemic change, tachycardia without chronic changes
- Echocardiography: Can diagnose acute and chronic cases by visualizing chordae tendineae, vegetations, wall motion abnormality, and estimating severity of disease
- Coronary catheterization: Indicated in acute cases to evaluate and treat ACS

TREATMENT

- ABCs, IV, O_2, monitor
- Nitrates, morphine, and diuretics for pulmonary edema, reducing afterload and regurgitant flow
- Antibiotics for infectious endocarditis (IE)
- Catheterization and emergency mitral valve reconstruction for ischemic rupture
- Digitalis, long-acting nitrates, and salt restriction for chronic disease

Artificial Valves

- Mechanical: Bileaflet hinged disk, tilting disk, or caged-ball prostheses:
    - Patients require lifelong anticoagulation (ASA and coumadin)
    - Monitor INR (should be > 2)
    - "Mechanical murmur" systolic with loud, closing machine-like sound
    - Complications: Chronic low-grade hemolysis from turbulent flow and subsequent anemia, valve failure, thrombosis, systemic emboli, bleeding from high INR, risk for IE (contamination and bacteremic)
- Bioprosthetic: Bovine or porcine:
    - ASA only anticoagulation
    - Mitral bioprosthesis has diastolic rumble.
    - Complications: 30 to 70% failure rate at 10 years, risk for IE (contamination and bacteremic), valve failure, thrombosis, systemic emboli
    - Immunosuppressive agents required to prevent rejection

HEART TRANSPLANT

Things to Keep in Mind

- Denervated hearts have no native sympathetic and parasympathetic tone, responding only to circulating catecholamines and medications, so don't try any vagal maneuvers or atropine (which inhibits vagal tone).
- All transplant patients are immunocompromised. If they present with fever, diagnose and treat aggressively with broad-spectrum antibiotics.
- With piggyback heart transplant, you may see two separate independent P waves in the ECG, one from the old heart and one from the new heart.
- Before prescribing anything for the transplant patient as an outpatient, find out if it will interact with his or her immunosuppressant medication.
- Dysrhythmias, atypical fatigability, and exertion intolerance should be treated as acute rejection until proven otherwise. If hemodynamically unstable because of the dysrhythmias, acute rejection regimen should be instituted (methylprednisolone 1 gm IV), and modified ACLS protocols should be followed.
- Atrial dysrhythmias are treated with digoxin or Ca^{2+} channel blockers.
- Ventricular dysrhythmias are treated with lidocaine.
- Refractory bradycardia is treated with IV theophylline or isoproterenol, or transcutaneous/transvenous pacing.

AORTIC ANEURYSM

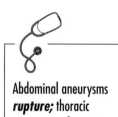

Abdominal aneurysms *rupture;* thoracic aneurysms *dissect.*

Abdominal Aortic Aneurysm (AAA)

PATHOPHYSIOLOGY

- Atherosclerotic, thinned tunica media has decreased elastin fibers and forms aneurysm from HTN.
- The larger the aneurysm, the weaker the wall, and therefore gradual enlargement of AAA.

RISK FACTORS

- Age > 60
- Male gender
- HTN
- Cigarette smoking
- Coronary artery disease
- Peripheral vascular disease
- Family history of AAA in first-degree relative

SIGNS AND SYMPTOMS

- Abdominal pain (77%)
- Pulsatile abdominal mass (70%)
- Back/flank pain (60%)
- Tender abdomen (41%)
- Nausea/vomiting (25%) with blood (5%)
- Syncope (18%)
- Nonpalpable distal pulses (6%)
- Known history of AAA (5%)

DIAGNOSIS

- CXR: Can be normal
- Abdominal x-ray: May see calcified outline of AAA
- ECG: Tachycardia ± ischemic changes
- Ultrasound: Ideal for the unstable patient because of machine portability; however, bowel gas and obesity may obscure visualization.
- Computed tomography (CT) scan: Only for hemodynamically stable patients. Contrast allows full evaluation for both aneurysmal size and possible dissection.
- Aortography: Rarely done because of CT scan's availability and rapid ultrasound. Also, used only in the hemodynamically stable patient.
- Magnetic resonance imaging (MRI): Best for the asymptomatic patient

TREATMENT

- ABCs, IV access (two large bore), O_2, monitor
- IV fluid if in a shock state
- Rapid transport to OR with vascular surgeon

Thoracic Aortic Aneurysm

DEFINITION

A tearing of the aorta due to hypertensive "shearing forces" on an atherosclerotic vessel that infiltrate through the intima and track or "dissect" between the intima and adventitial layers. Dissection can occur proximally or distally and can involve other vessels (carotids, renals, iliacs, pericardium).

CLASSIFICATION

- DeBakey classification (anatomic):
  - Type I: Ascending and descending
  - Type II: Ascending only
  - Type III: Descending only

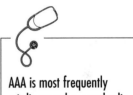

AAA is most frequently misdiagnosed as renal colic.

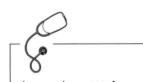

The mortality is 50% for those who rupture and get to the OR.

Typical scenario:
A 73-year-old male who is a 2-pack-per-day smoker with HTN and peripheral vascular disease presents with severe midabdominal and left flank pain. He states he had this same pain 1 week ago, and that it got so bad he passed out. Physical exam reveals bruits over the abdominal aorta and a tender pulsatile mass. *Think: AAA.*

- Stanford classification:
  - Type A: Ascending aorta
  - Type B: Descending aorta

RISK FACTORS

- HTN
- Connective tissue disease (Marfan's, Ehlers–Danlos)
- Male gender (three times more affected than women)
- Congenital heart disease
- Third-trimester pregnancy
- Turner's syndrome
- Cocaine use

SIGNS AND SYMPTOMS

- Abrupt onset of pain that is maximal at onset and migrates:
  - Type I: Pain begins in anterior chest and radiates to jaw, neck, or arms.
  - Type II: Pain begins between the scapulae and radiates to the abdomen and lumbar area.
- Elevated BP
- Tachycardia
- Shock
- Focal neurological deficits:
  - Stroke-like syndrome if carotid involvement
  - Hoarse voice if there is compression of recurrent laryngeal nerve
  - Horner's syndrome if superior cervical sympathetic ganglion is compressed
- ≥ 20 mm Hg BP difference between upper and lower extremities
- Aortic insufficiency murmur
- May present with cold pulseless extremity

DIAGNOSIS

- ECG: LVH with strain pattern, ± ischemic change if dissection into coronaries or if MI, low voltage if effusion, electrical alternans if tamponade
- CXR: Mediastinal widening (75%) (see Figure 8-16), calcification of aortic arch, displacement of trachea and/or nasogastric tube to one side
- TEE: Diagnostic study of choice with almost 100% sensitivity and specificity. Can differentiate between true and false lumens. Minimally invasive, does not require IV contrast. May not however, be readily available
- MRI: Also close to 100% sensitivity and specificity, but is time consuming, allows limited access to patient during scan. Noninvasive, no contrast dye needed
- CT scan: Rapid dynamic scans of multiple levels of chest immediately following IV bolus of contrast (95% specificity and sensitivity)
- Aortography: Used to be gold standard. Invasive, requires contrast dye. About 90% sensitive and specific. Can miss thrombosed false lumens. Time consuming, takes patient out of ED suite

TREATMENT

- ABCs, IV access (two large bore), O₂, monitor
- Antihypertensive medications (decrease shearing force), labetalol IV

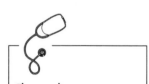

Typical scenario:
A 67-year-old male with history of HTN presents with a sudden-onset excruciating chest pain radiating to the left jaw. Physical exam reveals an aortic insufficiency murmur, a BP of 217/110, and cool clammy skin. *Think: Thoracic dissection (type I).*

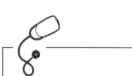

Thoracic dissections are most frequently misdiagnosed as AMIs.

Always get at least a chest film when you suspect MI: Some of these patients will have aortic dissection, and thrombolysis may kill them.

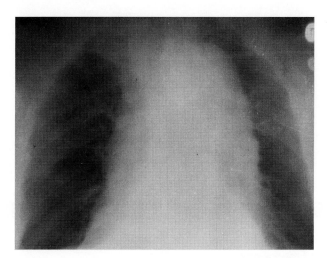

FIGURE 8-16. CXR of widened mediastinum.

(Reproduced, with permission, from Tintinalli JE, Kelen GD, Stapczynski JS. *Emergency Medicine: A Comprehensive Study Guide,* 5th ed. New York: McGraw-Hill, 2000: 415.)

0.25 mg/kg (or 20 mg) over 2 minutes and then nitroprusside 0.3 to 10 μg/kg/min

- Immediate surgical consultation: Go to OR for repair if patient is unstable or hypotensive.
- Ascending involvement = repair
- Descending involvement = BIG OR risk

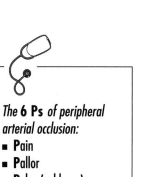

The most specific CXR sign for thoracic dissection is extension of the aortic shadow by more than 5 mm beyond its calcified aortic wall.

PERIPHERAL ARTERIAL OCCLUSION

PATHOPHYSIOLOGY

- A blockage in arterial flow compromises all tissue distally, resulting in irreversible cell death within 4 to 6 hours.
- Without rapid aggressive treatment, it can lead to gangrene, limb amputation, and death.
- Embolic sources (e.g., thrombus of cardiac origin breaks off and travels distally) and nonembolic sources (e.g., atherosclerosis and plaque rupture with thrombus occlusion, vasospasm, and/or arteritis)

RISK FACTORS

- HTN
- Smoking
- High cholesterol
- Diabetes
- Recent MI or A-fib

CLINICAL FINDINGS

- Abrupt onset of pain in leg known to have poor circulation
- The 6 Ps may not all be present.
- Use handheld Doppler to try finding nonpalpable pedal pulse.

*The **6 Ps** of peripheral arterial occlusion:*
- **Pain**
- **Pallor**
- **Polar (coldness)**
- **Pulselessness**
- **Paresthesias**
- **Paralysis**

DIAGNOSIS

- ECG: A-fib or atrial flutter, or sinus rhythm, LVH
- CXR: ± Cardiomegaly

TREATMENT

- ABCs
- Immediate consult of vascular surgery consult
- IV heparinization if no contraindications

HTN

Hypertensive Emergency

DEFINITION

HTN that causes end-organ damage

SIGNS AND SYMPTOMS

Signs of end-organ damage:
- Brain:
    - Hypertensive encephalopathy—loss of integrity of the blood–brain barrier and resulting cerebral edema
    - Intracerebral hemorrhage—a result of long-standing HTN, vascular disease, or aneurysm rupture
- Eye: Hypertensive retinopathy—"cotton-wool" spots (focal ischemia), hemorrhage, and papilledema (optic disc edema from hypoxia)
- Heart:
    - LV failure and pulmonary edema due to too much afterload for the pump to handle
    - ACS—not enough blood flow to meet the pump's O_2 demand
- Kidney: Acute renal failure—causes and is caused by HTN:
    - Pregnancy: Eclampsia (see obstetrics section)
    - Vascular: Aortic dissection (see above)

DIAGNOSIS

- Labs: Elevated BUN and Cr, urinalysis (for red blood cells [RBCs], protein, and casts), cardiac enzymes if chest pain or pulmonary edema, CBC, electrolytes
- CXR: ± Pulmonary edema, ± cardiomegaly
- ECG: LVH, ischemic change
- CT head: ± Bleed/edema

TREATMENT

Reduce the mean arterial pressure by no more than one third. Common intravenous agents include:
- Nitroglycerin
- Nitroprusside
- Labetalol
- Phentolamine for pheochromocytoma
- Hydralazine for preeclampsia-related HTN

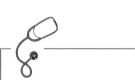

The *mean arterial pressure* is: (2DBP + SBP)/3

Nitroprusside can cause cyanide toxicity.

Hypertensive Urgency

- SBP ≥ 180 mm Hg, DBP ≥ 110 mm Hg without evidence of end-organ damage
- Most common cause is noncompliance with medications.
- Treatment: Oral agents

Typical scenario:
A 47-year-old female presents with BP of 200/130. She is a known hypertensive but admits to being noncompliant with her medications. Physical examination is unremarkable. *Think: Hypertensive urgency.*

VENOUS INSUFFICIENCY

PATHOPHYSIOLOGY

- Incompetent valves in peripheral venous system (~90% lower extremities) cause "venous stasis" of peripheral blood, microextravasation of RBCs, and fluid causing pigment (hemosiderin) deposition in local tissues (stasis dermatitis) and pitting edema.
- Stasis in turn can lead to poor wound healing and intravascular thrombosis (see below).

TREATMENT

- Advise avoidance of prolonged periods of standing/working on feet.
- Elevate legs when resting.
- Wear gradient compression hose.
- A mild diuretic in a low dose may be helpful.

THROMBOPHLEBITIS

DEFINITIONS

- DVT: Involves the deep venous system, typically calf, popliteal, femoral, common femoral, and iliac
- Superficial thrombophlebitis can be present at the same time as DVT and can occur in any superficial vein. Varicose veins are a predisposing factor.

PATHOPHYSIOLOGY

- Intravascular (intravenous) spontaneous clot (thrombosis) and concurrent surrounding inflammatory response to that clot
- Clot can dissolve, propagate, or embolize to a distal site (creating pulmonary embolus or a paradoxic CVA through ASD/VSD).

RISK FACTORS

- Prior DVT
- Pregnancy or postpartum state
- Malignancy
- Prolonged immobility
- IV drug abuse
- Recent trauma or burns
- Coronary artery disease
- Polycythemia vera
- Thrombocytosis
- Antithrombin III, protein C or S deficiency

Typical scenario:
A 39-year-old female who arrived home from her 18-hour car ride the previous evening presents with right calf swelling and pain. Physical exam reveals the right calf to be 4 cm larger than the left, and it is warm to the touch. *Think: DVT.*

- Aquired immune deficiency syndrome
- Autoimmune disease (e.g., systemic lupus erythematosus)
- Indwelling catheter

CLINICAL FINDINGS

- Unilateral swelling and pitting edema of a lower extremity
- Redness, pain, heat (very similar to cellulitis in appearance)
- Palpable pulses in extremity
- Palpable cord if superficial enough

DEFINITION

- Labs: PT and PTT should be normal. D-dimer may be elevated but is nonspecific.
- Ultrasound of affected lower extremity: Looking at venous system and its compressibility is the most readily available imaging study, while venography is the gold standard.

TREATMENT

- Anticoagulation with heparin if DVT or PE present: 80 U/kg IV bolus followed by 18 U/kg/hr infusion. LMWH can be used for DVT without PE.
- Inferior vena caval filter (Greenfield) for patients with malignancy, already on oral anticoagulation, or who have a contraindication to anticoagulation (frequent falls in elderly)
- Consider thrombolytics for massive iliofemoral thrombosis.

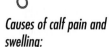

Causes of calf pain and swelling:
- DVT
- Baker's cyst
- Hematoma
- Abscess

Gastrointestinal Emergencies

ESOPHAGUS

Varices

DEFINITION

Dilated submucosal veins

EPIDEMIOLOGY

- Found in 50% of patients with cirrhosis
- Usually develop due to portal hypertension
- Thirty percent of patients with varices develop upper gastrointestinal (GI) bleeds.

CLINICAL FINDINGS

- Asymptomatic until rupture
- Bleeding is usually massive.
- Present with spontaneous emesis of either bright red blood or coffee ground material

TREATMENT

- Volume replacement with normal saline (NS) and packed red blood cells
- Nasogastric (NG) suction
- Intravenous (IV) vasopressin or octreotide to control bleeding
- Emergent endoscopy to localize bleeding for possible sclerotherapy or rubber band ligation of varices
- Consider tamponade with Sengstaken–Blakemore tube for persistent bleeding.
- GI consult
- Hospital admission for all unstable cases

Boerhaave's Syndrome

DEFINITION

Spontaneous full-thickness distal esophageal perforation that usually results from violent retching

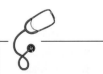

Higher morbidity and mortality rate than any other source of upper GI bleed

Many patients with varices have coagulopathy due to underlying cirrhosis.

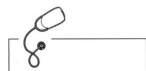

Beta-blocker therapy may reduce rebleeds by decreasing portal hypertension.

165

RISK FACTORS

Alcohol ingestion

CLINICAL FINDINGS

- Severe epigastric and retrosternal chest pain with radiation to back, neck, and shoulders
- Subcutaneous emphysema

DIAGNOSIS

- Chest x-ray (CXR) may be normal or demonstrate mediastinal widening, pleural effusion, mediastinal emphysema, or left pneumothorax.
- Water-soluble oral contrast (Gastrografin) confirms the diagnosis.

TREATMENT

Tube thoracostomy and immediate repair is indicated to prevent mediastinitis, which can cause shock and sepsis.

Esophageal Foreign Body (FB) Ingestion

SITES OF IMPACTION

- The most common site in children is at the cricopharyngeus muscle (C5).
- The most common site in adults is at the lower esophageal sphincter (LES) (T10).

EPIDEMIOLOGY

- Eighty percent of obstructions occur in children and are due to coins, marbles, buttons, etc.
- Twenty percent of obstructions occur in adults and are due to meat impaction.

SIGNS AND SYMPTOMS

- Dysphagia
- Gagging
- Throat pain
- FB sensation
- Vomiting
- Anorexia
- Anxiety

DIAGNOSIS

- CXR and soft-tissue films of the neck to look for:
  - The flat surface of a coin or other such FB will be seen when it is lodged in the esophagus.
  - The edge will be seen when located in the trachea.
- If radiographs do not demonstrate FB, then consider esophagogram with contrast or endoscopy.

TREATMENT

- If FB is in the upper third of the esophagus (cervical esophagus, top 5 cm), it can be removed with a Magill forceps and a laryngoscope.

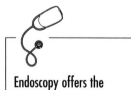

Subcutaneous and mediastinal emphysema may be noted by Hamman's sound—rice crispies in milk.

Adults with esophageal meat impactions almost always have underlying pathology such as carcinoma or strictures.

Endoscopy offers the advantage of being able to visualize and *remove* FB.

- For meat impactions in the distal (last 3 cm) esophagus:
  - IV glucagon or sublingual nitroglycerin can be used to relax smooth muscle and decrease LES tone.
  - Carbonated beverages and other gas-forming agents may be useful to push the meat impaction down into the stomach by raising the intraluminal pressure.
- Most FB that pass into the stomach may be managed expectantly (observed) for passage into the stool (takes 3 to 5 days).
- Approximately 1% of impacted FB cannot be removed by direct visualization or do not pass into the stomach and must be removed surgically.
- Endoscopic removal is required for sharp objects and objects larger than 2 cm wide or 5 cm long.
- Removal of these objects before they pass the pylorus decreases chance of perforation.

Most alkaline batteries will pass into the stomach and can be managed expectantly. However, 10% of button batteries will lodge in the esophagus, and these must be removed because they are highly corrosive (alkali causes liquefaction necrosis).

Gastroesophageal Reflux Disease (GERD)

DEFINITION

Reflux of acidic gastric contents into the esophagus

CAUSES

- Relaxed or incompetent LES
- Hiatal hernia
- Decreased esophageal motility
- Delayed gastric emptying
- Diabetes mellitus
- Gastroparesis
- Gastric outlet obstruction
- Anticholinergic use
- Fatty foods

CAUSES OF LOWERED LES TONE

- Coffee
- Cigarettes
- Alcohol
- Chocolate
- Peppermint
- Anticholinergics
- Progesterone
- Estrogen
- Nitrates
- Calcium channel blockers

SIGNS AND SYMPTOMS

- Substernal burning pain
- Dysphagia
- Hypersalivation (water brash)
- Cough

A majority of patients with asthma have associated GERD.

DIAGNOSIS

Barium swallow, esophagoscopy, mucosal biopsy

TREATMENT

- Elevate head of bed.
- Discontinue foods that decrease LES tone.
- Oral antacids
- H$_2$ blocker or proton pump inhibitor
- Patients with hiatal hernia may be candidates for Nissen fundoplication (the stomach is wrapped around the distal esophagus to create a "new sphincter").

COMPLICATIONS OF GERD

- **Esophagitis:** Esophageal damage, bleeding, and friability due to prolonged exposure to gastric contents
- **Peptic stricture:** Occurs in about 10% of patients with GERD
- **Barrett's esophagus:** Transformation of normal squamous epithelium to columnar epithelium, sometimes accompanied by an ulcer or stricture
- **Esophageal cancer:** Upper two thirds squamous, lower one third adenocarcinoma

Barrett's esophagus carries a 2 to 5% risk of development of esophageal adenocarcinoma, which carries a < 5% chance of 5-year survival.

STOMACH

Mallory–Weiss Tear

DEFINITION

A **partial-thickness** tear at the gastroesophageal junction associated with hematemesis, usually self-limited

Note partial tear as opposed to full tear of Boerhaave's.

RISK FACTORS

- Alcoholism
- Hiatal hernia
- Gastritis

CLINICAL FINDINGS

- Prior history of vomiting, retching, or straining
- Endoscopy establishes diagnosis.

TREATMENT

Usually self-limited

Things that cause gastritis:
SPIT BANDS
Shock states
Pancreatic juice
Infection with *Helicobacter pylori*
Tobacco

Bile
Alcohol
Nonsteroidal anti-inflammatory drugs (NSAIDs)
Drug-induced
Steroids, stress

Acute Gastritis

DEFINITION

- Inflammation of the stomach

ETIOLOGIES

- Stress gastritis is due to severe medical or surgical illness including trauma, burns, hypotension, sepsis, central nervous system (CNS) injury (Cushing ulcer), mechanical respiration, and multiorgan failure.
- Corrosive gastritis is most commonly seen with alcohol.

CLINICAL FINDINGS

- Most asymptomatic unless ulcers or other complications develop
- Symptomatic: Abdominal pain, nausea/vomiting, GI bleed
- Typically diagnosed at endoscopy for complaints of dyspepsia or upper GI bleed

TREATMENT

- Avoid alcohol, cigarettes, caffeine, and citrus and spicy foods for 6 weeks.
- Prophylaxis with H_2 blocker

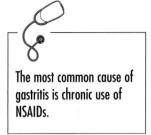

The most common cause of gastritis is chronic use of NSAIDs.

Upper GI Bleed

DEFINITION

Bleeding that is proximal to ligament of Treitz

ETIOLOGY

- Peptic ulcer (45%)
- Gastric erosions (23%)
- Varices (10%)
- Mallory–Weiss tear (7%)
- Esophagitis (6%)
- Duodenitis (6%)

NSAID use, steroids, or dyspepsia: *Think: Peptic ulcer disease (PUD).*

CLINICAL FINDINGS

- Most common presentation is hematemesis (bright red blood or "coffee grounds") or melena (dark tarry stool) with or without abdominal pain.
- Hematochezia (bright red bloody stool) usually indicates lower GI bleed, but may also be present in massive upper GI bleeds.
- Check for hypotension, tachycardia, weakness, pallor, syncope, and diaphoresis.
- Ear, nose, and throat exam should be done to rule out nosebleeds, which can mimic upper GI bleed (swallowed blood).

Chronic liver disease: *Think: Esophageal varices or portal hypertension.*

DIAGNOSIS

- Routine labs: Complete blood count (CBC), prothrombin time, partial thromboplastin time, type and crossmatch 4 to 6 units, electrolytes, liver function tests (LFTs)
- Abdominal radiograph (AXR): Usefulness very limited but may rule out free air

Heavy alcohol ingestion or retching: *Think: Mallory–Weiss tear.*

TREATMENT

- Rapid assessment and management with ABCs (airway, breathing, and circulation) supporting airway, IV (NS or lactated Ringer's solution), O_2, and monitor
- Blood products for continued active bleeding or failure to improve vitals. Consider use of IV vasopressin or octreotide.
- NG lavage looking for coffee grounds or fresh blood
- GI consult for identification of bleeding sites with endoscopy

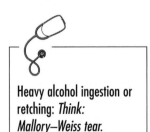

Initial hematocrit is a poor indicator of the severity of acute bleeding because it takes 24 to 72 hours to equilibrate.

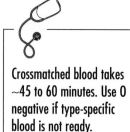

Crossmatched blood takes ~45 to 60 minutes. Use O negative if type-specific blood is not ready.

Pain is visceral in nature and is therefore vague and midline.

Adverse effects of cimetidine:

- Increases levels of drugs cleared via P450 system (e.g., warfarin, phenytoin, diazepam, propranolol, lidocaine, theophylline, tricyclic antidepressants)
- CNS dysfunction in the elderly
- Thrombocytopenia
- Painful gynecomastia

- Surgical consultation and intervention is indicated if patient does not respond to medical or endoscopic treatment.
- Admit all unstable patients.

SMALL INTESTINE

PUD

DEFINITION

Disruption of the mucosal defensive factors by acid and pepsin, which causes ulceration of the mucosa beyond the muscularis

RISK FACTORS

- Infection with *H. pylori*
- Cigarette use
- Ethanol use
- NSAIDs (prostaglandin depletion)
- Steroids
- Hepatic cirrhosis
- Renal failure
- Familial predisposition to ulcers

CLINICAL FINDINGS

- Classically, the pain is described as burning, gnawing, dull, or hunger-like.
- Gastric ulcer pain begins shortly after eating.
- Duodenal ulcer pain occurs 2 to 3 hours after meal.
- Ulcers are most commonly located along the lesser curvature of the stomach or the first portion of duodenum.
- Simple bleeding (most common cause of upper GI bleed):
  - Most stop spontaneously.
  - Posterior ulcer erodes into the gastroduodenal artery.

DIAGNOSIS

- Most peptic ulcer disease is not definitively diagnosed in the emergency department, but rather treated empirically.
- Endoscopy is 95% accurate for diagnosis.

TREATMENT

- Treatment is primarily outpatient unless complications occur.
- Advise patient to avoid substances that exacerbate ulcers.
- Pain relief with antacids given 1 hour before and 3 hours after meal (poor compliance due to frequency of therapy)
- H_2 receptor antagonists (cimetidine, ranitidine, famotidine, or nizatidine) are mainstay of therapy.
- Proton pump inhibitors such as omeprazole and lansoprazole are used for ulcers refractory to H_2 blockers.
- Eradicate *H. pylori* disease.
- Patients who demonstrate any complication should be stabilized and admitted.

COMPLICATIONS OF PUD

Perforation

Signs and Symptoms
- Sudden onset of generalized abdominal pain associated with a rigid abdomen often radiating to back
- Vomiting involved in 50%

Diagnosis
- AXR and upright chest to look for free air: Useful for 70% of anterior perforations (most common type). Does not pick up posterior perforations because the posterior duodenum is retroperitoneal

Treatment
IV fluids, NG drainage, antibiotics, immediate surgery

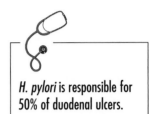

Severe sudden abdominal pain with history of ulcer: *Think: Perforation* (common board case). Patients usually lie still and avoid movement.

Gastric Outlet Obstruction

Pathophysiology
Healing ulcer may scar and block the antral or pyloric outlet.

H. pylori is responsible for 50% of duodenal ulcers.

Signs and Symptoms
- History of vomiting undigested food shortly after eating
- Succussion splash: Splashing sound made when abdomen is gently rocked
- Early satiety
- Weight loss

Diagnosis
- Characteristic electrolyte abnormalities (hypokalemia, hypochloremia, and metabolic alkalosis)
- AXR will show dilated stomach with large air–fluid level.

Treatment
- NG suctioning
- Correction of electrolyte abnormalities
- Hospital admission

Inflammatory Bowel Disease (IBD)

Definition
A chronic, inflammatory disease affecting GI tract. Two major types are Crohn's disease (CD) and ulcerative colitis (UC).

Epidemiology
- More common in people of Caucasian and Jewish background
- Peak incidence in ages 15 to 35
- Occurs with familial clustering
- Incidence: UC = 2 to 10/100,000; CD = 1 to 6/100,000
- UC more common in women
- CD more common in men
- Associated risk of colon cancer is 10 to 30 times for UC and 3 times for CD

Crohn's: Lower incidence, lower risk of cancer, more common in men

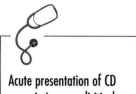

Acute presentation of CD can mimic appendicitis due to inflammation of the distal ileum.

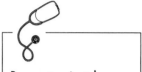

Recurrent perirectal abscesses may be the presenting complaint in a young person with undiagnosed CD.

Signs and Symptoms

UC	CD
Bloody diarrhea (more prominent than in CD)	■ Fever
Rectal pain	■ Malaise
	■ Weight loss
	■ Crampy abdominal pain
	■ Tender right lower quadrant (RLQ) mass

Extraintestinal Manifestations

Extraintestinal manifestations affect 20% of patients with IBD (see Table 9-1).

Pathology

UC	CD
Inflammation of the **mucosa only** (exudate of pus, blood, and mucus from the *"crypt abscess"*)	Inflammation involves **all bowel wall layers,** which may lead to fistulas and abscesses
Always **starts in rectum** (up to one third don't progress)	Rectal sparing in 50%

Diagnosis (Colonoscopy Findings)

UC	CD
Continuous lesions	**Skip lesions:** Interspersed normal and diseased bowel
Rare	**Aphthous ulcers**
Lead pipe colon appearance due to chronic scarring and subsequent retraction and loss of haustra	**Cobblestone** appearance from submucosal thickening interspersed with mucosal ulceration

Complications

UC	CD
Perforation	Abscess
Stricture	Fistulas
Megacolon	Obstruction
	Perianal disease

Treatment

Supportive Care

Antidiarrheals
■ Decrease frequency of stool
■ Loperamide and diphenoxylate are used for patients with fatty acid–induced diarrhea.
■ Cholestyramine is used for patients without fatty acid–induced diarrhea.
■ Contraindicated in severe colitis due to risk of toxic megacolon

Anticholinergics
■ Reduce abdominal cramping, pain, and urgency
■ Opium–belladonna combination works well to control diarrhea and pain.

Early institution of NG suction, IV fluids, and steroids to reduce inflammation in suspected bowel obstruction

HIGH-YIELD FACTS

Gastrointestinal Emergencies

TABLE 9-1. Extraintestinal Manifestations of Inflammatory Bowel Disease

Eye involvement	■ Uveitis	CD > UC
		Uveitis, erythema nodosum, and colitic arthritis are commonly seen together.
	■ Episcleritis	
Dermatologic	■ Erythema nodosum	CD > UC, especially in children Parallels disease course (gets better as IBD improves)
	■ Pyoderma gangrenosum	UC > CD May or may not follow disease course
	■ Aphthous ulcers	CD
Arthritis	■ Colitic arthritis	CD > UC Parallels disease course
	■ Ankylosing spondylitis	30 times more common in UC Unrelated to disease course
Hematologic	■ Anemia ■ Thromboembolism	
Hepatobiliary	■ Fatty liver ■ Hepatitis ■ Cholelithiasis ■ Primary sclerosing cholangitis	UC > CD
Renal	■ Secondary amyloidosis leading to renal failure	CD Unrelated to disease course

Specific Therapy

Sulfasalazine
- Consists of 5-acetylsalicylic acid (ASA) (active component) and sulfapyridine (toxic effects are due to this moiety)
- How it works in IBD is unknown (because other NSAIDs do not work), but its mechanisms of action include:
  - Altering action of microbial agents
  - Inhibition of leukocyte motility
  - Free radical scavenger
  - Inhibition of prostaglandin and leukotriene synthesis
- Side effects include GI distress in one third of patients (give enteric-coated preparation), decreased folic acid absorption, and male infertility (reversible).
- Drug appears safe in children and pregnant women.

> Sulfasalazine is also used to treat rheumatoid arthritis, but in this case, it is the sulfapyridine component that is the active one.

Corticosteroids
- Early phase of action blocks vascular permeability, vasodilation, and infiltration of neutrophils.
- Late phase of action blocks vascular proliferation, fibroblast activation, and collagen deposition.
- May be given as enemas (decreases systemic absorption)

> Drugs with only the 5-ASA component are not effective in IBD.

Antibiotics (used for CD)
- Three-week courses of metronidazole and ciprofloxacin have been used to induce disease remission with some success.

- Mechanism of action is unknown because other antibiotics with a similar antimicrobial spectrum have not been shown to be effective.

Immunomodulators
- Used in refractory cases, especially in CD
- Include azathioprine, 6-mercaptopurine, and methotrexate

Experimental Therapy
- Includes anti-tumor necrosis factor alpha (TNFα) antibodies, recombinant anti-TNF cytokines

Mesenteric Ischemia

DEFINITION

Lack of perfusion to bowel with high mortality rate usually due to delay of diagnosis

RISK FACTORS

- Age > 50
- Valvular or atherosclerotic heart disease
- Arrhythmias (especially atrial fibrillation)
- Congestive heart failure
- Recent myocardial infarction (MI)
- Critically ill patients with sepsis or hypotension
- Use of diuretics or vasoconstrictive drugs
- Hypercoagulable states

CLINICAL FINDINGS

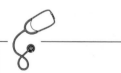

A diagnosis of mesenteric ischemia requires a high index of suspicion.

Gas in the bowel wall is known as *pneumatosis intestinalis.*

- Severe acute midabdominal **pain out of proportion to findings** (i.e., patient complains of severe pain but is not very tender on exam)
- Sudden onset suggests arterial vascular occlusion by emboli, consistent with acute ischemia.
- Insidious onset suggests venous thrombosis or nonocclusive infarction (intestinal angina), consistent with chronic ischemia.
- As infarct develops, peritoneal signs develop suggestive of dead bowel.

DIAGNOSIS

- AXR may reveal dilated loops of bowel, air–fluid level, irregular thickening of the bowel wall (thumbprinting), and gas in the bowel wall or portal system.
- Computed tomography (CT) scan may demonstrate air in the bowel wall, mesenteric portal vein gas, and bowel wall thickening.
- Angiography makes the definitive diagnosis and should not be delayed.

TREATMENT

- IV fluid to correct fluid and electrolyte abnormalities
- Supplemental O_2
- NG tube to decompress bowel
- Antibiotics to cover gut flora
- Selective vasodilator infusion (e.g., papaverine) during angiography
- Surgery to remove emboli or dead bowel

Hernias

Definitions

- Protrusion of a structure through an opening that is either congenital or acquired
- Reducible hernia: Protruding contents can be pushed back to their original location.
- Incarcerated hernia: An irreducible hernia may be acute and painful or chronic and asymptomatic.
- Strangulated hernia: Incarcerated hernia with vascular compromise

Risk Factors

- Obesity
- Chronic cough
- Pregnancy
- Constipation
- Straining on urination
- Ascites
- Previous hernia repair

Clinical Findings of Inguinal Hernias

Direct
- Protrudes through floor of Hesselbach's triangle
- Frequency increases with age.
- Rarely incarcerates

Indirect
- Protrudes lateral to the inferior epigastric vessels
- Most commonly occurring hernia
- Frequently incarcerates
- History of palpable, soft mass that increases with straining (patient bears down and coughs while you pass digit in external canal)
- Bowel sounds may be heard over hernia if it contains bowel.

Diagnosis

- Can be made from physical exam
- Abdominal radiograph to look for air–fluid levels (obstruction) or free air under the diaphragm (perforation)

Treatment

- May attempt reduction of incarcerated hernia with outpatient referral for surgery. Advise patient to refrain from straining.
- A strangulated hernia requires immediate surgery. Do not attempt to reduce dead bowel into abdomen!

Intussusception

Definition

The telescoping of one segment of bowel into another, the most common being the ileocecal segment

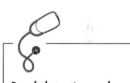

Incarcerated hernias are the second most common cause of small bowel obstruction (SBO) (after adhesions).

Bowel obstruction can be the first presenting sign of a hernia.

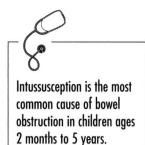

Intussusception is the most common cause of bowel obstruction in children ages 2 months to 5 years.

RISK FACTORS

Fifty percent have recent viral infection.

CLINICAL FINDINGS

- Classic triad:
  - Colicky abdominal pain
  - Vomiting
  - Currant jelly stool (late finding)
- Elongated mass may be palpable in right upper quadrant (RUQ).

DIAGNOSIS

Diagnosis by air or barium enema—"coiled spring" appearance of bowel

TREATMENT

Air or barium enema leads to reduction in 60 to 70%. Remaining cases require surgery.

SBO

Inspect for scars and hernias and ask about past surgical history (risk for adhesions).

ETIOLOGIES

- Adhesions (most common)
- Hernia (second most common)
- Neoplasms
- Intussusception
- Gallstones
- Bezoars
- IBD
- Abscess

CLINICAL FINDINGS

In proximal obstruction, bilious vomiting can occur early with minimal distention.

- Intermittent crampy abdominal pain
- Vomiting
- Abdominal distention
- Absence of bowel movements or flatulence for several days
- Hyperactive high-pitched bowel sounds **(borborygmi)** (become hypoactive and eventually absent as the obstruction progresses)

DIAGNOSIS

AXR may demonstrate stepladder appearance of air–fluid levels, thickening of small bowel wall, or loss of markings (haustra).

TREATMENT

- IV fluids, NG suction, and early surgical consult
- May consider antibiotics if infection present

LIVER

Hepatitis

DEFINITION

Inflammation of the liver secondary to a number of causes

ETIOLOGIES

- Alcohol:
  - Most common precursor to cirrhosis
  - May develop after several decades of alcohol abuse or within 1 year of heavy drinking
- Autoimmune: Little is known at this time.
- Toxins: Acetaminophen, carbon tetrachloride, heavy metals, tetracyclines, valproic acid, isoniazid, amiodarone, phenytoin, halothane, methyldopa
- Viruses:
  - Hepatitis A (HAV): Fecal–oral transmission via contaminated water or food, endemic areas; no carrier state; does not cause chronic liver disease
  - Hepatitis B (HBV): Sexual and parenteral transmission; has a carrier state and causes chronic disease; effective vaccine available
  - Hepatitis C (HCV): Sexual and parenteral transmission; has a carrier state and causes chronic disease; no vaccine available
  - Hepatitis D: Sexual and parenteral transmission; incomplete virus—requires coinfection with HBV
  - Hepatitis E (HEV): Similar to HAV but higher incidence of fulminant liver failure; no serologic marker
  - Cytomegalovirus
  - Herpes simplex virus
- Parasites:
  - *Entamoeba histolytica* abscess presents with RUQ pain, fever, and diarrhea.
  - *Clonorchis sinensis* (liver fluke)

CLINICAL FINDINGS

- RUQ tenderness (due to distention of liver capsule)
- Alcoholic:
  - Can range from mild liver disease to acute liver failure
  - May present with liver enlargement, weakness, anorexia, nausea, abdominal pain, and weight loss
  - Dark urine, jaundice, and fever are frequent complaints.
  - Physical exam may reveal jaundice, pedal edema, gynecomastia, palmar erythema, and spider angiomata.
  - Complications: Ascites, portal hypertension, esophageal varices, spontaneous bacterial peritonitis (SBP), hepatic abscess, hepatorenal syndrome, hepatic encephalopathy
- Viral:
  - Prodrome of anorexia, nausea, vomiting, malaise, and flulike symptoms
  - History of travel to endemic area for HAV and HEV
  - Serologic studies may be ordered in emergency department, but results are not immediately available.
- Parasites: History of travel to endemic area

DIAGNOSIS

- Thrombocytopenia
- Elevated bilirubin
- Serum glutamate pyruvate transaminase (SGPT) > serum glutamic-oxaloacetic transaminase (SGOT) suggestive of viral hepatitis
- PT usually normal

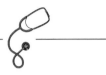

HBV and HCV are more contagious than human immunodeficiency virus (HIV). Always use universal precautions.

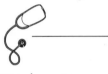

Concurrent HBV/HCV infection is common and exacerbates liver disease. Both carry increased risk of cirrhosis and hepatocellular carcinoma.

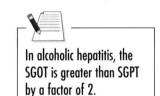

HCV is the most common cause of viral hepatitis in the United States.

In alcoholic hepatitis, the SGOT is greater than SGPT by a factor of 2.

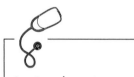

Admit hepatitis if:
- Encephalopathic
- Excessive bleeding
- INR > 3
- Intractable vomiting
- Immunosuppressed
- Due to alcohol
- Hypoglycemic
- Bilirubin > 25

TREATMENT

- Supportive care is the mainstay of therapy.
- Alcohol:
  - Hospital admission for all but the mildest cases
  - Correct electrolyte abnormalities.
  - Supplement thiamine and folate.
  - High-calorie/high-protein diet
- HBV: Interferon-alpha, ribavirin
- Acetaminophen poisoning: N-acetylcysteine (best if given within 24 hours of ingestion, but usually no hepatitis by then; can give up to 1 week after ingestion)
- Parasites:
  - Metronidazole/albendazole
  - Occasionally needle aspiration and decompression or surgical decontamination

Hepatic Encephalopathy

DEFINITION

A manifestation of hepatic failure, the final common pathway

TREATMENT

- Correction of fluids and electrolyte abnormalities
- Lactulose and neomycin to clear the gut of bacteria and nitrogen products
- Liver transplant may be lifesaving.

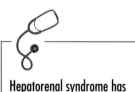

Reye's syndrome: Acute hepatic encephalopathy associated with ASA use in children

Hepatorenal Syndrome

DEFINITION

Acquired renal failure in association with liver failure; cause unknown

CLINICAL FINDINGS

- Hypotension
- Ascites:
  - Portal hypertension (high hydrostatic pressure)
  - Hypoalbuminemia (low oncotic pressure)

DIAGNOSIS

- Azotemia, oliguria, hyponatremia, low urinary sodium
- Sodium retention by kidneys from increase renin and angiotensin levels
- Impaired liver clearance of aldosterone (all hormones)

TREATMENT

- Low-salt diet
- Fluid restriction
- Diuretics (spironolactone and furosemide or hydrochlorothiazide)
- Paracentesis: Therapeutic in massive ascites with respiratory compromise; low risk of bleeding, infection, or bowel perforation

Hepatorenal syndrome has a bad prognosis. Mortality is almost 100%.

SBP

ETIOLOGY

- Bacterial breach of intestinal barrier to peritoneum
- *Escherichia coli*, pneumococci (anaerobes rare)

CLINICAL FINDINGS

- SBP should be suspected in cirrhotics with fever, abdominal pain, worsening ascites, and encephalopathy.
- Paracentesis:
  - Total white blood cell (WBC) count > 500 cells/mL
  - > 250 polymorphonuclear neutrophil/mL, very specific for SBP
  - Total protein > 1 g/dL
  - Glucose < 50 mg/dL
  - Cultures positive in 80 to 90%

TREATMENT

Hospital admission for IV antibiotics (third-generation cephalosporin)

Hepatic Abscess

ETIOLOGY

- Ascending cholangitis:
  - Most common cause of hepatic abscess
  - Frequent organisms include *E. coli, Proteus vulgaris, Enterobacter aerogenes*, and anaerobes.
- Parasites (e.g., *E. histolytica, Echinococcus*): Travel history
- Idiopathic

GALLBLADDER

Cholangitis

DEFINITION

Obstruction of the biliary tract and biliary stasis leading to bacterial overgrowth and infection

ETIOLOGY

- Common duct stone is the most common cause.
- 1° sclerosing cholangitis

CLINICAL FINDINGS

- **Charcot's triad:** RUQ pain, jaundice, fever/chills
- **Reynold's pentad:** Charcot's triad + shock and mental status change
- Labs: Elevated WBC, bilirubin (direct > indirect), and alkaline phosphatase ultrasound (95% sensitivity) reveals ductal dilatation and gallstones.

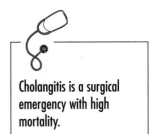

A high index of suspicion is necessary for diagnosis of SBP, as symptoms can be very mild.

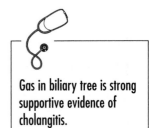

Cholangitis is a surgical emergency with high mortality.

Gas in biliary tree is strong supportive evidence of cholangitis.

TREATMENT

- ABCs
- IV hydration
- Correction of electrolytes
- Antibiotics
- Surgery consult
- Endoscopic retrograde cholangiopancreatography (ERCP) may be effective in decompression (high morbidity).

Cholelithiasis and Cholecystitis

DEFINITIONS

- Cholelithiasis is a stone in the gallbladder.
- Choledocholithiasis is a stone in the common bile duct.
- Biliary colic: Transient gallstone obstruction of cystic duct causing intermittent RUQ pain lasting a few hours after a meal. No established infection.
- Acute cholecystitis is the obstruction of the cystic duct with pain lasting longer, fever, chills, nausea, and positive Murphy's sign.

DIAGNOSIS

- Labs: Alkaline phosphatase, bilirubin, LFTs, electrolytes, blood urea nitrogen (BUN), creatinine, amylase, lipase, CBC
- Plain films may reveal radiopaque gallstones (10 to 15%).
- Ultrasound to look for: Presence of gallstones, thickened gallbladder wall, positive sonographic Murphy's sign, gallbladder distention, fluid collection:
  - Presence of gallstones, thickened gallbladder wall, and pericholecystic fluid has a positive predictive value of > 90%.
- Hepato-iminodiacetic acid *(the study of choice)*: For this test, technetium-99m–labeled iminodiacetic acid is injected IV and is taken up by hepatocytes. In normals, the gallbladder is outlined within 1 hour.

TREATMENT

- Uncomplicated biliary colic may go home.
- Acute cholecystitis should be admitted to the surgical service.
- Poor surgical candidates may receive oral bile salts to promote dissolution of the stones: Second-line therapy.

Risk factors for cholelithiasis: **8 Fs**
Female
Fat
Fertile
Forty
Fibrosis, cystic
Familial
Fasting
F-Hgb (sickle cell disease)
Also:
Diabetes
Oral contraceptives

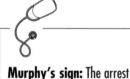

Murphy's sign: The arrest of inspiration while palpating the RUQ. This test is > 95% sensitive for acute cholecystitis, less sensitive in the elderly.
Sonographic Murphy's sign: The same symptom when the ultrasound probe is placed on the RUQ.

Gallstone composition:
- Cholesterol (70%): Radiolucent
- Pigment (20%): Radiodense
- Mixed (10%)

Acute Pancreatitis

DEFINITION

Inflammation and self-destruction of the pancreas by its digestive enzymes

RISK FACTORS

- Gallstones and alcohol account for 85% of all cases.
- Pancreatic tumor (obstructing common duct)
- Hyperlipidemia
- Hypercalcemia
- Trauma
- Iatrogenic (ERCP)
- Ischemia
- Drugs (thiazide, diuretics, steroids)
- Familial
- Viral (coxsackievirus, mumps)

CLINICAL FINDINGS

- Abrupt onset of deep epigastric pain with radiation to the back
- Positional preference—leaning forward
- Nausea, vomiting, anorexia, fever, tachycardia, and abdominal distention with diminished bowel sounds
- Jaundice with obstructive etiology

DIAGNOSIS

- Leukocytosis, elevated amylase and lipase (lipase more specific)
- AXR: Sentinel loop, colon cutoff (distended colon to midtransverse colon with no air distally)
- Ultrasound: Good for pseudocyst, abscess, and gallstones
- CT preferred diagnostic test

PROGNOSIS

Ranson's criteria: Mortality rates correlate with the number of criteria present. Presence of more than three criteria equals a 1% mortality rate, while the presence of six or more criteria approaches a 100% mortality rate:

- At presentation:
  - Age > 55
  - WBC > 16000
  - Glucose > 200
  - Lactic dehydrogenase > 350
  - SGOT > 250
- During initial 48 hours:
  - Hematocrit decrease > 10 points
  - BUN increase > 5
  - Serum Ca^{2+} < 8
  - Arterial PO_2 < 60
  - Base deficit > 4
  - Fluid sequestration > 6 L

Typical scenario:
A 45-year-old obese woman complains of fever, RUQ pain, and nausea that is worse when she eats. *Think: Cholecystitis.*

Hypercalcemia can cause pancreatitis, and pancreatitis can cause hypocalcemia.

A sentinel loop is distention and/or air–fluid levels near a site of abdominal distention. In pancreatitis, it is secondary to pancreatitis-associated ileus.

Typical scenario:
A 50-year-old male alcoholic presents with midepigastric pain radiating to the back. He is leaning forward on his stretcher and vomiting. *Think: Pancreatitis.*

Typical scenario:
A 66-year-old female with hypertension and seizures for which she is on furosemide and valproic acid presents with abdominal pain, back pain, and fever. Her nonfasting glucose is noted to be 300. *Think: Pancreatitis.*

TREATMENT

- Fluid resuscitation
- Electrolyte correction
- Prevention of vomiting with NG suction and antiemetics
- Analgesia
- Nothing by mouth (NPO) (pancreatic rest)

Pancreatic Pseudocyst

DEFINITION

- Encapsulated fluid collection with high enzyme content in a pseudocyst protruding from the pancreatic parenchyma
- Most common complication of pancreatitis (2 to 10%)

CLINICAL FINDINGS

- Symptoms of pancreatitis
- CT and ultrasonography (US) both have a sensitivity of 90%.

TREATMENT

- Surgical creation of fistula between cyst and stomach allowing for continuous decompression is most effective. Cyst eventually resolves without further intervention.
- Drain in 6 weeks when walls mature to reduce secondary infection, hemorrhage, or rupture.

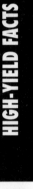

Suspect a pancreatic pseudocyst when patients with pancreatitis fail to resolve.

Pancreatic Abscess

DEFINITION

Extensive necrosis of fat and mesentery with inflamed pancreas

ETIOLOGY

Most commonly enteric organisms (50% polymicrobial)

CLINICAL FINDINGS

- Presents 1 to 4 weeks after acute pancreatitis
- Fever, abdominal pain, tenderness, distention, paralytic ileus, and leukocytosis
- CT is diagnostic study of choice.

TREATMENT

- Antibiotics
- Surgical debridement

Appendicitis is the most common surgical emergency.

Appendicitis

DEFINITION

Inflammation of the appendix

PATHOPHYSIOLOGY

- The inciting event is obstruction of the lumen of the appendix.
- This leads to an increase in intraluminal pressure with vascular compromise of the wall of the appendix.
- The environment is now ripe for bacterial invasion.

ETIOLOGY

- Fecalith (most common cause)
- Lymphoid hyperplasia
- Worms
- Granulomatous disease
- Inspissated barium
- Tumors
- Adhesions
- Dietary matter such as seeds

CLINICAL FINDINGS

- Usually begins as vague periumbilical pain, then migrates to the RLQ where it becomes more intense and localized (McBurney's point)
- Retrocecal appendicitis can present as right flank pain.
- Anorexia
- Nausea, vomiting
- Low-grade fever
- RLQ pain with rebound tenderness and guarding
- **Rovsing's sign:** Pain in RLQ when palpation pressure is exerted in left lower quadrant (LLQ)
- **Iliopsoas sign:** Pelvic pain upon flexion of the thigh while the patient is supine
- **Obturator sign:** Pelvic pain upon internal and external rotation of the thigh with the knee flexed

DIAGNOSIS

- Labs: Leukocytosis, hematuria, pyuria
- If the diagnosis is clear-cut, no imaging studies are necessary.
- AXR may demonstrate fecalith (5% of time) or loss of psoas shadow.
- US will show noncompressible appendix.
- CT scan with contrast may demonstrate periappendiceal streaking. CT is 90 to 95% sensitive for appendicitis.

TREATMENT

- NPO
- IV hydration
- Antibiotics
- Surgery

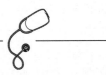

Appendicitis in late pregnancy presents with RUQ pain due to displacement of appendix by gravid uterus.

Appendicitis:
Do not delay the diagnosis. Mortality of perforation is about 3%.

Conditions that mimic appendicitis: **CODE APPY CD**
Ovarian cyst
Diverticulitis
Ectopic pregnancy

Adenitis of the mesentery
Pelvic inflammatory disease
Pyelonephritis
Yersinia gastroenteritis

LARGE INTESTINE

Large Bowel Obstruction

ETIOLOGIES

- Tumor (most common)

- Diverticulitis
- Volvulus (sigmoid and cecal)
- Fecal impaction (especially elderly and mentally retarded)

CLINICAL FINDINGS

- Intermittent crampy abdominal pain, vomiting, abdominal distention
- Absence of bowel movements or flatulence for several days

DIAGNOSIS

AXR may demonstrate stepladder appearance of air–fluid levels, thickening of bowel wall, or loss of colonic markings (haustra).

TREATMENT

- IV fluids, NG suction, and early surgical consult
- May consider antibiotics if infection present
- Sigmoidoscopy may be done to decompress bowel.

Ogilvie's Syndrome

DEFINITION

Colonic pseudo-obstruction due to marked cecal dilatation

RISK FACTORS

- Use/abuse of opiates, tricyclic antidepressants, anticholinergics
- Prolonged bed rest

DIAGNOSIS

AXR reveals cecal dilatation. A cecum diameter > 12 cm is a risk for perforation.

TREATMENT

- Decompression with enemas
- If unsuccessful, colonoscopic decompression

Diverticular Disease

DEFINITIONS

- Diverticula are saclike herniations of colonic mucosa (most common at sigmoid) occurring at weak points in the bowel wall (insertions of arteries) with increased luminal pressures.
- Diverticulosis is the presence of diverticula, most commonly associated with massive painless bleeding.
- Diverticulitis (diverticula + inflammation) is the most common complication of diverticulosis. Fecal material lodges in diverticula, leading to inflammation and ischemia and mucosa erosion.

EPIDEMIOLOGY

- Prevalent in 35 to 50% of general population
- Increased in the elderly and industrialized nations

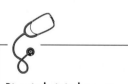

Due to its small radius, the cecum is normally the site of highest pressure in the GI tract.

Diverticulosis is the most common cause of painless lower GI bleeding in older patients.

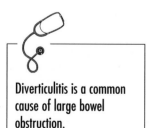

Diverticulitis is a common cause of large bowel obstruction.

ETIOLOGIES

- Low-fiber diet
- Chronic constipation
- Family history

CLINICAL FINDINGS

- Diverticulosis:
    - Rectal bleeding
    - Anemia
    - Hematochezia
- Diverticulitis:
    - Constant severe LLQ pain with guarding
    - Abdominal distention
    - Fever
    - Diarrhea
    - Anorexia
    - Nausea

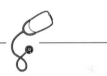

Typical scenario:
A 70-year-old male presents with LLQ pain, diarrhea, fever, and guaiac-positive stool. AXR shows an ileus. *Think: Diverticulitis.*

DIAGNOSIS

- AXR: Ileus, air–fluid levels, free air if perforation
- CT: Study of choice
- Colonoscopy and barium enema are relatively contraindicated in acute diverticulitis due to risk of perforation.

Barium enema and colonoscopy should be avoided in acute cases of diverticulitis due to risk of perforation.

TREATMENT

- ABCs
- Treat any hemodynamic compromise associated with massive GI bleeding.
- Diverticulosis: High-fiber diet and stool softeners to decrease luminal pressure and prevent constipation
- Diverticulitis: IV fluids, NPO, NG suction (for ileus), and broad-spectrum antibiotics. Admit with surgical consult if severe.

COMPLICATIONS

Abscesses, obstruction, fistula, stricture, and perforation

Lower GI bleed

DEFINITION

Bleeding distal to the ligament of Treitz (small intestine or colon)

ETIOLOGIES

- Diverticulosis (70%)
- Angiodysplasia
- Colon cancer
- Hemorrhoids
- Trauma
- IBD
- Ischemic colitis
- Inappropriate anticoagulation
- Irradiation injury

Angiodysplasia is the most common cause of lower GI bleeding in younger patients.

CLINICAL FINDINGS

- Hematochezia
- Abdominal pain
- Weakness
- Anorexia
- Melena
- Syncope
- Shortness of breath

DIAGNOSIS

- NG lavage to rule out upper source (if blood is not seen and bile is aspirated, an upper source is unlikely)
- CBC (note acute blood loss will not be reflected in hematocrit)
- Colonoscopy to localize and possibly limit bleeding
- If colonoscopy fails to reveal source, consider angiography or nuclear bleeding scan.

TREATMENT

- ABCs
- Treat any hemodynamic compromise associated with massive GI bleeding similar to upper GI bleeding (stabilize first).
- Anoscopy and sigmoidoscopy for evidence of anorectal disease
- Surgery if unstable or refractory to medical therapy

RECTUM/ANUS

Anal Fissure

DEFINITION

Linear tear of the anal squamous epithelium

ETIOLOGIES

- Most benign fissures occur in posterior or anterior line.
- Fissures in other location or multiple sites are associated with CD, infection, and malignancy.

CLINICAL FINDINGS

- Perianal pain during or after defecation with blood-streaked toilet paper
- Diagnosis made by visual inspection

TREATMENT

Sitz baths, stool softener, high-fiber diet, hygiene, and analgesics

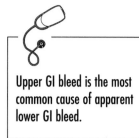

Upper GI bleed is the most common cause of apparent lower GI bleed.

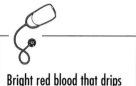

Bright red blood that drips into the toilet or streaks stool suggests anorectal source.

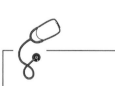

Anal fissures are the most common cause of anorectal pain (especially in children).

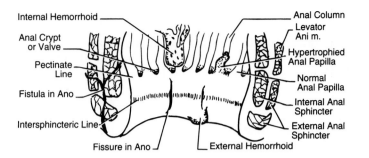

FIGURE 9-1. Anatomy of internal and external hemorrhoids.
(Reproduced, with permission, from DeGowin RL, Brown DD. *DeGowin's Diagnosis Examination*, 7th ed. New York: McGraw-Hill, 2000: 592.)

Hemorrhoids

DEFINITION

Dilated veins of the hemorrhoidal plexus (see Figure 9-1):
- Internal—arise above the dentate line and usually insensitive
- External—below the dentate line, well innervated, painful!

CLINICAL FINDINGS

External hemorrhoids present with painful thrombosis.

TREATMENT

If pain is severe, then excision of clot under local anesthesia followed by sitz baths and analgesics. Otherwise manage expectantly with hydrocortisone cream, local anesthetic ointment, and sitz baths.

Perirectal Abscess

DEFINITION

An abscess in any of the potential spaces near the anus or rectum (perianal, ischiorectal, submucosal, supralevator, and intersphincteric); begins with infection of the anal gland as it drains into the anal canal

CLINICAL FINDINGS

Extreme pain and mass on rectal exam

TREATMENT

- Superficial abscesses close to the skin may be excised and packed in the emergency department.
- Deep abscesses like the intersphincteric and supralevator may need to be excised in the operating room.

As with all abscesses, the treatment is drainage, and routine use of antibiotics is not warranted.

Perianal and Pilonidal Abscesses

ETIOLOGY

Ingrowing hair induces abscess formation.

CLINICAL FINDINGS

- Pain, swelling, redness, presence of fluctuant mass
- Perianal is the most common anorectal abscess (40 to 50%).
- Pilonidal abscesses occur in the midline upper edge of the buttock.

TREATMENT

Incision and drainage followed by later surgical excision

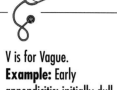

V is for Vague.
Example: Early appendicitis; initially dull, periumbilical pain

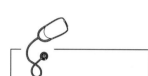

P is for Pinpoint.
Example: Late appendicitis; local inflammation leads to tenderness in the RLQ.

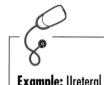

Example: Ureteral obstruction can produce pain in the ipsilateral testicle.

Typical scenario:
A 26-year-old woman complains of severe LLQ pain, vaginal bleeding, weakness, and light-headedness. Last menstrual period was 6 weeks ago. *Think: Ectopic pregnancy.*

ABDOMINAL PAIN: GENERAL PRINCIPLES

Abdominal Pain

VISCERAL PAIN

- Vague, dull, and poorly localized pain
- Midline location due to bilateral innervation of organs based on their embryological origin
- Associated with stretching, inflammation, or ischemia, involving bowel walls or organ capsules

PARIETAL PAIN

- Sharp, well-localized pain; peritonitis associated with rebound and involuntary guarding
- Pain location correlates with associated dermatomes:
  - Occurs commonly with inflammation, frank pus, blood, or bile in or adjacent to the peritoneum

Peritonitis is associated with rebound tenderness and involuntary guarding.

REFERRED PAIN

- Pain stimuli generated at an afflicted location are perceived as originating from a site in which there is no current pathology.
- These sites are usually related by a common embryological origin.
- The pain can sometimes be perceived in both locations.

CAUSES OF ABDOMINAL PAIN (BY QUADRANTS)

Right Upper Quadrant	Left Upper Quadrant
Gastric ulcer	*Gastric ulcer*
Peptic ulcer	*Gastritis*
Biliary disease	*Pancreatitis*
Hepatitis	*Splenic injury*
Pancreatitis	
Retrocecal appendicitis	
Renal stone	Renal stone
Pyelonephritis	Pyelonephritis
MI	MI
Pulmonary embolus	Pulmonary embolus
Pneumonia	Pneumonia

Right Lower Quadrant	Left Lower Quadrant
Appendicitis	*Diverticulitis*
Ovarian cyst	*Ovarian cyst*
Mittelschmerz	*Mittelschmerz*
Pregnancy (ectopic or normal)	*Pregnancy (ectopic or normal)*
Tubo-ovarian abscess	*Tubo-ovarian abscess*
Pelvic inflammatory disease	*Pelvic inflammatory disease*
Ovarian torsion	*Ovarian torsion*
Cystitis	Cystitis
Prostatitis	Prostatitis
Ureteral stone	Ureteral stone
Testicular torsion	Testicular torsion
Epididymitis	Epididymitis
Diverticulitis	Diverticulitis
Abdominal aortic aneurysm	Abdominal aortic aneurysm

Note: *All premenopausal women with abdominal pain must have a pregnancy test, even if they say they are not sexually active.*

OTHER CAUSES OF ABDOMINAL PAIN

Abdominal Wall
- Hernia
- Rectus sheath hematoma

Metabolic
- Diabetic ketoacidosis
- Acute intermittent porphyria
- Hypercalcemia

Infectious
- Herpes zoster
- Mononucleosis
- HIV

Drugs/Toxins
- Heavy metal poisoning
- Black widow spider envenomation

Other
- Sickle cell anemia
- Mesenteric ischemia

ABDOMINAL PAIN IN THE ELDERLY

Elderly patients who present with abdominal pain must be treated with particular caution. Common problems include:
- Difficulty communicating
- Comorbid disease
- Inability to tolerate intravascular volume loss
- Unusual presentation of common disease
- May not mount a WBC count or a fever
- Complaint often incommensurate with severity of disease

Note: Up to 2% of elderly patients with an MI will present with abdominal pain.

> **Typical scenario:**
> A 28-year-old woman presents with diffuse abdominal pain, nausea, and confusion. She is not pregnant. She currently takes a stained-glass class. *Think: Lead poisoning.*

> In elderly patients with abdominal pain, always consider vascular causes, including:
> - Abdominal aortic aneurysm
> - Mesenteric ischemia
> - MI

Renal and Genitourinary Emergencies

ACUTE RENAL FAILURE (ARF)

DEFINITIONS

Classified as prerenal, intrinsic, or postrenal

Prerenal ARF

ETIOLOGY

- Hypovolemia (blood loss, vomiting, diarrhea, burns)
- Decreased cardiac output
- Sepsis
- Third spacing
- Hypoalbuminemia
- Drugs (nonsteroidal anti-inflammatory drugs [NSAIDs], angiotensin-converting enzyme [ACE] inhibitors)
- Renal artery obstruction

DIAGNOSIS

- Urine sodium excretion is < 10 and fractional excretion of sodium (FeNa) is < 1%.
- $FeNa = \dfrac{(Urine\ Na) \times (Plasma\ creatinine) \times 100}{(Plasma\ Na) \times (Urine\ creatinine)}$

TREATMENT

- Volume replacement
- Diuretics for congestive heart failure (CHF)
- Positive inotropics (e.g., dobutamine) or afterload reduction (e.g., ACE inhibitors) for pump failure
- Mobilize third-space fluid.

Postrenal ARF

DEFINITION

Obstruction anywhere from renal parenchyma to urethra

> Oliguria is the production of < 500 mL of urine in 24 hours.

> Most cases of prerenal failure will need FLUID, FLUID, and more FLUID.

ETIOLOGY

- Nephrolithiasis
- BPH
- Neurogenic bladder
- Bladder neck obstruction
- Urethral strictures
- Substances causing renal tubular obstruction: Acyclovir, methotrexate, uric acid, oxalate, myeloma (Bence Jones) proteins

TREATMENT

- Foley catheter
- Percutaneous nephrostomy tubes for obstructing renal stones
- Urology consult
- Aggressive hydration may be necessary if tubular obstruction is suspected.

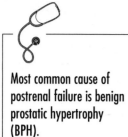

Most common cause of postrenal failure is benign prostatic hypertrophy (BPH).

Intrinsic ARF

DEFINITION

Insult to the kidney parenchyma from disease states, drugs, or toxins

ETIOLOGY

- Acute tubular necrosis:
  - Intravenous (IV) contrast
  - Acute ischemia
  - Myoglobinuria from rhabdomyolysis
  - Drugs (aminoglycoside antibiotics, ACE inhibitors, NSAIDs)
- Glomerulonephritis (GN):
  - Antecedent streptococcal (group A, beta-hemolytic)
  - Systemic lupus erythematosus
  - Wegener's granulomatosis
  - Polyarteritis nodosa
  - Goodpasture's
  - Henoch–Schönlein purpura
  - Drugs (gold, penicillamine)
  - Immunoglobulin A nephropathy (Berger's disease)
  - Idiopathic
- Acute interstitial nephritis

TREATMENT

- Treat underlying cause.
- Discontinue any offending agents.
- Increase urine output in oliguric patients with hydration and diuretics (mannitol, furosemide).
- Increase renal perfusion with dopamine if needed.
- Consider dialysis for severe cases.

An accurate history is imperative. Drugs, medical history, and family history are all important to help determine a cause of renal failure.

Typical scenario:
An 81-year-old woman is brought in by ambulance. She was found lying on the floor of her apartment after sustaining a fall 3 days ago. Her creatine kinase is 12,500. Her blood urea nitrogen/creatinine (BUN/Cr) is 100/45. *Think: Rhabdomyolysis.*

OVERVIEW

- Patients developing CRF are treated with diet and medications first and progress to use of intermittent dialysis and finally chronic dialysis.
- Uremia, electrolytes, anticoagulants, immunosuppression, vascular access, and cardiovascular stress with hemodialysis all contribute to potential problems.

EMERGENCIES

- Arrhythmias: Due to electrolyte imbalances and drug toxicities:
  - Hyperkalemia is the most common when dialysis appointments are missed.
  - Others include hypocalcemia, hypokalemia (during or immediately after dialysis), and hypermagnesemia.
- Hypertension: Due to increased intravascular volume:
  - Need dialysis but may temporize with IV nitroprusside, hydralazine, or labetalol
- Hypotension: Due to ultrafiltration during dialysis:
  - Give IV fluid and pressors as necessary.
- Neurological:
  - Lethargy, seizures, coma, headache, and confusion all may occur.
  - Electrolytes, hypoglycemia, and concurrent illness (e.g., sepsis) all may be contributing factors.
  - Must rule out intracranial bleed (especially if projectile vomiting or focal neurological exam) because of use of IV heparin during hemodialysis. Most common intracranial bleed here is subdural hematoma.
  - "Hemodialysis disequilibrium" occurs usually after the first hemodialysis treatment due to osmotic shifts; symptomatic treatment leads to complete recovery by the next day.
- Gastrointestinal (GI):
  - Upper GI bleeds from anticoagulation, uremic gastritis, and peptic ulcer disease are more common than in the general population.
  - Bowel obstruction may occur due to use of oral phosphate binders. Avoid Mg^{2+}-containing antacids and Fleet enemas (contain phosphate).
- Vascular:
  - External vascular access devices or internal shunts and grafts may become clotted or infected.
  - Strictures, aneurysms, vascular steal syndromes, or excessive bleeding may occur in the extremity where the graft is.
  - Take care to avoid blood draws, blood pressure measurements, or other procedures in that extremity.
- Genitourinary:
  - Uremia: Discussed below

EMERGENT HEMODIALYSIS

Indications
- Electrolyte abnormalities: Hyperkalemia is the most common and potentially the most dangerous even at moderate levels.

Typical scenario:
A 23-year-old man presents with hypertension and hematuria. He reports having a sore throat 2 weeks ago. His BUN/Cr is 34/2.0. *Think: Poststreptococcal GN.*

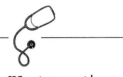

CRF patients are sick. Anything out of the ordinary in these patients should be investigated.

HIGH-YIELD FACTS

Renal and Genitourinary Emergencies

- Volume overload and its various manifestations—the patient may be oliguric; also may have uncontrollable hypertension
- Intractable acidosis; $HCO_3^- < 10$
- Severe uremia
- Dialysis may also be necessary to treat drug overdoses.

PERITONEAL DIALYSIS

Problems occur with the intraperitoneal catheter:
- It can become clogged or kinked, resulting in fluid overload and abdominal distention.
- Adhesions may form in the peritoneal space, decreasing fluid drainage.
- If aseptic technique is not followed, peritonitis may occur manifested by abdominal tenderness and GI symptoms:
  - If systemic symptoms are present, IV antibiotics are necessary. Otherwise, antibiotic infusion into the peritoneum suffices as treatment.

HEMATURIA

ETIOLOGY

- GN
- BPH
- Vascular:
  - Renal vessel thrombosis
  - Abdominal aortic aneurysm (AAA)
  - Arteriovenous malformation
- Urologic cancer:
  - Bladder cancer
  - Renal cell carcinoma
  - Rhabdomyosarcoma
- Urolithiasis/nephrolithiasis
- Acute GN
- Pseudohematuria:
  - Vegetable dyes (e.g., beets, rhubarb)
  - Phenolphthalein
  - Phenazopyridine
  - Porphyria
  - Contamination from menstrual blood
- Sickle cell disease
- Trauma
- Infection:
  - *Schistosoma haematobium*
  - Sexually transmitted disease (STDs)
  - Urinary tract infection (UTI)

CLINICAL FINDINGS

- Start with a urinalysis and go from there.
- Timing of hematuria:
  - At initiation of the stream suggests a urethral source.
  - At the end of the stream suggests prostate or bladder neck problems.
  - Continuous hematuria has a renal, bladder, or ureteral source.

- "Brown" or "Coca-Cola" urine has a renal source: Hematuria, GN, and myoglobinuria.

PROTEINURIA

DEFINITION

> 150 mg/24 hours in adult patients

CLINICAL FINDINGS

- Tubular source (impaired reabsorption) has > 2 g/day excretion (e.g., diabetic or hypertensive nephropathy).
- Glomerular source (diffusion across glomerular membrane) may have up to 10 g/day excretion (e.g., nephrosis).
- These criteria apply if proteinuria is isolated. A nephritic picture will have proteinuria but other urinalysis findings as well (e.g., casts).

NEPHROLITHIASIS

EPIDEMIOLOGY

- 2 to 5% incidence
- Peak incidence in midlife

PATHOPHYSIOLOGY

- ~90% of stones are radiopaque.
- Stone composition:
  - Caoxalate: 75%, radiopaque
  - Struvite: 15%, radiopaque
  - Urate: 10%, radiolucent
  - Cystine: 1%, radiopaque
- Stones partially obstruct at five different places where the most pain occurs:
  - Renal calyx
  - Ureteropelvic junction
  - Pelvic brim
  - Ureterovesicular junction (tightest space)
  - Vesicular orifice
- Stone passage:
  - Rarely fully obstruct the ureter due to their shapes
  - < 5-mm stones—almost always pass freely
  - 5- to 8-mm stones—15% will pass freely
  - > 8-mm stones—only 5% will pass freely

RISK FACTORS

- Medications (hydrochlorothiazide, acetazolamide, allopurinol, antacids, excess vitamins)
- Male gender
- Dehydration

- Hot climate
- Family history
- Inflammatory bowel disease
- Gout
- Hyperparathyroidism
- Immobilization
- Sarcoidosis
- Malignancy

CLINICAL FINDINGS

- Pain:
  - Flank, abdominal, or back pain, with radiation to groin
  - Patients are very restless and cannot sit (opposite of patients with peritonitis who tend to lie perfectly still).
  - Waxes and wanes
- Possibly: Nausea, vomiting, ileus, hematuria (micro- or macroscopic), low-grade fever, urinary urgency/frequency

DIAGNOSIS

- Intravenous pyelogram (IVP) is considered the gold standard, but it requires contrast dye, which can be nephrotoxic.
- Ultrasound and computed tomographic (CT) scan are being used more and more since contrast is not necessary for either when ruling out stones—useful when renal failure may be an issue.
- In most emergency departments (EDs), noncontrast abdominal CT is the first-line test.
- KUB (kidney, ureter, and bladder) may be able to detect a stone, but it is not helpful to determine pyelonephritis or hydronephrosis. It may be a good screening tool if other abdominal pathology cannot be ruled out.
- Testing is necessary in first-time presentations and in the elderly.

TREATMENT

- Analgesia
- Hydration
- Nephrostomy tubes may be necessary to relieve severe hydronephrosis.
- Extracorporeal shockwave lithotripsy, cystoscopy, and ureteroscopy may be necessary to mobilize obstructing stones.
- Admit for:
  - Obstructing stone
  - Infected stone
  - Intractable pain
  - Patient with single kidney

Typical scenario:
A 34-year-old man presents with left flank pain radiating to his left testicle. The pain does not change with movement or position and is colicky in nature. Urine dip is positive for blood. *Think: Renal colic.*

It is unusual to see first-time presentation of kidney stone in the elderly. Even when the story seems classic, investigate symptoms in the elderly carefully. The most commonly missed diagnosis is AAA.

NEPHROTIC SYNDROME

DEFINITION

Protein-losing nephropathy with protein loss > 3.5 g/day

ETIOLOGIES

- Membranous nephropathy most common cause in adults
- Minimal change disease most common cause in children

Typical scenario:
An 8-year-old boy presents with facial edema. Urine dipstick reveals large protein. *Think: Nephrotic syndrome.*

CLINICAL FINDINGS

- Peripheral edema
- Ascites
- Anasarca
- Hypertension

DIAGNOSIS

- Urinalysis shows oval fat bodies (tubular epithelial casts with cholesterol)
- Hypoalbuminemia
- Hypercholesterolemia
- Chest x-ray may demonstrate pleural effusion.

TREATMENT

- Steroids
- Bedrest
- Other immunosuppressive agents possible for refractory cases

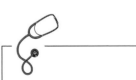

Patients can develop a hypercoagulable state due to nephrotic loss of antithrombin III.

TESTICULAR TORSION

DEFINITION

Twisting of a testicle on its root

EPIDEMIOLOGY

Most common in infants under age 1 and in young adults

CLINICAL FINDINGS

- Usually occurs during strenuous activity (e.g., athletic event), but sometimes occurs during sleep
- Pain may be in the lower abdomen, inguinal canal, or testicle. No change in pain with position
- Twisting is usually in a horizontal direction.
- Physical exam alone is not sufficient to exclude the diagnosis.

DIAGNOSIS

Doppler ultrasound to look for flow to testicle: No flow is highly suggestive of torsion.

TREATMENT

- Immediate urology consult
- Attempt manual correction of the torsion—untwist from medial to lateral (i.e., patient's right testicle gets rotated counterclockwise and the left clockwise).
- If Doppler ultrasound is equivocal and manual detorsion does not work, immediate exploratory surgery is necessary to prevent death of the testicle.
- Time is testicle! (The longer the delay to definitive treatment, the lower the chance of salvaging the testicle.)

Typical scenario:
A 19-year-old man presents with severe pain to the right testicle, which occurred suddenly while he was playing baseball. Physical exam reveals a tender, swollen, firm testicle with a transverse lie. There is no cremasteric reflex on that side. *Think: Testicular torsion.*

Manual detorsion is like "opening the book." Imagine a book standing on its spine and the front and back covers are the right and left testes, respectively. "Open" the front cover to untwist the right and likewise for the left.

TORSION OF APPENDIX TESTIS OR APPENDIX EPIDIDYMIS

DEFINITION

Both the testis and epididymis have a small appendix that can become twisted.

CLINICAL FINDINGS

"Blue dot" sign: Palpation of a tender nodule on transillumination of the testes

TREATMENT

- Get an ultrasound/Doppler to look for blood flow to testes (need to rule out testicular torsion).
- If normal, then appendix testis can be allowed to degenerate.
- Analgesia as needed

ORCHITIS

DEFINITION

Inflammation of the testicles

ETIOLOGIES

- Mumps
- Syphilis

CLINICAL FINDINGS

- Presents with history of bilateral testicular pain
- Usually will remit after a few days

TREATMENT

- Treat symptomatically (pain management).
- Disease-specific treatment (e.g., antibiotics for syphilis)

HYDROCELE

DEFINITION

Fluid accumulation in a persistent tunica vaginalis due to obstruction, which impedes lymphatic drainage of the testicles

ETIOLOGY

- Trauma
- Neoplasia
- Congenital
- Infection: Elephantiasis
- CHF

CLINICAL FINDINGS

- May cause much discomfort and pain when distended
- Other scrotal masses must be ruled out (e.g., torsion).
- Transilluminates on physical exam

TREATMENT

- Surgical follow-up for drainage
- Reassurance is usually necessary.

VARICOCELE

DEFINITION

Varicose vein in scrotal sac

ETIOLOGY

Caused by venous congestion in the spermatic cord

CLINICAL FINDINGS

- Palpating "a bag of worms" in the testis
- Accentuated by Valsalva maneuver and supine position
- Usually asymptomatic, but persistence has been implicated in sterility.

TREATMENT

May be surgically excised to improve spermatogenesis (elective procedure)

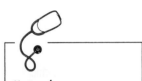

Varicocele:
Not a life- or limb- (testis) threatening emergency

EPIDIDYMITIS

DEFINITION

Inflammation of the epididymis

ETIOLOGY

- Bacterial infection
- Congenital abnormalities with reflux
- STDs with urethral stricture

CLINICAL FINDINGS

- Gradual onset of lower abdominal or testicular pain
- Dysuria
- There may be isolated firmness or nodularity on the testis.
- May spread to epididymo-orchitis

TREATMENT

- Antibiotics for infection
- Bed rest
- Scrotal elevation (scrotal support when ambulating)

Typical scenario:
A 27-year-old man presents with lower left abdominal pain and left testicular pain for 2 weeks. Palpation of the testes is normal except for isolated tenderness of the epididymis. Cremasteric reflex is normal. *Think: Epididymitis.*

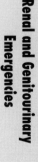

HIGH-YIELD FACTS

Renal and Genitourinary Emergencies

- Cold compress
- NSAIDs
- Stool softener

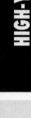

Typical scenario:
A 40-year-old diabetic man presents with severe perineal pain and fever of 103°F. Physical exam demonstrates crepitus over the medial thigh and widespread discoloration of the skin. *Think: Fournier's gangrene.*

The hallmark of Fournier's gangrene is pain of genital area out of proportion to physical exam.

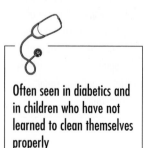

Typical scenario:
A 41-year-old man presents stating he heard his penis "crack" while having intercourse. Physical exam reveals an edematous, purplish penis. *Think: Penile fracture.*

Often seen in diabetics and in children who have not learned to clean themselves properly

FOURNIER'S GANGRENE

DEFINITION

Rapidly progressive gangrene of groin

ETIOLOGY

- Usually polymicrobial origin from skin, rectum, or urethra
- Subcutaneous spread becomes virulent and causes end-artery thrombosis and extensive necrosis in scrotal, medial thigh, and lower abdominal areas.

EPIDEMIOLOGY

Especially prevalent in diabetic and other immunocompromised patients

TREATMENT

- Broad-spectrum IV antibiotics
- Surgical debridement
- Hyperbaric oxygen therapy shown to be of benefit

FRACTURE OF PENIS

CLINICAL FINDINGS

- "Snapping sound" during sexual intercourse due to tearing of the tunica albuginea
- Penis is tender, swollen, and discolored.
- Urethra is usually spared.

TREATMENT

Surgery necessary to evacuate hematoma and to repair the tunica

BALANOPOSTHITIS

DEFINITION

Inflammation of the glans penis and foreskin:
- Balanitis = inflammation of glans
- Posthitis = inflammation of foreskin

ETIOLOGY

- Allergy to latex condoms
- Diabetes mellitus

- Infection—most commonly with *Candida albicans*
- Drugs—sulfonamides, tetracyclines, phenobarbital

CLINICAL FINDINGS

Areas are purulent, excoriated, malodorous, and tender.

TREATMENT

- Preventative therapy with adequate cleaning and drying
- Topical therapy useful
- Consider circumcision, especially if recurrent.
- Look for phimosis/paraphimosis.

PEYRONIE'S DISEASE

DEFINITION

Gradual or sudden dorsal curvature of the penis

ETIOLOGY

- Due to thickened plaque on tunica—may be associated with Dupuytren contractures in the hand
- May be painful and preclude sexual intercourse

TREATMENT

Spares urethra and not emergent; reassurance and referral

PHIMOSIS

DEFINITION

Inability to retract foreskin over glans

ETIOLOGY

May be from infection, poor hygiene, old injury with scarring

CLINICAL FINDINGS

May cause urinary retention secondary to pain or obstruction of urethra

TREATMENT

Patient will need circumcision or dorsal slit to foreskin.

Do not force retraction of foreskin. May lead to paraphimosis.

PARAPHIMOSIS

DEFINITION

Inability to reduce proximal foreskin—"stuck" behind glans

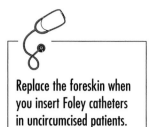

Replace the foreskin when you insert Foley catheters in uncircumcised patients.

PATHOPHYSIOLOGY

Leads to decreased arterial flow and eventual gangrene

TREATMENT

Attempt manual reduction or emergent circumcision.

PRIAPISM

DEFINITION

Pathologic erection

ETIOLOGY

- Sickle cell disease: Sickling in corpus cavernosum
- Drugs (e.g., prostaglandin E, papaverine, phentolamine, sildenafil, phenothiazines, trazodone)
- Leukemic infiltrate
- Idiopathic
- Spinal cord injury

CLINICAL FINDINGS

- Corpus cavernosum with stagnant blood—spongiosum and glans are usually soft

TREATMENT

- Intramuscular (IM) terbutaline (smooth muscle relaxer)
- Aspiration of blood from cavernosum
- Hydration, exchange transfusion, and hyperbaric oxygen for sickle cell disease

COMPLICATIONS

Urinary retention, infection, and impotence

BPH

DEFINITION

The prostate undergoes two growth spurts during life, the second of which begins at around 40 years. This second spurt focuses around the urethra and later in life may cause urinary obstruction.

CLINICAL FINDINGS

- Decreased urinary stream
- Hesitancy
- Dribbling
- Incomplete emptying of bladder
- Nocturia

- Overflow incontinence
- Chronic urinary retention
- Obstruction
- Enlarged prostate on rectal exam

ETIOLOGY

- Infection, drugs (e.g., alpha agonists), and alcohol may exacerbate symptoms to the point where patients are seen in the ED.

DIAGNOSIS

- Urinalysis to look for infection
- BUN/Cr to look for postrenal failure
- Prostate-specific antigen to monitor for prostate cancer (usually not done in the ED)
- Foley to check post voiding residual volume
- Sonogram to measure prostate size and look for hydronephrosis
- Urodynamic studies to determine effect of BPH on urinary flow (outpatient)
- Other outpatient studies such as cystoscopy and IVP are helpful for planning surgical procedures.

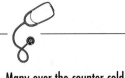

Many over-the-counter cold medications contain pseudoephedrine, which can cause complete obstruction.

TREATMENT

- Avoid things that exacerbate symptoms (e.g., caffeine).
- Leuprolide or finasteride to decrease testosterone levels (factor in growth), which result in decrease of prostate size
- Alpha blockers to decrease internal sphincter tone (doxazosin, terazosin, tamsulosin, prazosin)
- Transurethral resection of the prostate for definitive treatment

PROSTATITIS

DEFINITION

Inflammation of the prostate

ETIOLOGY

- UTI and STD pathogens

CLINICAL FINDINGS

- May present with chills, back pain, perineal pain
- Recurrent UTIs despite treatment
- Rectal exam will reveal a firm, warm, swollen, tender prostate.
- If exudate is expressed via the urethra, send it for culture.

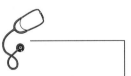

Do not massage the prostate on rectal exam if prostatitis is suspected due to increased risk of bacteremia.

TREATMENT

- Requires 1 month of total antibiotic therapy because of typically poor penetration into the prostate
- Acute prostatitis is susceptible to antibiotic treatment with usual UTI antibiotics since inflammation renders the prostate more penetrable.
- Chronically infected prostate without acute inflammation is a relatively

"protected" area. Choose your antibiotics wisely—fluoroquinolones have good penetration.

INGUINAL HERNIA

CLINICAL FINDINGS

- Presents as a palpable mass in the inguinal canal or as a scrotal mass
- The mass is usually reducible (either spontaneously or manually).
- Emergent situations occur when signs and symptoms of intestinal obstruction or severe pain or inability to reduce the mass lead to the diagnosis of incarcerated hernia.

TREATMENT

- Firmer manual reduction may be attempted in the ED, but if irreducible, surgical intervention is necessary.
- Reducible hernias should be referred for eventual repair to avoid incarceration.

Inguinal hernia is a common cause of scrotal or inguinal mass. Listen for bowel sounds over the mass. Transilluminate to rule out hydrocele. When you're convinced, try to reduce.

Typical scenario:
A 25-year-old man presents with right-sided groin pain that occurred after he attempted to lift a refrigerator. On physical exam, there is a bulge in the inguinal canal. Bowel sounds can be heard over the canal. *Think: Inguinal hernia.*

URETHRAL STRICTURE

DEFINITION

Fibrotic narrowing of urethral lumen

ETIOLOGY

- Often due to STDs (urethral inflammation → fibrosis)
- Urethral instrumentation

CLINICAL FINDINGS

- Urinary retention, difficulty voiding
- Difficulty placing Foley or coudé catheter

TREATMENT

Catheterization or expansion of urethra with filiform rods

Urethral stricture:
Differential includes voluntary tightening, bladder neck contraction, and BPH.

URINARY RETENTION

DEFINITION

Inability to void completely

ETIOLOGY

- BPH
- Drugs (anticholinergics, antihistamines, antispasmodics, alpha-adrenergic agonists, antipsychotics, tricyclic antidepressants)

204

- Mechanical: Stenosis of urethral meatus, bladder neck contracture, urethral stricture
- Cancer (bladder and prostate)
- Neurogenic bladder

CLINICAL FINDINGS

- Inability to void for > 7 hours
- Hesitancy
- Decreased urinary stream
- Lower abdominal pain
- Distended bladder

DIAGNOSIS

- Urinalysis to look for infection
- BUN/Cr to evaluate renal function

TREATMENT

- Catheterization is both diagnostic and therapeutic. Patients can be discharged after observation for a few hours with outpatient urology referral.
- Antibiotics for concurrent UTI

COMPLICATIONS

- Patients with chronic urinary retention can develop post obstructive diuresis when retention is relieved by Foley.
- Post obstructive diuresis is characterized by massive urine output, which can lead to hypotension due to hypovolemia and electrolyte imbalances.

UTI

DEFINITION

- Infection anywhere from kidney parenchyma (pyelonephritis) to urethral orifice (urethritis)

ETIOLOGY

- UTIs in men often due to anatomical defect
- Usual culprits are gram-negative aerobes (e.g., *E. coli*) but spectrum varies: *Staphylococcus saprophyticus*, *Proteus* (alkaline urine), *Klebsiella*, *Enterobacter*

EPIDEMIOLOGY

- Women: 10 to 20% lifetime incidence
- Men: 1 to 10% lifetime incidence
- Institutionalized patients: 50% incidence

CLINICAL FINDINGS

- Presentation varies with sites of involvement.
- Pyuria
- Bacteriuria
- Dipstick may be positive for leukocyte esterase and nitrites.

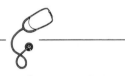

Consider nosocomial infections with *Pseudomonas* and methicillin-resistant *Staphylococcus aureus* in institutionalized or recently hospitalized patients.

- Microscopic or gross hematuria
- Urine culture and sensitivity
- White blood cells (WBC) in urinary sediment (> 5 to 10 WBC/hpf)

DIAGNOSIS

- Imaging studies (IVP, ultrasound, CT scan, retrograde urogram) necessary for:
  - All children under 5 (rule out pyelonephritis)
  - All male children (rule out anatomic defect)
  - Recurrent UTIs in women
  - Fever for more than 3 days with treatment
  - Recurrent pyelonephritis
- In severely ill patients: Must rule out things such as perinephric abscess and pyoureter

TREATMENT

- Trimethoprim–sulfamethoxazole, fluoroquinolones, and aminopenicillins have all been used and are effective; may need culture to streamline treatment.
- Patients with chronic Foley catheters can have asymptomatic bacteruria and need not be treated; if symptomatic, change catheter and treat (probably need admission for IV antibiotics; also beware of fungal infection in these patients if unresponsive to therapy).
- Stable pyelonephritis (no signs and symptoms of sepsis) may be treated as an outpatient with close follow-up.
- In pregnant patients, all bacteriuria must be treated and all pyelonephritis must be admitted for IV antibiotics; higher risk of miscarriage with UTI.

STDs

Gonorrhea

ETIOLOGY

Neisseria gonorrhoeae

SIGNS AND SYMPTOMS

- Purulent discharge
- Dysuria, epididymitis, inguinal lymphadenitis, proctitis (in homosexuals)
- Oral or pharyngeal lesions may be present if acquired through oral sex.
- Systemic infection may present as fever, rash, or monoarticular arthritis (usually the knee).

TREATMENT

- Ceftriaxone 125 mg single IM injection

or

- Cefixime 400 mg orally once

or

- Ciprofloxacin 500 mg orally once

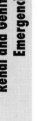

Due to a high rate (~60%) of concurrent chlamydia infection, treatment for chlamydia should always be included with that for gonorrhea.

- Ofloxacin 400 mg orally once
- Azithromycin 2 g orally once

Chlamydia

ETIOLOGY

Specific serotypes of *Chlamydia trachomatis*

SIGNS AND SYMPTOMS

- Dyspareunia
- Pelvic pain
- Yellow mucopurulent discharge
- Friable, erythematous cervix
- Tender epididymis if causing epididymitis

TREATMENT

- Azithromycin 1 g orally once

or

- Doxycycline 100 mg orally twice a day for 7 days

or

- Ofloxacin 300 mg orally twice a day for 7 days

or

- Erythromycin 500 mg orally four times a day for 7 days

Lymphogranuloma Venereum (LGV)

ETIOLOGY

Specific serotypes of *Chlamydia trachomatis* (different from the ones that cause chlamydia)

SIGNS AND SYMPTOMS

- Initial small painless papule that quickly disappears
- Inguinal lymphadenopathy appears 2 to 6 weeks later, which may suppurate through the skin—these remain painless.
- Extensive scarring and strictures may result.

TREATMENT

3 weeks of doxycycline or erythromycin

Chancroid

ETIOLOGY

Haemophilus ducreyi

SIGNS AND SYMPTOMS

- Painful inguinal adenopathy
- Tender, shallow ulcers with irregular reddish borders
- Inguinal mass/abscess from coalesced nodes (bubo)

Due to a high rate (~60%) of concurrent gonorrhea infection, treatment for gonorrhea should always be included with that for chlamydia.

PainFUL ulcers:
- Chancroid
- Herpes

PainLESS ulcers:
- LGV
- Syphilis

Urethral discharge:
- *Gonococcus*
- *Chlamydia*
- *Trichomonas*

- Azithromycin 1 g orally once

or

- Ceftriaxone 250 mg IM once

or

- Erythromycin 500 mg orally four times a day for 7 days

or

- Ciprofloxacin 750 mg orally once

Syphilis

ETIOLOGY

Treponema pallidum

1° Stage

- Painless ulcer (chancre), which is highly ineffective; ulcers heal spontaneously 3 to 6 weeks after primary infection.

2° Stage

- Fever, sore throat, rash (trunk with spread to palms and soles), malaise, warts (condylomata lata), aseptic meningitis, lymphadenopathy; also spontaneously resolves

3° Stage

- May occur after many years of latency
- Various manifestations in multiple systems:
  - *Argyll Robertson pupil* (small pupil that reacts to accommodation but not light)
  - *Tabes dorsalis* (posterior column disease presenting with loss of position, deep pain and temperature sensation, ataxia, decreased or absent deep tendon reflexes, wide-based gait, urinary retention or incontinence, impotence, and sharp leg pain)
  - *Gumma* (granulomatous, necrotic lesions on the skin and submucosa involving the palate, nasal septum, or other organ)
  - Thoracic aortic aneurysm/dissection (due to spirochetes in aortic vasa vasorum)

TREATMENT

For 1° and 2°
- Benzathine penicillin G 2.4 million units IM once
- If penicillin-allergic, consider desensitization or doxycycline or tetracycline orally for 2 weeks.

For Neurosyphilis
- Aqueous penicillin G 2.4 million units every 4 hours for 10 to 14 days

or

- Ceftriaxone 1 g IV/IM daily for 14 days

Human Papillomavirus (HPV)

ETIOLOGY

HPV

SIGNS AND SYMPTOMS

- Genital and anal warts causing discomfort but not pain
- Condylomata acuminata when warts coalesce

TREATMENT

- Cryotherapy
- Electrocautery
- 1% topical podophyllin solution (contraindicated in pregnancy)

Trichomoniasis

ETIOLOGY

Trichomonas vaginalis

SIGNS AND SYMPTOMS

- Copious, foamy, yellow-green, malodorous discharge with pH > 5.5
- Punctate red spots on cervix or vaginal wall ("strawberry cervix")
- Labial irritation or swelling
- Dyspareunia
- Dysuria
- Men may be asymptomatic.

TREATMENT

- Single-dose metronidazole (2 g) or 500 mg twice a day for 1 week. Abstain from alcohol while on drug.
- Clotrimazole for first-trimester pregnancy.

Herpes

ETIOLOGY

Herpes simplex virus

SIGNS AND SYMPTOMS

- Painful pustular or ulcerative lesions
- Initial infection more severe than recurrences
- May have systemic effects (fever, headache, myalgias), left axis deviation, aseptic meningitis
- Also a causative agent in encephalitis and esophagitis

TREATMENT

- Acyclovir (orally or IV depending if hospitalization is required or not)
- Acyclovir or valacyclovir can be chronically used for suppressive therapy—beware of superinfection.

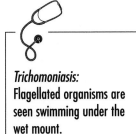

Trichomoniasis: Flagellated organisms are seen swimming under the wet mount.

"Whiff test": Two drops of KOH mixed with the discharge and heated onto a slide produces a fishy smell. This is characteristic of both *Trichomonas* and bacterial vaginosis.

HIGH-YIELD FACTS

Renal and Genitourinary Emergencies

EPIDEMIOLOGY

- An estimated 6% of crimes are rapes.
- Approximately one in eight women have been raped, with only 25% of cases reported.
- Two to 4% of rapes are committed against males.

CLINICAL FINDINGS

- The interviewer must determine from the patient the identity and number of persons involved, details on what happened (what kind of assault), areas of pain, how long ago it happened, what happened after the incident, last menstrual period, oral contraceptive use, last consensual intercourse, and allergies.
- Other signs of physical abuse:
  - Facial and extremity injuries are more common than actual injuries to the genitalia.
  - When males are sodomized, they may have thorax and abdomen abrasions because of the position they are in; also anal fissures and lacerations may be seen.
  - Decreased sphincter tone or severe hemorrhoids may indicate chronic sodomy.
- When examining a rape victim, most EDs use a standardized kit provided by the police:
  - All physical injuries (all lacerations and bruises) are documented.
  - A pelvic exam is done, and all mucosal surfaces (oral, vaginal, and anal) are sampled.
  - Testing for STDs is done.
  - Skin and fingernail scrapings are collected.
  - Semen can be sampled if found with the use of a Wood's lamp (fluoresces).

The most important aspect of dealing with sexual assault victims is to ensure their psychological well-being. This very traumatic experience could potentially be made worse by the victim's being surrounded and "interrogated" by hospital and police personnel, so every effort should be made to make the patient as comfortable as possible.

TREATMENT

- Addressing all physical injuries (admission if necessary)
- Tetanus prophylaxis
- STD and pregnancy testing (offer prophylaxis)
- Hepatitis B prophylaxis
- Human immunodeficiency virus counseling (offer prophylaxis)
- Most physicians will empirically treat for gonorrhea and chlamydia.
- Medical and psychiatric follow-up should be arranged within 2 weeks.

Hematologic and Oncologic Emergencies

COAGULATION CASCADE

Common pathway factors: I, II, V, X (see Figure 11-1)

Heparin

- Increases activated partial thromboplastin time (aPTT)
- Affects intrinsic pathway
- Decreases fibrinogen levels
- Primarily affects factors **VIII,** IX, X, XI, XII
- Low-molecular-weight heparins have 10 times activity against factor Xa.
- Safe in pregnancy
- Adverse effects include bleeding, thrombocytopenia, and osteoporosis.

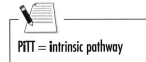

PiTT = intrinsic pathway

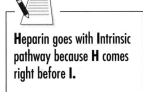

Heparin goes with Intrinsic pathway because **H** comes right before **I.**

Warfarin

- Increases prothrombin time (PT)
- Affects extrinsic pathway
- Decreased vitamin K
- Primarily affects II, V, **VII**
- Teratogenic
- Has an initial *procoagulant* effect, taking 48 to 72 hours to become anticoagulant. Concurrent coverage with heparin during this time is needed, and oral warfarin dose is titrated slowly.

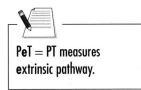

PeT = PT measures extrinsic pathway.

aPTT

- Tests extrinsic and common pathways
- Isolated elevation of aPTT (with normal PT) seen in:
  - Heparin therapy
  - Deficiencies of factors VIII (hemophilia A), factor IX (hemophilia B), factor XI, and factor XII (asymptomatic)

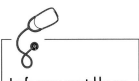

Leafy green vegetables are relatively contraindicated in patients on warfarin therapy due to their high vitamin K content.

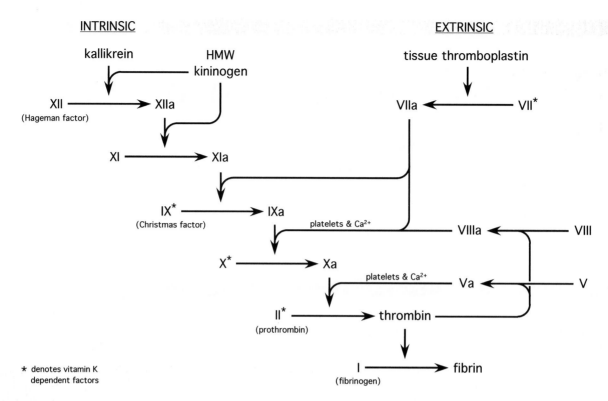

FIGURE 11-1. Common pathway factors.

PT

- Tests intrinsic and common pathways
- Isolated elevation of PT (with normal PTT) seen in:
  - Vitamin K deficiency
  - Warfarin therapy
  - Liver disease (decreased factor production)
  - Congenital (rare)

Thrombin Time

- Measures the time it takes to convert fibrinogen into a fibrin clot
- Elevated in:
  - Diffuse intravascular coagulation (DIC) (consumes fibrinogen)
  - Liver disease (decreased production of fibrinogen)
  - Heparin therapy (inhibits fibrinogen formation)
  - Hypofibrinogenemia (low fibrinogen to start)

Bleeding Time

- Measures time from start of skin incision to formation of clot (normal = 3 to 8 minutes)
- Independent of coagulation cascade
- Elevated in:
  - Thrombocytopenia
  - Qualitative platelet disorders
  - von Willebrand's disease (VWD)

HEMOPHILIA A

PATHOPHYSIOLOGY

Sex-linked recessive disease causing a deficiency of factor VIII

SIGNS AND SYMPTOMS

Dependent on amount of active factor:
- Five to 25% normal factor VIII activity (mild): Abnormal bleeding when subjected to surgery or dental procedures
- Two to 5% (moderate) and < 2% (severe) normal VIII activity: Deep tissue bleeding, intra-articular hemorrhages (usually knees), nerve impingement, intracranial bleeding (following trauma)

DIAGNOSIS

- Prolonged aPTT, normal bleeding time
- Clinical picture, family history, and the factor VIII coagulant activity level

TREATMENT

- Cryoprecipitate
- Recombinant factor VIII

> Unlike in VWD, bleeding time in hemophilia A is unaffected because no abnormality with platelets is present.

HEMOPHILIA B (CHRISTMAS DISEASE)

PATHOPHYSIOLOGY

X-linked recessive disease that causes a deficiency of factor IX

SIGNS AND SYMPTOMS

Identical to hemophilia A

DIAGNOSIS

Factor IX assay

TREATMENT

- Fresh frozen plasma (FFP)
- Recombinant factor IX

VWD

DEFINITION

- Type I: Partial quantitative deficiency of von Willebrand factor (VWF) (most common)
- Type II: Qualitative defect of VWF
- Type III: Almost total absence of VWF

> VWD is the most common inherited bleeding disorder.

PATHOPHYSIOLOGY

- VWF is a glycoprotein that is synthesized, stored, and secreted by vascular endothelial cells.
- It functions to allow platelets to adhere to the damaged endothelium and it carries factor VIII in the plasma.

ETIOLOGY

- Usually autosomal dominant inheritance

EPIDEMIOLOGY

- One in 100 live births have some defect in VWF.
- Only 1 in 10,000 manifests a clinically significant bleeding disorder.

SYMPTOMS AND SIGNS

- Epistaxis
- Gastrointestinal (GI) bleeding
- Menorrhagia
- Easy bruising
- Prolonged bleeding after dental extractions
- Ecchymoses

DIAGNOSIS

- Prolonged bleeding time
- Prolonged aPTT
- Normal PT
- Normal platelet count
- Definitive diagnosis made with abnormal assay of VWF, VWF:antigen, or factor VIII:C (usually not in the emergency department [ED])

TREATMENT

- Type I: Desmopressin
- Types II and III:
  - Factor VIII concentrates with large amounts of VWF:
    - Synthetic-treated product, no risk of infection
    - Provides VWF most efficiently, with the least amount of volume
  - Cryoprecipitate and FFP:
    - Will also work, but carry risk of infection and provide low concentration of VWF for given volume, resulting in volume overload for severe cases

THROMBOCYTOPENIA

DEFINITION

Platelet count < 140,000

ETIOLOGY

Increased Destruction
- Antibody-coated platelets removed by macrophages:
  - Idiopathic thrombocytopenic purpura (ITP)

---

*Causes of
thrombocytopenia:*
PLATELETS
Platelet disorders: TTP,
HUS, ITP, DIC
Leukemia
Anemia
Trauma
Enlarged spleen
Liver disease
EtOH
Toxins (benzene, heparins,
aspirin, chemotherapy
agents, etc.)
Sepsis

- Human immunodeficiency virus (HIV)-associated thrombocytopenia
- Transfusion reactions
- Some drug-induced thrombocytopenias
- Thrombin-induced platelet damage:
  - DIC (seen with obstetrical complications, metastatic malignancy, septicemia, and traumatic brain injury)
- Removal by acute vascular abnormalities:
  - Thrombotic thrombocytopenic purpura (TTP)
  - Hemolytic uremic syndrome (HUS)
  - Adult respiratory distress syndrome–induced thrombocytopenia

Decreased Production
- Decreased megakaryocytes in marrow:
  - Leukemia
  - Aplastic anemia
- Normal megakaryocytes:
  - Alcohol-induced reactions
  - Megaloblastic anemias
  - Some myelodysplastic syndromes

Sequestration in Spleen
- Cirrhosis with congestive splenomegaly
- Myelofibrosis with myeloid metaplasia

RISK FACTORS

- Drugs (chemotherapeutic agents, ethanol, thiazides)
- Prior thrombocytopenic episodes
- Underlying immunologic disorder
- Blood transfusion within 10 days
- Significant EtOH consumption
- Term pregnancy

SIGNS AND SYMPTOMS

- Petechiae
- Purpura
- Heme-positive stool
- Recurrent epistaxis, gingival bleeding, or menorrhagia
- Hepatosplenomegaly (jaundice, spider angiomas, and palmar erythema may be present if condition is due to EtOH abuse)

DIAGNOSIS

- Complete blood count (CBC) with platelet morphology and manual platelet count
- PT/PTT
- Bleeding time
- Liver function tests (LFTs)

TREATMENT

- Treat underlying disorder
- Platelet transfusion for actively bleeding patients with platelet count < 50,000/µL, and prophylactically for patients with < 10,000/µL
- Platelets are contraindicated in TTP.

Antiplatelet Therapy

- Platelets are significant components of the thrombotic response to damaged coronary and cerebral artery plaques.
- Prompt antiplatelet therapy can halt progression and significantly reduce morbidity/mortality from acute myocardial infarction and cerebrovascular accident.
- Platelet-rich thrombi are more resistant to endogenous thrombolysis and thrombolytic therapy (tissue plasminogen activato [tPA], streptokinase) than fibrin and red blood cell (RBC)-rich thrombi.
- Ongoing hemorrhage or high risk thereof is a contraindication to antiplatelet therapy.

ASPIRIN (ASA)

- Most cost-effective antiplatelet agent currently available
- Irreversibly acetylates platelet cyclooxygenase: As platelets have no biosynthetic machinery, it is inactivated for the lifespan of the platelet (8 to 10 days).
- Decreased platelet cyclooxygenase → decreased thromboxane A2, a proaggregatory agent.
- Decreased cyclooxygenase in the vascular endothelium → decreased prostacyclin—an antiaggregatory agent (this countertherapeutic effect contributes relatively little to the overall clinical effect of ASA).

TICLOPIDINE (TICLID)

- Irreversibly inhibits conversion of platelet surface receptor to its high-affinity binding state
- Prevents fibrinogen receptor expression
- Lasts for lifespan of platelet
- Reaches a maximal effect after 8 to 11 days of treatment
- More effective than ASA; slow onset of action relegates its use to preventive rather than acute therapy.
- Risk of neutropenia and agranulocytosis
- Expensive

CLOPIDOGREL (PLAVIX)

- Ticlopidine analog, similar mechanism
- Rapid onset of action, can be used acutely
- Intravenous (IV) administration possible
- Expensive

Common Agents with Antiplatelet Side Effects

- Nonsteroidal anti-inflammatory drugs (NSAIDs): Indomethacin, naproxen, ibuprofen
- Antimicrobials:
  - Penicillins: Penicillin G, ampicillin, methicillin, nafcillin
  - Cephalosporins: Cefotaxime
  - Nitrofurantoin

Antiplatelet drugs:
CAFE PORN
C⁴: Cardiovascular drugs
      Cholesterol-lowering drugs
      Cough suppressants
      Chemotherapy
A⁴: Antimicrobials
      Antihistamines
      Anticoagulants
      Anesthetics
 F: Food
 E: Ethanol

 P: Psychotropics
 O: Opiates
 R: Radiocontrast agents
 N: NSAIDs

- Antihistamines: Diphenhydramine
- Cough suppressants: Guaifenesin
- Opiates: Heroin
- Food and drink: EtOH, garlic, onion, vitamins C and E, ginger, cumin, turmeric, cloves
- Cardiovascular drugs:
  - Ca^{2+} channel blockers: Diltiazem, verapamil, nifedipine, nimodipine
  - Nitrates: Nitroglycerin, isosorbides, nitroprusside
  - Propranolol, quinidine
- Cholesterol lowering: Clofibrate
- Psychotropics:
  - Neuroleptics: Haloperidol, chlorpromazine
  - Tricyclics: Amitriptyline, imipramine
- Chemotherapy: Cisplatin, cyclophosphamide, vincristine, asparaginase, daunorubicin
- Radiographic contrast agents
- Anesthetics: Lidocaine, benzocaine, cocaine, halothane
- Anticoagulants: Heparin, tPA, protamine

ITP

DEFINITION

- A hematologic disorder not associated with a systemic disease or toxin exposure resulting in platelet destruction
- Usually chronic in adults and acute in children

ETIOLOGY

- Adult ITP usually results from antibody development against a structural antigen present on the platelet surface.
- Childhood ITP is thought to be triggered by a virus, which produces an antibody that cross-reacts with an antigen on the platelet surface.

PATHOPHYSIOLOGY

The antibody-coated platelets are removed from circulation by mononuclear phagocytes, thus decreasing the number of platelets in circulation.

DIAGNOSIS

- Peripheral blood smear should be unremarkable with the exception of decreased platelets.
- Bone marrow is normal with the exception of possibly increased megakaryocytes.

TREATMENT

Adults
- Initial treatment is prednisone 1 mg/kg/day. Platelet levels usually rise over the coming weeks, during which time the steroid dosage is tapered.
- Most patients fail to have a sustained response and will go on to have a splenectomy. This causes remission in 50 to 60% of patients.

Typical scenario:
A 42-year-old woman with no past medical history presents due to petechiae that have erupted over her arms and legs in the past 2 days. She also reports gingival bleeding. Physical exam reveals petechiae within the oral cavity as well. Labs demonstrate a platelet count of 7,000/mm³, normal PT/aPTT, and a prolonged bleeding time. *Think: ITP.*

Patients with ITP and Life-Threatening Bleeding

- Suppress mononuclear phagocyte clearance of platelets by administering IV immunoglobulin at 1 g/kg for 1 day. May cause platelet count to rise.
- High-dose methylprednisolone is less expensive and may result in the same increase in platelets.
- Platelet transfusion for life-threatening bleeding

TTP

DEFINITION

Severe disorder in which fibrin strands are deposited in multiple small vessels: This damages passing RBCs and platelets and results in thrombocytopenia and microangiopathic hemolytic anemia.

ETIOLOGY

Unknown

EPIDEMIOLOGY

- Female gender
- Age 10 to 45 years

RISK FACTORS

- Pregnancy, often indistinguishable from severe preeclampsia (see HELLP syndrome)
- Drugs: Quinine, cyclosporine, mitomycin C, ticlopidine, H_2 blockers, oral contraceptives, penicillin
- Autoimmune disorders (e.g., systemic lupus erythematosus)
- Infection (including *E. coli* O157: H7, *Shigella dysenteriae,* and HIV)
- Allogeneic bone marrow transplantation
- Malignancy

SIGNS AND SYMPTOMS

- Fever
- Waxing and waning mental status (correlates with lodging and dislodging of thrombus in cerebral vessels)
- Pallor
- Petechiae
- Colicky pain of various body parts (again due to thrombus in vessels)

DIAGNOSIS

- Diagnosis requires a combination of clinical suspicion and correlation with appropriate lab analyses.
- Peripheral blood smear: Schistocytes and helmet cells
- CBC: Anemia, thrombocytopenia, elevated reticulocyte count
- Blood urea nitrogen/creatinine (BUN/Cr): Azotemia
- Urinalysis: Hematuria, red cell casts, and proteinuria
- LFTs: Elevated lactic dehydrogenase, elevated bilirubin (unconjugated > conjugated), low haptoglobin

TTP diagnostic pentad:

- Fever
- Altered mental status
- Renal dysfunction
- Microangiopathic hemolytic anemia
- Thrombocytopenia

Typical scenario:
A 33-year-old woman is brought to the ED after her sister found her febrile and confused. Physical exam reveals fever, tachycardia, some mucosal bruising, a waxing and waning mental status, and trace heme-positive stool. Labs demonstrate a platelet count of 22,000/mm³, normal PT/aPTT, elevated bilirubin, and a BUN/Cr of 40/2.0. Peripheral smear shows schistocytes. *Think: TTP.*

TREATMENT

- **Do not transfuse platelets.**
- Plasmapheresis is mainstay of treatment (given daily, until platelet count rises to normal).
- May give FFP if plasmapheresis not available
- Transfuse packed RBCs if anemia is symptomatic (tachycardia, orthostatic hypotension, hypoxia).
- Consider corticosteroids, vincristine, antiplatelet agents, and splenectomy for refractory cases.
- Monitor for and treat acute bleeds (remember to look for intracranial bleed as well).
- Admit patients to the intensive care unit.

HUS

DEFINITION

Disorder thought to be on the same continuum as TTP (earlier) with renal dysfunction as its primary feature

ETIOLOGY

Unknown

EPIDEMIOLOGY

- Most common in childhood
- Adult form also seen

RISK FACTORS

- Infection with *E. coli* O157: H7 or *Shigella dysenteriae*
- Ingestion of undercooked meats and unpasteurized products

SIGNS AND SYMPTOMS

- Vomiting
- Diarrhea
- Abdominal pain
- Oliguria
- Pallor
- GI bleeding
- Seizures can result as a complication of renal failure, due to hypertension, hyponatremia, fluid overload, and electrolyte imbalances.

DIAGNOSIS

Same as TTP

TREATMENT

- Dialysis is the mainstay of therapy.
- Control hypertension.
- Replace electrolytes.
- Blood transfusion or erythropoietin for anemia

DO NOT transfuse platelets in patients with TTP, this could kill them.

TTP is a disease with high mortality when not diagnosed and treated early. Also, it is a disease that recurs, with each subsequent episode being slightly worse. Patients eventually die of multiple thrombi lodged in the brain, kidneys, and other organs.

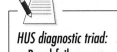

HUS diagnostic triad:
- **Renal failure**
- **Microangiopathic hemolytic anemia**
- **Thrombocytopenia**

Typical scenario:
A 6-year-old boy presents with abdominal pain, oliguria, diarrhea, and fever. Several kids from his school came down with the same thing after his birthday party at a local hamburger chain. Labs demonstrate acute renal failure. *Think: HUS.*

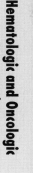

HIGH-YIELD FACTS

Hematologic and Oncologic Emergencies

Platelet transfusion is not contraindicated for HUS as it is for TTP.

- Platelet transfusion for active bleeding
- Plasmapheresis is sometimes used in adults.

PROGNOSIS

- The time for highest mortality is during the course of the disease, when central nervous system (CNS) complications can result.
- Most children recover without sequelae after the acute illness.
- Some children will have progressive renal dysfunction and hypertension and should be monitored for a period of at least 5 years.
- Adults do not recover so well and usually have residual renal failure.

DISSEMINATED INTRAVASCULAR COAGULATION (DIC)

DEFINITION

DIC is a coagulopathy that happens when both the fibrinolytic and coagulation cascades are activated.

RISK FACTORS

- Trauma:
  - Crush injuries, brain trauma, burns
- Obstetrical complications:
  - Abruptio placentae
  - Saline-induced therapeutic termination
  - Retained products of conception
  - Amniotic fluid embolism
- Infection: Usually from gram-negative organisms (endotoxin causes generation of tissue factor activity on the plasma membrane of monocytes and macrophages)
- Malignancy:
  - Mucin-secreting adenocarcinomas of pancreas and prostate
  - Acute promyelocytic leukemia
- Shock from any cause
- Snake bites
- Heat stroke
- Severe transfusion reaction
- Drugs
- Foreign bodies such as peritoneovenous shunts

Typical scenario:
A 27-year-old woman who is 39 weeks pregnant is the victim of a high-speed motor vehicle crash. She presents with vaginal bleeding and uterine irritability. A few hours later, she goes into shock and begins bleeding profusely from her multiple lacerations. Labs show prolonged PT/aPTT, thrombocytopenia, and fibrin split products. *Think: DIC due to abruptio placentae.*

PATHOGENESIS

- Results from generation of tissue factor in the blood or the introduction of tissue factor–rich substances into the circulation
- Tissue factor is the most fibrinogenic substance known, and it initiates coagulation.
- Coagulative activity is difficult to regulate once it is begun in this fashion, and soon the factors of coagulation have been exhausted, resulting in coagulopathy.

SIGNS AND SYMPTOMS

- Sites of recent surgery or phlebotomy bleed profusely and cannot be controlled with local measures.

- Ecchymoses form at sites of parenteral injections.
- Serious GI bleeding may ensue at sites of erosion of the gastric mucosa.

DIAGNOSIS

- Presence of fibrin split products
- Thrombocytopenia
- Markedly prolonged PT/PTT
- Low fibrinogen concentration
- Elevated plasma d-dimers (are the cross-linked fibrin degradation by products)
- Schistocytes on peripheral smear

TREATMENT

- Replacement of coagulation factors:
  - FFP, cryoprecipitate, and platelets
- Hemodynamic stabilization with fluids, blood, oxygen, and airway management as necessary
- Immediately identify and if possible correct the underlying cause:
  - Immediate broad-spectrum antibiotic coverage in the setting of gram-negative sepsis
  - Uterine evacuation in the setting of suspected retained products of conception
- Heparin has not been conclusively shown to increase survival. It should be considered if the underlying condition is a carcinoma or when a picture of thrombosis predominates.
- Antithrombin III may also be given (with or without heparin) to help interrupt the clotting cascade.

> PT/aPTT are normal in ITP, TTP, and HUS. They are abnormally elevated in DIC.

SICKLE CELL ANEMIA (SCA)

DEFINITION

- Genetic disease characterized by the presence of hemoglobin S in RBCs
- Hemoglobin S is formed by substitution of valine for glutamine in the sixth position of the β-hemoglobin chain.
- During periods of high oxygen consumption, this abnormal hemoglobin distorts and causes cell to sickle.
- Sickle cell trait: Heterozygous for sickle gene
- Sickle cell disease: Homozygous for sickle gene

EPIDEMIOLOGY

- More common in blacks than whites
- Increased incidence in populations from Africa, the Mediterranean, Middle East, and India

PATHOPHYSIOLOGY

- Deoxygenated hemoglobin S undergoes a conformational change with low O_2 tension.
- When enough hemoglobin S molecules change conformation, the hemoglobin molecules crystallize, forming a semisolid gel in the interior of the RBC.
- This causes the RBC to adopt a sickle shape.
- The distorted RBCs are inflexible and plug small capillaries, leading to occlusion and ischemia/infarction.

> *Features of SCA:*
> **SICKLE**
> **S**plenomegaly, sludging
> **I**nfection
> **C**holelithiasis
> **K**idney — hematuria
> **L**iver congestion, leg ulcers
> **E**ye changes

- The sickled cells also have an increased propensity to adhere to the capillary endothelium.
- The distortion also results in a weakening of the RBC membrane and the cells have a decreased lifespan in the circulation, causing the chronic hemolytic anemia.
- Early in the sickling process, the RBCs can resume their normal shape if O_2 tension is restored; later, the sickling becomes irreversible.
- Low RBC H_2O content can also trigger sickling.
- Early in life, the spleen removes most of the sickled cells from the circulation, causing splenomegaly. Eventually, the toll of continuous sequestration damages the spleen to the point of infarction. The spleen fibroses and shrivels to a fraction of its normal size, often termed *autosplenectomy*.
- Absence of splenic function renders these patients more susceptible to infections, particularly by encapsulated organisms (*Haemophilius influenzae, Pneumococcus, Meningococcus, Klebsiella*)

SIGNS AND SYMPTOMS

Vaso-occlusive Crisis

- Symptoms include arthralgias and pain.
- Caused by vascular sludging and thrombosis. These vaso-occlusive crises may cause organ failure (secondary to infarction), dehydration, fever, and leukocytosis.

Typical scenario:
A 24-year-old man with known sickle cell disease presents with pain in his lower back and knees. He is afebrile, has an O_2 saturation of 100%, and normal labs. *Think: Vaso-occlusive crisis of sickle cell disease.*

Acute Chest Syndrome

- Sudden onset of fever, chest pain, cough, shortness of breath, leukocytosis, and pulmonary infiltrates on chest radiograph
- Due to infection and occlusion of pulmonary microvasculature
- This is a major cause of mortality in patients > 5 years old.
- Arterial blood gas should be evaluated.
- Diagnosis of pulmonary embolism should usually be excluded with ventilation–perfusion scanning or computed tomographic (CT) angiography.

Aplastic Crisis

- Life-threatening complication characterized by severe pancytopenia
- Due to medullary sickling, common complication of infection with parvovirus B19

CNS Crisis

- This is the only type of vaso-occlusive crisis that is painless (no pain receptors).
- Cerebral vascular occlusion is more common in children, and cerebral hemorrhage is more common in adults.
- Evaluation should include CT scanning.
- Lumbar puncture should be performed if CT is negative and headache is present to exclude diagnosis of subarachnoid hemorrhage.

Priapism

Sickling in corpus cavernosum of penis causing protracted painful erection

Acute Splenic Sequestration

- Second most common cause of death in children with SCA (by adulthood, autosplenectomy will have disposed of this source of morbidity/mortality)
- Sickled cells block outflow from the spleen, causing pooling of blood and platelets in the spleen. In major sequestration crisis, the hemoglobin drops three points from baseline or to a level less than 6 g/dL.

Renal Papillary Necrosis

- Characterized by flank pain and hematuria
- Occurs because of the very high osmolalities in renal medulla needed to pull the water from the collecting ducts causing the RBCs to sickle

DIAGNOSIS

- All newborns at risk in the United States are screened for the disease.
- Peripheral smear: Howell–Jolly bodies (cytoplasmic remnants of nuclear chromatin that are normally removed by the spleen), sickled cells
- Blood tests show anemia, increased reticulocyte count, and increased indirect bilirubin.
- Hemoglobin electrophoresis will show hemoglobin S.

TREATMENT

- Vaso-occlusive crisis: Analgesia and hydration
- Aplastic crisis and splenic sequestration: Blood transfusion, circulatory support
- Acute chest syndrome: Oxygen, broad-spectrum antibiotics, and analgesia
- Priapism: Hydration, subcutaneous terbutaline (to relax smooth muscle)
- H. influenzae and pneumococcal vaccines for prophylaxis

Patients with SCA are prone to infection with encapsulated organisms. *Salmonella* osteomyelitis is most common among patients with SCA.

The best treatment for SCA patients is education about their disease, specifically, how to avoid vaso-occlusive crises.

GLUCOSE-6-PHOSPHATE DEHYDROGENASE (G6PD) DEFICIENCY

BIOCHEMISTRY

- G6PD is the first enzyme in the hexose monophosphate (HMP) shunt and the only entry point into this pathway from glycolysis.
- HMP shunt is only source of nicotinamide adenine dinucleotide phosphate (NADPH) in RBC (no mitochondria, glycolysis only)
- NADPH is the RBCs' primary defense against oxidative stressors.

METABOLISM

- Usual oxidants are superoxide (O_2^-) and hydrogen peroxide (H_2O_2).
- Oxidants react with hemoglobin and structural proteins → loss of function and lysis.
- Activity of G6PD decreases with normal RBC age. Half-life of single molecule is 62 days; in G6PD-deficient cell, half-life may be as low as 13 days.

G6PD deficiency is the most common metabolic disorder of RBCs.

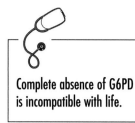

Complete absence of G6PD
is incompatible with life.

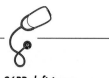

G6PD deficiency:
Think: Africa,
Mediterranean, Middle East,
Asia—all fairly contiguous
land masses with warm
climates.

Typical scenario:
A 35-year-old Italian man
presents complaining of
weakness, back pain, and
jaundice. He reports being
started on ciprofloxacin 2
days ago for pneumonia.
Think: G6PD deficiency.

GENETICS

- Gene on X chromosome, sex-linked trait
- Heterozygous females fare better than males.

PATHOLOGY

- Enzyme has reduced half-life or catalytic activity.
- Most patients have no anemia in the steady state.
- Most hemolysis is extravascular (liver and spleen), but some occurs intravascularly, causing hemoglobinemia and hemoglobinuria.
- Heinz bodies: Precipitates of oxidized hemoglobin bound to cell membrane

EPIDEMIOLOGY

- Worldwide prevalence:
  - African Americans: Milder form, 12% of men
  - Mediterraneans (Greeks, Italians, Arabs): More severe form, 20 to 30% of men
  - Kurdish and Sephardic Jews: 60 to 70% of men
- Correlated with incidence of *Plasmodium falciparum* malaria, conferring selective advantage in endemic areas

SIGNS AND SYMPTOMS

- Acute hemolysis:
  - Jaundice, dark urine, acute tubular necrosis (ATN) due to hemoglobinemia
  - Anemia: Pallor, tachycardia, systolic ejection murmur
  - Mesenteric and renal ischemia: Abdominal and back pain
  - Sudden drop of 3 to 4 g/dL in RBC hemoglobin
- Chronic hemolysis: Hepatosplenomegaly

TRIGGERS

- Infection (most common): Release of oxidants by macrophages
- Drugs: Antimalarials, quinolones, sulfa drugs, NSAIDs, nitrofurantoin, fava beans, vitamin C (acids)
- Diabetic ketoacidosis: Low pH is oxidative stress.

DIAGNOSIS

- Hemolysis:
  - CBC: Anemia, reticulocytosis, microcytosis, schistocytosis, Heinz bodies
  - Low haptoglobin, negative direct and indirect Coombs'
  - Elevated direct and indirect bilirubin
  - Urinalysis: Hemoglobinuria, elevated urobilinogen, ATN
- G6PD assay requires a 3-week wait after acute episode.

TREATMENT

- Volume loading—renal protection
- Removal of oxidative stressor if possible (discontinue drug, treat infection)
- RBC replacement as necessary; severe cases may require exchange transfusion.

- Acute crises will resolve spontaneously after ~1 week.
- Education is the most effective therapeutic measure.

TRANSFUSION REACTIONS

ABO Incompatibility

- Most common transfusion reaction
- Almost invariably due to **human error**
- Patients are immunized against A/B antigen (Ag) without prior exposure because endogenous bacteria produce glycoproteins with structures similar to the A/B Ag.
- Which antibody (Ab) form is actually determined by the patient's own A/B status.

Non-ABO Incompatibility

- Uncommon, occurring mostly in multitransfused patients
- One to 1.5% risk of red cell alloimmunization per unit transfused
- Fifteen to 20% incidence in multitransfused patients
- Most commonly Ab to Rh and Kell (K) Ag, less frequently Duffy (Fy) and Kidd (Jk) Ag
- Rh-negative mothers who give birth to Rh-positive children have a 15 to 20% chance of developing anti-Rh Ab due to fetal–maternal hemorrhage.
- Anti-Rh_o immune globulin is routinely given to Rh-negative mothers pre- and perinatally to prevent Rh immunization.

Rh immunoprophylaxis should be considered for all pregnant patients who sustain any abdominal trauma regardless of the amount of vaginal bleeding.

The Kleihauer–Betke test allows quantification of the amount of maternal–fetal blood mixing.

COMMON ED PRESENTATIONS OF CANCER COMPLICATIONS

Malignant Pericardial Effusions

- Seen with cancers of lung and breast, Hodgkin's and non-Hodgkin's lymphoma, leukemia, malignant melanoma, and postradiation pericarditis
- Large effusions can lead to cardiac tamponade (see Trauma chapter).

Syndrome of Inappropriate Antidiuretic Hormone (SIADH)

- Most commonly associated with small cell carcinoma
- Other cancers that can cause SIADH are brain, thymus, pancreas, duodenum, prostate, and lymphosarcoma.
- See Diagnostics chapter for description.

Adrenal Crisis

- Seen with malignant melanoma and cancers of breast, lungs, and retroperitoneal organs
- See Endocrine Emergencies chapter for description.

Neutropenic Sepsis

- Defined as fever and absolute granulocyte count < 500/mm^3
- Patients are at great risk of developing overwhelming sepsis.
- Treated with hydration, broad-spectrum antibiotics, and reverse isolation

Superior Vena Cava (SVC) Syndrome, Acute Spinal Cord Compression, and Tumor Lysis Syndrome

See individual sections below.

SVC SYNDROME

DEFINITION

Acute or subacute obstruction of the SVC due to compression, infiltration, or thrombosis

EPIDEMIOLOGY

- ~90% of cases due to malignancy:
  - External compression by tumor
  - Direct infiltration by tumor
  - SVC thrombosis due to partial obstruction related to above; often augmented by hypercoagulability of malignancy
  - Causative tumors:
    - Small cell lung cancer: 65%
    - Breast cancer: 10 to 15%
    - Testicular cancer: 10 to 15%
- ~10% of cases due to "benign" causes:
  - Thoracic aortic aneurysm
  - Goiter
  - Pericardial constriction
  - 1° SVC thrombosis
  - Idiopathic sclerosing aortitis
  - Tuberculous mediastinitis
  - Central venous catheters
- ~5% incidence in lung cancer and lymphoma patients

PHYSIOLOGY

- Blood flow: Internal jugular and subclavian veins → brachiocephalic (innominate) veins → SVC ← azygous vein ← bronchial veins
- Blockade above the azygous vein manifests less severely, as chest wall collaterals allow bypass of the obstruction and because unobstructed drainage of the bronchial veins avoids many of the pulmonary problems.
- Due to lack of gravitational assistance with drainage, many symptoms are more severe in the recumbent position and in the morning after sleep.
- Slow-growing tumors allow more time for collateral development, and thus a less severe picture, than rapidly growing ones.

> **Typical scenario:**
> A 53-year-old female with known breast cancer presents with facial and upper extremity edema and distended neck veins. She states the symptoms are worse in the morning. She is afebrile; her lungs reveal mild crackles bilaterally to auscultation. *Think: SVC syndrome.*

SIGNS AND SYMPTOMS

- Distended neck veins (67%)
- Isolated upper extremity edema, particularly periorbital and facial (56%)
- Pulmonary manifestations (40%): Shortness of breath, tachypnea, cyanosis, crackles, rales
- Less commonly, sequelae of increased intracranial pressure (ICP): Papilledema, cerebral edema, altered mental status, visual disturbances, headache, seizures, coma, cerebral hemorrhage, death
- Can be mistaken for congestive heart failure or pericardial tamponade

DIAGNOSIS

- Chest x-ray: Pleural effusion, mass apparent in only 10% of cases
- Chest CT/magnetic resonance imaging (MRI) for mass
- If mass detected, biopsy for definitive diagnosis

TREATMENT

- Supportive measures
- Increased ICP may require emergent surgical resection.
- Definitive treatment depends on etiology of obstruction.

SPINAL CORD COMPRESSION

DEFINITION

Malignancy metastasizing to and destroying vertebral bodies, causing cord impingement

ETIOLOGY

- Most common malignancies: Lymphoma, lung, breast, prostate
- Other causes: Melanoma, myeloma, renal cell cancer, vertebral subluxation, epidural hematomas, and intramedullary metastasis

SIGNS AND SYMPTOMS

- Metastases almost always remain epidural.
- Spinal distribution:
  - 15% cervical
  - 68% thoracic
  - 19% lumbosacral
- Back pain:
  - 95% incidence
  - Usually localized to level of tumor
  - Variable radicular involvement
  - Acute or insidious onset
  - May be exacerbated by percussion, neck flexion, straight leg raises, or Valsalva
- Weakness, usually symmetric (75%)
- Autonomic or sensory involvement (50%)

- Motor deficits follow usual pattern of cord injury: Early flaccidity/hyporeflexia (spinal shock), later spasticity/hyperreflexia

DIAGNOSIS

- Diagnostic study of choice is MRI.
- Myelography can also be used. Positive myelogram shows dye obstruction at level of lesion.
- Plain films of spine (90% show evidence of tumor, but not whether it is compressing the spinal cord)

TREATMENT

- High-dose steroids to control inflammation/edema
- Oncology consult
- Radiation is usual therapy of choice, but depends on the radiosensitivity of the tumor.
- Surgery is indicated if a biopsy is required, the spine is unstable, or the involved area has already been maximally irradiated.

TUMOR LYSIS SYNDROME

DEFINITION

Acute life-threatening condition arising from massive release of lysed tumor cell cytosol and nucleic acids

PATHOLOGY

- Usually occurs 1 to 5 days after instituting antineoplastic therapy (chemotherapy or radiation)
- Likelihood of syndrome increases with tumor bulk and sensitivity to antineoplastic therapy.
- Generally low risk with solid tumors
- Most common with hematologic malignancies: Acute leukemias, lymphomas (particularly Burkitt's)
- Manifestations largely due to electrolyte disturbances
- Prior renal impairment increases risk.
- Acute renal failure from urate and Ca^{2+} crystal deposition also contributes to electrolyte disturbances.

CLINICAL MANIFESTATIONS

- Hyperuricemia:
  - Due to DNA breakdown
  - Due to urate nephropathy
- Hyperkalemia:
  - Due to release of cytosol
  - Cardiac dysrhythmias
- Hyperphosphatemia:
  - Due to protein breakdown
  - Nephropathy due to precipitation of calcium phosphate crystals
- Hypocalcemia:
  - Due to hyperphosphatemia driving renal excretion of Ca^{2+}
  - Neuromuscular symptoms: Muscle cramps, tetany, convulsions

- ■ Cardiac dysrhythmias
- ■ Confusion
- ■ Uremia:
  - ■ Due to protein breakdown

TREATMENT

- ■ Treat rapidly and aggressively.
- ■ Oncology consult
- ■ Discontinue antineoplastic therapy if possible.
- ■ Frequent monitoring of electrolytes, calcium, and phosphorus
- ■ Hyperuricemia: Hydration, allopurinol, alkalinization of the urine, diuretics
- ■ Hyperkalemia/hypocalcemia: Calcium carbonate, other standard measures may be used if necessary.
- ■ Consider emergent hemodialysis to lower uric acid, potassium, phosphate, and urea.
- ■ Prognosis in setting of preexisting renal failure is often grave.

Gynecologic Emergencies

OVARIAN DISORDERS

Ovarian Cysts

TYPES

Follicular Cysts
- First 2 weeks of menstrual cycle (most common)
- Pain secondary to stretching of capsule/rupture of cyst
- Usually regress spontaneously in 1 to 3 months

Corpus Luteum Cysts
- Last 2 weeks of menstrual cycle (less common)
- Bleeding into cyst cavity may cause stretching or rupture of capsule.
- Usually regress at end of menstrual cycle

Polycystic Ovaries (PCO)
- Endocrine disorder: Hyperandrogenism and anovulation
- Menses occur infrequently but are heavy and painful.
- Ovarian cysts possibly secondary to chronic anovulation
- Long-term management is with oral contraceptives.

SIGNS AND SYMPTOMS

Cysts are usually asymptomatic unless complicated by rupture, torsion, or hemorrhage.

DIAGNOSIS

Ultrasound is useful for visualizing cysts and signs of rupture (free fluid in pelvis).

TREATMENT

Most complications are treated surgically.

> *PCO classic triad:*
> - Obesity
> - Hirsutism
> - Oligomenorrhea

Ovarian Torsion

DEFINITION

Twisting of the ovary on its stalk

EPIDEMIOLOGY

- Most common in the mid-20s

PATHOPHYSIOLOGY

- Venous drainage is occluded, but arterial supply remains patent.
- Ovarian edema, hemorrhage, and necrosis may occur rapidly.

SIGNS AND SYMPTOMS

- Sudden onset of severe unilateral pelvic pain
- Over 90% occur in the presence of enlarged ovary (tumor, cyst, abscess, or hyperstimulated with fertility drugs).
- Patients often give history of similar pain that resolved spontaneously (twisting/untwisting).
- Unilateral adnexal tenderness on pelvic exam

DIAGNOSIS

- Doppler ultrasound reveals decreased or absent flow to ovary and can demonstrate location of an adnexal mass.

TREATMENT

- Laparotomy/laparoscopy usually successful early on
- Advanced cases may require oophorectomy.

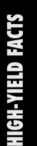

Adnexal torsion is a gynecologic emergency.

The most common ovarian tumor is a benign cystic teratoma (dermoid cyst).

Ovarian Tumors

- Malignant tumors are less common than benign ones but have the highest mortality of all gynecologic malignancies.
- They usually present late in course with abdominal distention (secondary to massive ascites).

VAGINAL DISORDERS

Bacterial Vaginosis

DEFINITION

Most common vulvovaginitis

ETIOLOGY

- Marked decrease in numbers of lactobacilli (protective)
- Infection with organisms such as *Peptostreptococcus* species, *Bacteroides* species, and *Gardnerella vaginalis*

SIGNS AND SYMPTOMS

Fishy-smelling itchy discharge

DIAGNOSIS

Via wet mount of vaginal smear

Lactobacilli are abundant in yogurt. A Yoplait a day keeps vaginitis away.

Diagnostic Criteria for Bacterial Vaginosis

- White, noninflammatory vaginal discharge (relative absence of white blood cells [WBCs])
- Clue cells (epithelial cells coated by bacteria) on microscope (Figure 12-1)
- pH > 4.5
- "Whiff test" (fishy odor to discharge after adding KOH)

TREATMENT

- For nonpregnant patients, metronidazole can be given several ways:
  - 500 mg PO bid × 7 days
  - Single 2 g PO dose (causes extreme nausea)
  - .75% gel intravaginally bid × 5 days
- For pregnant patients, oral clindamycin 300 mg PO bid × 7 days
- Encourage treatment of sexual partners as well.

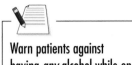

Warn patients against having *any* alcohol while on metronidazole (not even a teaspoonful of alcohol-containing mouthwash). It can cause a disulfiram-like reaction when co-ingested with alcohol, resulting in severe retching.

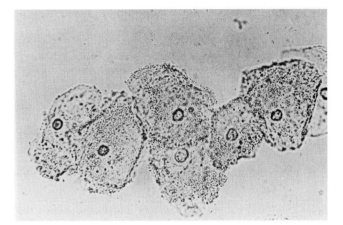

FIGURE 12-1. Clue cells in bacterial vaginosis.

(Reproduced, with permission, from Knoop K, Stack LB, and Storrow AB. *Atlas of Emergency Medicine.* New York: McGraw-Hill, 1997: 488.)

Trichomoniasis

DEFINITION

Sexually transmitted vulvovaginitis

ETIOLOGY

Trichomonas vaginalis, a flagellated protozoan

SIGNS AND SYMPTOMS

- Copious, yellow-green, malodorous, foamy vaginal discharge (pH > 5.5)
- Punctate hemorrhages on cervix or vaginal wall ("strawberry cervix")
- Dyspareunia
- Dysuria
- Labial irritation or swelling
- Ninety percent of infected men are asymptomatic. The trichomonads live in the seminal fluid.

T. vaginalis is the most common cause of vaginitis worldwide.

DIAGNOSIS

Presence of motile trichomonads on wet mount (Figure 12-2)

TREATMENT

- Metronidazole (see options above)
- For pregnant patients: Clotrimazole 100 mg intravaginally once daily × 14 days

COMPLICATIONS

Associated with increased risk of:
- Premature rupture of membranes
- Preterm delivery
- Postpartum endometritis

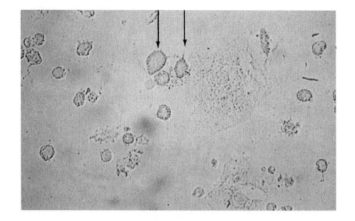

FIGURE 12-2. Trichomonads.

(Reproduced, with permission, from Knoop K, Stack LB, and Storrow AB. *Atlas of Emergency Medicine.* New York: McGraw-Hill, 1997: 488.)

Candidiasis

DEFINITION

Most common fungal infection

ETIOLOGY

Candida albicans

RISK FACTORS

- Diabetes mellitus
- Stress
- Human immunodeficiency virus
- Post antibiotic therapy
- Pregnancy
- Oral contraceptive therapy

SIGNS AND SYMPTOMS

- White "cottage cheese" discharge (pH < 4.5)
- Beefy red swollen labia
- Pruritus

Typical scenario:
A woman presents with a recurrent vaginal candidiasis that is refractory to treatment. *Think: Diabetes mellitus.* Get a blood glucose.

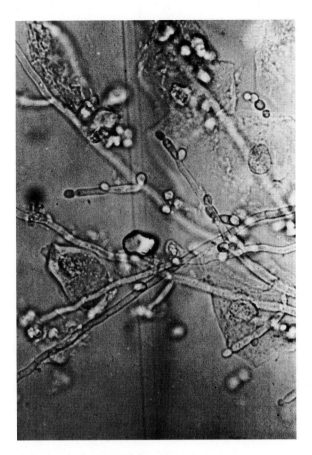

FIGURE 12-3. Pseudohyphae seen in candidiasis.
(Reproduced, with permission, from Pearlman MD, Tintinalli JE, eds. *Emergency Care of the Woman.* New York: McGraw-Hill, 1998: 544.)

DIAGNOSIS

Presence of pseudohyphae on 10% KOH prep (Figure 12-3)

TREATMENT

Multiple antifungal preparations (oral and intravaginal) are available.

Contact Vulvovaginitis

DEFINITION

Vulvovaginitis caused by exposure to chemical irritant or allergen (douches, soaps, tampons, underwear, topical antibiotics)

SIGNS AND SYMPTOMS

- Erythema and edema of labia
- Clear watery discharge

TREATMENT

- Removal of offending substance
- Sitz baths for mild cases
- Topical steroids for severe cases

Atrophic Vaginitis

DEFINITION

Decreased estrogen stimulation of vagina leads to mucosal atrophy.

ETIOLOGY

- Pregnancy and lactation
- Postmenopause

SIGNS AND SYMPTOMS

- Red, dry-appearing labial mucosa
- Atrophic vagina is predisposed to ulceration and superinfection.

TREATMENT

- Topical vaginal estrogen cream
- Hormone replacement therapy for postmenopausal women

UTERINE DISORDERS

Endometriosis

DEFINITION

Presence of endometrial glands/stroma outside the uterus that may affect ovaries, fallopian tubes, bladder, rectum, or appendix

PATHOPHYSIOLOGY

Most commonly accepted hypothesis is "retrograde menstruation":
- During menses, uterus contracts against partially closed cervix.
- Menstrual flow passes retrograde into fallopian tubes and pelvic cavity.
- Ectopic endometrial tissue then responds to cyclic hormonal influence.

SIGNS AND SYMPTOMS

- Pain most often occurs just before and during menses.
- Classic triad of endometriosis:
  - Dysmenorrhea
  - Dyspareunia
  - Dyschezia

DIAGNOSIS

Is suspected clinically, confirmed by direct visualization (laparoscopy)

TREATMENT

- Analgesia for acute episodes (nonsteroidal anti-inflammatory drugs or opiates)
- Hormonal therapy (suppress normal menstrual cycle) for long-term control
- Surgery for cases refractory to medical management

Every woman who presents with abdominal/pelvic pain or vaginal bleeding should have a documented β-hCG test. All women are pregnant until proven otherwise.

236

Dysfunctional Uterine Bleeding

TYPES AND CAUSES

- Ovulatory regular menstrual periods with intermenstrual bleeding:
  - Causes include oral contraceptives, persistent corpus luteum, and uterine fibroids.
- Anovulatory chronic estrogen stimulation without cyclic progesterone:
  - Hyperstimulated endometrium thickens and sheds irregularly.
  - Most common during menarche and menopause
  - Increased risk of endometrial hyperplasia/adenocarcinoma
- Miscellaneous:
  - Carcinoma, polyps, condylomata, lacerations (trauma), retained foreign bodies, endometriosis, blood dyscrasias, anticoagulant use

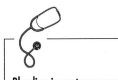

Bleeding in postmenopausal women (over 6 months after cessation of menopause) may represent early signs of cervical or endometrial neoplasia and should be referred for urgent gynecologic follow-up.

TREATMENT

- Treatment in the hemodynamically stable, nonpregnant patient is primarily supportive.
- Oral contraceptive pills (several regimens) will stop the bleeding and may be useful to "jump start" a regular cycle, although still anovulatory.
- Refer for gynecologic follow-up.

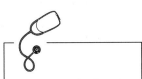

Warn patients that heavy withdrawal bleeding may follow cessation of oral contraceptive therapy.

CERVIX

Anatomy

- The cervix is the lowest portion of the uterus, composed primarily of collagen with 10% smooth muscle.
- Cervical dysplasia may occur secondary to infection, inflammation, or neoplasia.
- Abnormalities noted on speculum exam should be referred for gynecologic follow-up.

Cervicitis

DEFINITION

Inflammation of the cervix, most often due to infection

ETIOLOGY

- *Neisseria gonorrhoeae*
- *Chlamydia trachomatis*
- *Trichomonas vaginalis*

RISK FACTORS

Unsafe sexual practices

SIGNS AND SYMPTOMS

- Yellow mucopurulent discharge
- Dysuria
- Friable cervix

DIAGNOSIS

- Culture of discharge
- Wet mount to look for WBCs or motile trichomonads

TREATMENT

For Gonorrhea
- Ceftriaxone 125 mg single IM injection
- Cefixime 400 mg PO once
- Ciprofloxacin 500 mg PO once
- Ofloxacin 400 mg PO once
- Azithromycin 2 g PO once

For Chlamydia
- Azithromycin 1 g PO once
- Doxycycline 100 mg PO bid × 7 days
- Ofloxacin 300 mg PO bid × 7 days
- Erythromycin 500 mg PO qid × 7 days

For Trichomonas
- Metronidazole

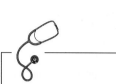

Due to the high rate of concurrent chlamydia and gonorrhea infection, treatment for both is given when either is suspected.

BARTHOLIN'S GLAND ABSCESS

PATHOPHYSIOLOGY

- Bartholin's (vestibular) gland lies at 5 and 7 o'clock positions of vestibule.
- Secretions normally provide lubrication during intercourse.
- Obstruction of gland leads to cyst formation, which may develop into abscess.

ETIOLOGY

Most common pathogens:
- *Neisseria gonorrhoeae*
- *Chlamydia trachomatis*
- Anaerobes
- Normal vaginal flora

TREATMENT

- Incision and drainage (usually under conscious sedation)
- Once the abscess cavity is drained, a balloon catheter is left in the cavity for continuous drainage while healing (6 weeks). The patient may engage in all activities including intercourse while it is in place.
- Antibiotics
- Definitive surgical excision may be indicated for recurrent abscesses.

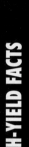

There is a high rate of recurrence of Bartholin's abscess secondary to fistulous tract formation.

DEFINITION

Ascending infection of the vagina, fallopian tubes, and ovaries

PATHOPHYSIOLOGY

Bacterial infection involving female upper reproductive tract cases are presumed to originate with a sexually transmitted disease of the lower genital tract, resulting in inflammation and scarring.

RISK FACTORS

- Previous PID
- Multiple sexual partners
- Intrauterine device use
- Douching
- Instrumentation of cervix

ETIOLOGY

- The most common pathogens are *Neisseria gonorrhoeae* and *Chlamydia trachomatis*.
- Anaerobes, gram-negatives, and mycoplasma are less common.

DIAGNOSIS

Major Criteria (Usually All Three Present)
- Lower abdominal tenderness
- Cervical/uterine tenderness (cervical motion tenderness)
- Adnexal tenderness

Minor Criteria (Usually at Least One Present)
- Fever
- Elevated WBC
- Elevated erythrocyte sedimentation rate
- Gram stain showing gram-negative diplococci

Other Helpful Tests
- Positive antibody test for chlamydia
- Purulent aspirate on culdocentesis
- Adnexal mass on exam/ultrasound consistent with abscess

CENTERS FOR DISEASE CONTROL GUIDELINES FOR INPATIENT ADMISSION

- Uncertain diagnosis
- Suspected tubo-ovarian abscess (TOA)
- Fever > 102.2°F
- Failure of outpatient therapy
- Pregnancy
- First episode in a nulligravida
- Inability to tolerate PO intake
- Inability to follow up in 48 hours
- Immunosuppressed patient

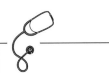

PID is a leading cause of female infertility.

PID is a risk factor for infertility, chronic pelvic pain, and ectopic pregnancy.

The most accurate way to diagnose PID is via laparoscopy.

Typical scenario:
A 19-year-old woman presents with bilateral abdominal pain, fever (101°F), nausea, vomiting, and general malaise. Her last menstrual period was 3 days ago. Pelvic exam reveals exquisite cervical motion and bilateral adnexal tenderness. *Think: PID.*

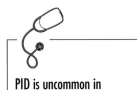

PID is uncommon in pregnancy due to the plug formed by the fusion of the chorion and decidua, providing an additional natural barrier to infection.

HIGH-YIELD FACTS

Gynecologic Emergencies

- Other considerations for admission:
  - Pediatric patient
  - Presence of infected foreign body

TREATMENT

Inpatient Therapy (Parenteral)
- Cefotetan or cefoxitin plus doxycycline

or

- Clindamycin plus gentamicin

Outpatient Therapy (14-Day Course)
- Ceftriaxone or cefoxitin IM plus doxycycline

or

- Ofloxacin plus metronidazole

COMPLICATIONS

- TOA
- Fitz-Hugh–Curtis syndrome
- Septic abortion
- Intrauterine growth retardation
- Premature rupture of membranes
- Preterm delivery

> The most common organism in TOA is *Bacteroides*.

TOA

- Common and potentially fatal complication of PID
- Intravenous antibiotics curative in 60 to 80% of cases
- Surgical drainage or salpingectomy/oophorectomy in resistant cases
- Ruptured TOA presents with shock and 15% mortality rate.

Fitz-Hugh–Curtis Syndrome

- "Perihepatitis" secondary to ascending gonorrhea/chlamydia infection (infection tracks up fallopian tubes into paracolic gutters)
- Mild elevations of liver function tests with symptoms of diaphragmatic irritation
- "Violin string" adhesions are classic anatomic findings.
- Treatment with intravenous antibiotics (as for PID) is usually curative.

Obstetric Emergencies

- Complex interaction between hypothalamus, pituitary, ovaries, endometrium
- Follicular phase begins with onset of menses and ends with preovulatory luteinizing hormone (LH) surge.
- Luteal phase begins with LH surge and ends with onset of menses.
- Gonadotropin-releasing hormone: Secreted by hypothalamus, stimulates release of follicle-stimulating hormone (FSH)/LH by pituitary
- FSH: Stimulates follicular growth and estradiol secretion during follicular phase
- LH: Surge just prior to midcycle is responsible for ovulation.
- Estradiol: Peaks once during follicular phase, again during luteal phase
- Progesterone: Corpus luteum secretes progestin during luteal phase.

Human Chorionic Gonadotropin (hCG)

- Presence of beta subunit of hCG is used as criteria for positive pregnancy test.
- Produced by trophoblastic tissue ~8 to 9 days after ovulation
- Maintains corpus luteum (which maintains progesterone production)
- After 6 to 8 weeks, progesterone production shifts to placenta.

Human Placental Lactogen (hPL)

- Produced by placenta, increases throughout pregnancy
- Antagonizes insulin → increased glucose levels.

Prolactin

- Rises in response to increasing maternal estrogen
- Stimulates milk production

Progesterone

- Produced by the ovaries (up to 8 weeks) and placenta (after 8 weeks)
- Prevents uterine contractions

Estrogens

- Produced by both fetus and placenta
- Limited role in monitoring course of pregnancy and fetal well-being

Cortisol

- Both maternal and fetal adrenal production
- Responsible for differentiation of type II alveoli → surfactant production
- Antagonizes insulin → increased glucose levels.

MATERNAL PHYSIOLOGY

Cardiovascular

- Plasma volume increases to ~150% of pre-gestational levels.
- Increase in red blood cell (RBC) mass less than plasma volume → hemoglobin/hematocrit will drop slightly ("anemia of pregnancy")
- Heart rate and stroke volume both rise → increased cardiac output.
- Systolic BP/diastolic BP/mean arterial pressure all decrease until 20 weeks, then rise again.
- Gravid uterus obstructs venous return from lower extremities.
- Increased blood flow to kidneys (waste) and skin (heat)

> Patients in second and third trimester of pregnancy may experience a significant drop in blood pressure (BP) when lying down. This "supine hypotensive syndrome" is relieved by turning onto the left side, taking weight of the uterus off the vena cava.

Respiratory

- Functional residual capacity decreases due to effects of gravid uterus.
- Increased tidal volume and minute ventilation
- Hyperventilation leads to chronic respiratory alkalosis.

Renal

- Progesterone causes smooth muscle dilatation (ureters, bladder).
- Renal bicarbonate excretion compensates for respiratory alkalosis.
- Both renal plasma flow and glomerular filtration rate increase.
- Renin levels are elevated → increased angiotensin levels.

Metabolic

- By 10th week, increased insulin levels and anabolic activity
- Insulin resistance and hPL/cortisol activity → elevated glucose levels

Endocrine

- Estrogen stimulates thyroxine-binding globulin → increased T_3/T_4 levels.

- Both adrenocorticotropic hormone and cortisol levels increased after 3 months.

PRENATAL CARE

Routine Tests

- Blood tests (blood counts, type and screen, Rh factor, glucose screen)
- Syphilis, rubella, hepatitis B
- Serum alpha-fetoprotein (between 16 and 20 weeks)
- Ultrasonography (around 16 to 20 weeks)
- Cervical cultures for gonorrhea, chlamydia, group B strep, and cytology

Monitoring

- Weight gain (26 to 28 pounds is average)
- Urinalysis (glucose, protein)
- BP
- Fundal height (after 22 weeks) approximates age of fetus.
- Fundal height above pubic symphysis in centimeters approximates weeks gestation
- Fetal assessment: Attitude, lie, presentation, position
- Nonstress test (NST): Assess for fetal heart rate accelerations in response to movement.
- Amniotic fluid index (AFI): Assess for oligohydramnios (AFI < 5 cm).
- Reactive NST and adequate AFI with normal fetal movement constitutes a normal biophysical profile.

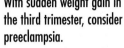

With sudden weight gain in the third trimester, consider preeclampsia.

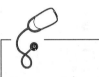

Asymptomatic bacteriuria in the pregnant woman is treated with antibiotics (e.g., nitrofurantoin).

COMPLICATIONS OF PREGNANCY

Ectopic Pregnancy

PATHOPHYSIOLOGY

- Zygote implants outside uterus (95% in fallopian tubes).
- Aborts when vascular supply to abnormal placenta disrupted, but may rupture as well

RISK FACTORS

- History of pelvic inflammatory disease (PID)
- History of tubal surgeries
- Previous ectopics
- Intrauterine device contraceptives
- Fertility drugs
- In vitro fertilization

SIGNS AND SYMPTOMS

Classic triad:
- Abdominal pain
- Vaginal bleeding
- Amenorrhea

Typical scenario:
A 29-year-old woman with history of PID presents due to abdominal pain and vaginal spotting. Her last menstrual period was 10 weeks ago. No intrauterine pregnancy (IUP) can be detected on ultrasonography. *Think: Ectopic pregnancy (EP).*

Spectrum anywhere from asymptomatic up to hemorrhagic shock

DIAGNOSIS

β-hCG

- Sensitivity of pregnancy tests: Urine positive > 20 mIU/mL
- Serum normal pregnancy—β-hCG doubles every 2 days
- Ectopic pregnancy—β-hCG increases ~⅔ every 2 days

Progesterone in the Presence of Classic Triad

- < 5 ng/mL highly suggestive of EP
- > 25 ng/mL highly suggestive of IUP

Ultrasound

- Used to establish presence or absence of IUP (Figure 13-1)
- Presence of echogenic adnexal mass and pelvic free fluid is highly suggestive of EP (Figure 13-2).
- Can usually visualize IUP (gestational sac) by transvaginal sonogram at β-hCG > 1,500 (approximately 5 weeks) and by transabdominal sonogram at 6,500
- Incidence of coexisting EP/IUP (heterotopic) is 1/30,000, but increases to 1/8,000 in women on fertility drugs.

IUP sono findings:
Fetal pole (β-hCG
~10,500 to 17,000)
Yolk sac (β-hCG ~7,500)

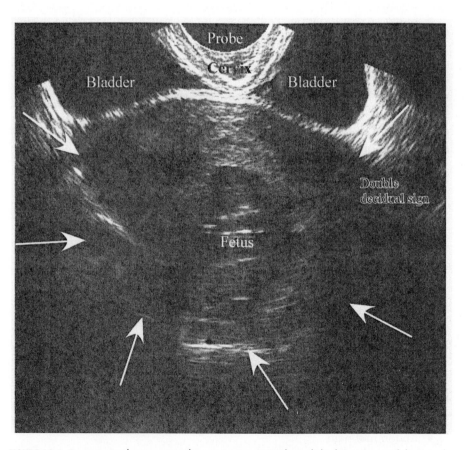

FIGURE 13-1. Transvaginal sonogram demonstrating IUP. The solid white arrows delineate the uterus.

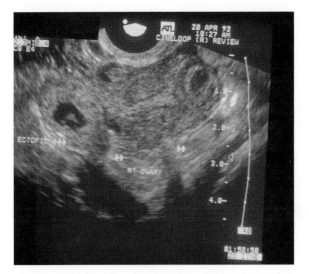

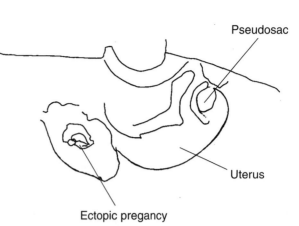

FIGURE 13-2. Transvaginal sonogram of an EP. Note the pseudosac, which lacks the double sign and the eccentric location of the "pregnancy" in relation to the uterus.

(Reproduced, with permission, from Knoop K, Stack LB, and Storrow AB. *Atlas of Emergency Medicine.* New York: McGraw-Hill, 1997: 261.)

TREATMENT

- Laparoscopy for nondiagnostic sonogram (if clinically suspicious for EP)
- Medical management: Methotrexate for termination
- Surgery for hemodynamic instability or if medical management not feasible

Hyperemesis Gravidarum

DEFINITION

- Syndrome of intractable nausea and vomiting in a pregnant woman
- Usually occurs early in pregnancy and resolves by end of first trimester

Eating small frequent meals and things such as toast and crackers may help the ease the nausea and vomiting and keep some food down.

TREATMENT

- Fluid and electrolyte abnormalities are common and should be replaced as indicated.
- Metoclopramide is class B and effective treatment for nausea and vomiting.

Rhesus (Rh) Isoimmunization

DEFINITION

Immunologic disorder that affects Rh-negative mothers of Rh-positive fetuses

PATHOPHYSIOLOGY

- Occurs with maternal exposure to fetal Rh-positive blood cells in the setting of transplacental hemorrhage (typically occurs during delivery, may also occur with abortions and trauma)
- Initial exposure leads to primary sensitization with production of immunoglobulin M antibodies.

245

- In subsequent pregnancies, maternal immunoglobulin G antibody crosses placenta and attacks Rh-positive fetal RBCs.

PREVENTION

- Prevention of Rh isoimmunization is by administering Rh_o immune globulin (RhoGAM) to mothers during time of potential antigen exposure (amniocentesis, threatened abortion, trauma, delivery, etc.).
- RhoGAM is also administered prophylactically to all Rh-negative mothers ~28 weeks' gestation.

Threatened Abortion

DEFINITION

Abdominal pain or vaginal bleeding in first 20 weeks' gestation

SIGNS AND SYMPTOMS

- Closed cervix
- No passage of fetal tissue by history or exam

DIAGNOSIS

β-hCG and ultrasound to confirm IUP and rule out EP

TREATMENT

- Bed rest for 24 hours
- Avoid intercourse, tampons, and douching until bleeding stops.
- Arrange outpatient follow-up for repeat β-hCG/sonogram in 24 to 48 hours.
- Rh isoimmunization prophylaxis as needed

Inevitable Abortion

DEFINITION

Vaginal bleeding with open cervical os but no passage of fetal products

TREATMENT

- Dilation and curettage (D&C, evacuation of pregnancy)
- Rh isoimmunization as needed

Incomplete Abortion

DEFINITION

Incomplete passage of fetal products

SIGNS AND SYMPTOMS

- Open cervical os
- Pain and bleeding

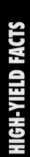

First-trimester vaginal bleeding occurs in approximately 40% of first-time pregnancies, one half of which will eventually result in miscarriage.

HIGH-YIELD FACTS

Obstetric Emergencies

246

TREATMENT

- D&C
- Rh isoimmunization prophylaxis as needed

Complete Abortion

DEFINITION

Complete passage of fetal products and placenta

SIGNS AND SYMPTOMS

- Closed cervical os
- Uterus contracts
- Pregnancy-induced changes begin to resolve.

TREATMENT

- Supportive management with outpatient follow-up for ultrasound-confirmed complete abortion
- D&C if unsure all products have been passed
- Rh isoimmunization prophylaxis as needed

Septic Abortion

DEFINITION

Uterine infection during any stage of an abortion

CAUSES

Bowel and genital flora are most often implicated.

SIGNS AND SYMPTOMS

- Fever
- Bleeding
- Cramping pain
- Purulent discharge from cervix
- Boggy, tender, enlarged uterus

TREATMENT

- Prompt evacuation
- Broad-spectrum antibiotics
- Rh isoimmunization prophylaxis as needed

Missed Abortion

DEFINITION

Uterine retention of dead fetal products for several weeks after abortion

SIGNS AND SYMPTOMS

May progress to spontaneous abortion with expulsion of products

TREATMENT

- D&C
- Rh isoimmunization prophylaxis as needed
- Complications may occur secondary to infection or coagulopathy.

THIRD-TRIMESTER BLEEDING (28+ WEEKS)

Abruptio Placentae

DEFINITION

Premature separation of normally implanted placenta from uterine wall (usually third trimester)

RISK FACTORS

- Previous abruptio placentae
- Abdominal trauma
- Hypertension
- Cocaine use
- Smoking
- Multiparity
- Advanced maternal age

Hypertension is the most common risk factor for abruptio placentae.

SIGNS AND SYMPTOMS

- Vaginal bleeding with dark clots
- Abdominal pain
- Uterine pain/irritability
- Uterus may be soft or very hard.

DIAGNOSIS

- Ultrasound is not useful in the diagnosis of abruptio placentae.

TREATMENT

- Emergent obstetrical consultation for maternal/fetal monitoring and possible delivery
- Rh isoimmunization prophylaxis as needed

COMPLICATIONS

- Fetal distress
- Diffuse intravascular coagulation
- Amniotic fluid embolism
- Maternal/fetal death

Placenta Previa

DEFINITION

Implantation of placenta overlying internal cervical os

RISK FACTORS

- Previous placenta previa
- Prior C-section
- Multiple gestations
- Multiple induced abortions
- Advanced maternal age

SIGNS AND SYMPTOMS

- Painless vaginal bleeding
- Soft, nontender uterus

DIAGNOSIS

Ultrasonography will confirm placental location.

TREATMENT

- Pelvic/cervical exam is *not* performed in the emergency department, as this can precipitate massive bleeding. It is done in the operating room where emergency C-section can be performed if massive bleeding does occur.
- Emergent obstetrical consultation for maternal/fetal monitoring and possible delivery
- Rh isoimmunization prophylaxis as needed

PREGNANCY-INDUCED HYPERTENSION

Defined as BP > 140/90, increase in systolic BP > 20, or increase in diastolic BP > 10

Preeclampsia and Eclampsia

DEFINITIONS

- Preeclampsia is a syndrome of hypertension, proteinuria, and generalized edema that occurs in weeks 20 to 24 of pregnancy.
- Eclampsia is preeclampsia plus seizures.

RISK FACTORS

- Primigravida
- Very young or advanced maternal age
- History of hypertension or kidney disease
- Diabetes mellitus
- Hydatidiform mole
- Multiple gestations
- Family history of pregnancy-induced hypertension

SIGNS AND SYMPTOMS

- Weight gain > 5 lbs/wk
- Headache, visual disturbances
- Peripheral edema
- Pulmonary edema
- Oliguria

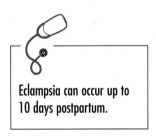

Eclampsia can occur up to 10 days postpartum.

HELLP *syndrome complicates ~10% of preeclampsia:* **H**emolysis, **E**levated **L**iver enzymes, **L**ow **P**latelets

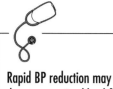

DIAGNOSIS

Diagnostic Triad
- Hypertension as defined above
- Proteinuria > 300 mg/24 hr
- Generalized edema

Laboratory Findings
- Elevated uric acid, serum creatinine, liver function tests, and bilirubin
- Thrombocytopenia

TREATMENT

- Absolute bed rest
- Left lateral decubitus position to increase blood flow to uterus
- Hydralazine for BP control (labetalol for refractory cases)
- Magnesium sulfate for seizure and secondary BP control (phenytoin or diazepam for refractory cases). Watch for signs of magnesium toxicity.
- Maintain urine output at 30 cc/hr, as many of the drugs used are cleared through the kidney.
- Definitive treatment is delivery of the fetus.

HYDATIDIFORM MOLE

Definition

- "Molar pregnancy" secondary to overproduction of chorionic villi
- Partial mole: Triploid (two sets paternal, one maternal), presence of fetal parts, higher tendency to progress to choriocarcinoma
- Complete mole: Diploid (two sets maternal), absence of fetal parts

RISK FACTORS

- Previous history of molar pregnancy
- Very young or advanced maternal age

SIGNS AND SYMPTOMS

- Severe nausea and vomiting
- Uterus larger than expected for dates
- Passage of grapelike clusters of vesicles through vagina
- Intermittent vaginal bleeding during early pregnancy
- Preeclampsia before 20 weeks' gestation

DIAGNOSIS

- Anemia
- β-hCG higher than expected
- Snowstorm appearance on ultrasound (Figure 13-3)

TREATMENT

- D&C
- Follow-up to monitor for choriocarcinoma

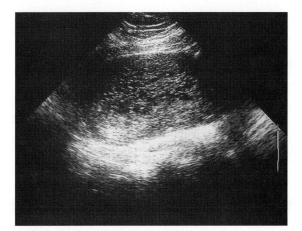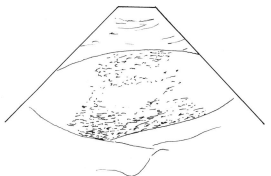

FIGURE 13-3. Sonogram of a hydatidiform mole.
(Reproduced, with permission, from Pearlman MD, Tintinalli JE, eds. *Emergency Care of the Woman.* New York: McGraw-Hill, 1998: 657.)

NORMAL LABOR AND DELIVERY

- Progressive cervical effacement and/or dilatation in the presence of uterine contractions occurring < 5 minutes apart and lasting 30 to 60 seconds at a time (Table 13-1)
- "False" labor—during last 4 to 8 weeks of pregnancy, contractions (Braxton Hicks) occur in the absence of cervical dilatation or effacement.

First Stage

- Starts with onset of labor, ends with complete dilatation (10 cm) of cervix
- "Latent" phase—effacement with minimal dilatation
- "Active" phase—accelerated rate of cervical dilatation

Second Stage

- Starts with complete cervical dilatation, ends with delivery of baby
- Six cardinal movements of labor: Descent, flexion, internal rotation, extension, external rotation, expulsion

TABLE 13-1. Duration of the Stages of Labor

	Primiparous	Multiparous
First stage	6–18 hours	2–10 hours
Cervical dilatation (active phase)	1.0 cm/hr	1.2 cm/hr
Second stage	0.5–3.0 hours	5–20 minutes
Third stage	0–30 minutes	0–30 minutes
Fourth stage	~1 hour	~1 hour

Third Stage

- Starts with delivery of baby, ends with delivery of placenta
- Assess external genitalia for signs of perineal/rectal tears.

Fourth Stage

- Starts with delivery of placenta, ends with stabilization of mother
- Monitor for hemodynamic instability and postpartum hemorrhage.

Premature Rupture of Membranes (PROM)

DEFINITION

Rupture of fetal membranes before labor begins

SIGNS AND SYMPTOMS

Leakage of amniotic fluid prior to onset of labor at any stage of gestation

DIAGNOSIS

- Pooling of amniotic fluid in vaginal fornix
- Nitrazine paper test: Turns blue in presence of amniotic fluid (false positive seen with use of lubricant)
- Ferning pattern on microscopic paper (false negative seen with blood) (Figure 13-4)

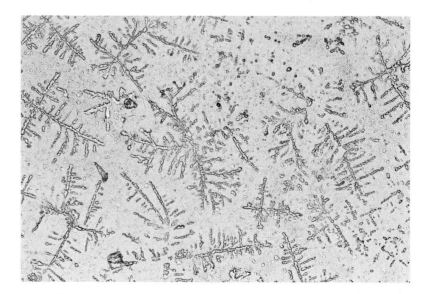

FIGURE 13-4. "Ferning" pattern of amniotic fluid when exposed to air. Can be useful for diagnosing PROM.

(Reproduced, with permission, from Knoop K, Stack LB, and Storrow AB. *Atlas of Emergency Medicine.* New York: McGraw-Hill, 1997: 265.)

- If fetus > 37 weeks, delivery within 24 hours
- If fetus < 37 weeks, timing of delivery is weighed against risks of fetal immaturity.

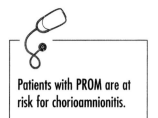

Patients with PROM are at risk for chorioamnionitis.

Preterm Labor

DEFINITION

Defined as labor occurring after 20 weeks' and before 37 weeks' gestation

DIAGNOSIS

Diagnosed by regular uterine contractions in the presence of cervical dilatation/effacement

TREATMENT

- Hydration and bed rest (successful in ~20% cases)
- Glucocorticoids (Celestone) to accelerate fetal lung maturity
- Tocolysis with magnesium sulfate, beta blockers (terbutaline, ritodrine), and prostaglandin synthetase inhibitors (indomethacin)
- Contraindications to tocolysis:
  - Severe preeclampsia
  - Severe bleeding from placenta previa or abruptio placentae
  - Chorioamnionitis

Strategies for Assessing Potential Fetal Distress

1. Assess for short-term (beat-to-beat) and long-term variability of fetal heart rate (normal).
2. Assess for response of fetal heart rate to uterine contractions:
   - Accelerations are a normal response to uterine contractions.
   - Early decelerations are usually related to head compression (normal).
   - Variable decelerations may be related to intermittent cord compression.
   - Late decelerations are often related to uteroplacental insufficiency.
3. Fetal tachycardia may be a sign of maternal fever or intrauterine infections.
4. Presence of "heavy" meconium in amniotic fluid increases risk of aspiration.

POSTPARTUM COMPLICATIONS

Postpartum Hemorrhage

DEFINITION

- Classified as early (within 24 hours of delivery) or late (up to 1 to 2 weeks postpartum)
- > 500 mL blood loss (vaginal delivery) or 1,000 mL (cesarean delivery)

HIGH-YIELD FACTS

Obstetric Emergencies

CAUSES OF EARLY POSTPARTUM HEMORRHAGE

- **Uterine atony:** Most common cause (overdistended uterus, prolonged labor, oxytocin use)
- **Genital tract trauma:** Vaginal or rectal lacerations
- **Retained products of conception:** Acts as a wedge preventing uterine contractions, leading to increased bleeding
- **Uterine inversion:** Uterus turns inside out, leading to vasodilatation and increased bleeding

CAUSES OF LATE POSTPARTUM HEMORRHAGE

- Endometritis
- Retained products of conception

SIGNS AND SYMPTOMS

- Vaginal bleeding
- Soft, atonic uterus

TREATMENT

- Repair any lacerations.
- Manually remove placenta if it does not pass.
- Bimanual massage and/or intravenous oxytocin to stimulate uterine contractions
- Metyhylergonovine for refractory cases

Endometritis

DEFINITION

Infection of the endometrium

CAUSES

Majority of infections are caused by normal vaginal/cervical flora (enterococci, streptococci, anaerobes).

SIGNS AND SYMPTOMS

- Fever
- Tender, swollen uterus
- Foul-smelling lochia

DIFFERENTIAL

In patients who do not respond to antibiotic therapy, consider:
- Pelvic abscess (requires surgical drainage)
or
- Pelvic thrombophlebitis (requires anticoagulation)

TREATMENT

- Broad-spectrum antibiotics
- Hospitalization

Musculoskeletal Emergencies

SPRAINS AND STRAINS

DEFINITIONS

Sprain
- A partial or complete rupture of the fibers of a ligament
- First degree: Joint is stable; integrity of the ligament is maintained with a few fibers torn.
- Second degree: Joint stability is maintained but ligamentous function is decreased.
- Third degree: Joint instability with complete tearing of ligament

Strain
- A partial or complete rupture of the fibers of the muscle–tendon junction
- First degree: Mild
- Second degree: Moderate, associated with a weakened muscle
- Third degree: Complete tear of the muscle–tendon junction with severe pain and inability to contract the involved muscle

ETIOLOGY

Trauma: Indirect or direct, causing the ligaments of any joint to stretch beyond their elastic limit

SIGNS AND SYMPTOMS
- Pain and swelling over area involved
- Patient may have experienced a snap or pop at time of injury.

TREATMENT

For First- and Most Second-Degree Sprains
- Rest, ice, compression, and elevation for 24 to 36 hours ("RICE" therapy)
- Weight bearing as tolerated in the case of lower extremity sprain
- Pressure dressing can also be applied.
- Crutches as needed
- Orthopedic follow-up is not always necessary.
- Analgesia (e.g., ibuprofen—to be taken with food to decrease gastric irritation)

RICE *therapy:*
Rest
Ice
Compression (splint)
Elevation

For Third-Degree Sprains
- Splint that prevents range of motion (ROM) of joint
- Crutches: Provide non–weight-bearing status in lower extremity injuries
- RICE and pain medications
- Orthopedic follow-up for appropriate treatment, which usually includes operative repair in the young

General Complications of Orthopedic Trauma

- Compartment syndrome (see below)
- Rhabdomyolysis
- Malunion
- Nonunion
- Avascular necrosis (AVN) (see below)
- Fat embolism (especially with fracture of long bone)
- Hemorrhage (especially with pelvic fracture)
- Neurovascular injury

Compartment Syndrome

DEFINITION

- Compartment syndrome results when the pressure in a compartment exceeds the arterial perfusion pressure.
- This normally occurs at pressures > 20 mm Hg.
- It occurs at lower pressures when the arterial pressure is lower than normal, such as in prolonged systemic shock.
- The excess compartment pressure causes muscle and nerve necrosis due to ischemia.

ANATOMY

Major compartments include:
- Hand: Associated with crush injury
- Forearm: Associated with supracondylar fracture of the humerus
- Thigh: Associated with crush injury
- Leg: Associated with tibial fracture
- Foot: Associated with calcaneus fracture

RISK FACTORS

- Crush injuries
- Circumferential burns
- Constrictive devices (military antishock trousers suit, casts, clothing)
- Hemorrhage
- Edema
- Patients with altered mental status who cannot report compartment pain

Compartment syndrome is most common in the lower extremity.

High-Yield Facts

Musculoskeletal Emergencies

Signs and Symptoms

Earlier Findings
- Pain out of proportion to the injury
- Pain with passive flexion
- Decreased two-point sensory discrimination
- Paresthesia or hypesthesia
- Tenseness of compartment

Late Findings
- Pallor of skin
- Absence of pulses
- Cold extremity

Diagnosis

Made by measuring compartment pressure, which can be done with a commercial device (the Stryker®) or with an 18G needle connected to a manometer and a water piston via a three-way stopcock

Treatment

- Remove any constricting devices.
- Fasciotomy for pressures > 30 mm Hg

AVN of the Hip

Etiology

- The medial and lateral circumflex arteries supply the femoral head and then circle closely around the head of the femur, rendering them vulnerable.
- These arteries may become occluded as in sickle cell disease or during immobilization.
- AVN is also frequently a complication following fractures of the neck of the femur or dislocation of the head.
- It may occur at any time postop up to 20 years later.

Signs and Symptoms

- Aching of joint early on
- Difficulty sitting for prolonged periods
- Weakness of hip
- Limp

Diagnosis

- Radiographs may not show signs of the disease until it is more advanced so that the femoral head has started to flatten and become irregularly shaped.
- Later films show evidence of osteoarthritis (OA).

Treatment

- In less severe cases, physical therapy can provide a strengthening and mobility program and assistive devices for protective weight bearing.

6 Ps *of compartment syndrome:*
Pain
Paresthesia (most reliable)
Paralysis
Pallor
Pulselessness
Poikilothermia

The presence of pulses does *not* rule out compartment syndrome.

257

- More severe cases require total hip replacement followed by physical therapy.
- There is a worse prognosis in older patients compared to the young who are still growing.

Anterior Shoulder Dislocation

ETIOLOGY

Forcible external rotation and abduction of the arm

SIGNS AND SYMPTOMS

- Shoulder pain
- Patient maintains shoulder in elevated position.
- Difficulty with internal rotation of arm
- Axillary nerve palsy:
    - Decreased sensation over deltoid
    - Decreased ability to abduct shoulder

DIAGNOSIS

See Figure 14-1.

TREATMENT

- Closed reduction under conscious sedation
- Sling and swathe for 4 weeks

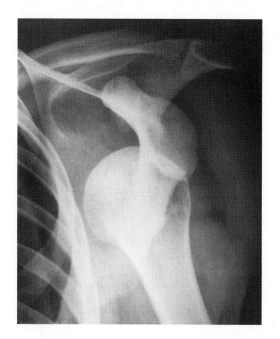

FIGURE 14-1. Anterior shoulder dislocation.

(Reproduced, with permission, from Schwartz DT, Reisdorff EJ. *Emergency Radiology.* New York: McGraw-Hill, 2000: 109.)

- ROM exercises
- Surgical repair for nonreducible dislocations

COMPLICATIONS

Associated fractures (occur about 40% of the time):
- Bankart: Fracture of glenoid margin
- Hill–Sachs: Fracture of humeral head

Posterior Shoulder Dislocation

RISK FACTORS

- Lightening injury
- Seizures

SIGNS AND SYMPTOMS

Arm is internally rotated and adducted.

DIAGNOSIS

- Lightbulb sign: Lightbulb appearance of internally rotated proximal humerus (Figure 14-2)

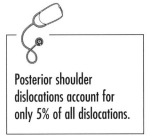

Posterior shoulder dislocations account for only 5% of all dislocations.

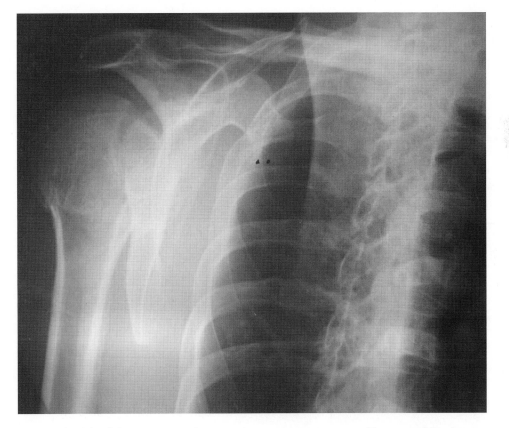

FIGURE 14-2. Posterior shoulder dislocation. Note the "ice cream cone sign," so named because of the characteristic appearance of the neck and head of the humerus.

(Reproduced, with permission, from Simon RR, Koenigsknecht SJ. *Emergency Orthopedics: The Extremities,* 4th ed. New York: McGraw-Hill, 2001: 325.)

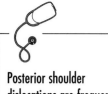

Posterior shoulder dislocations are frequently missed. Surgical fixation is necessary when the diagnosis is delayed for 2 weeks or more.

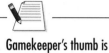

Gamekeeper's thumb is commonly associated with ski pole injury.

Carpal tunnel syndrome is the most common entrapment neuropathy.

TREATMENT

- Closed reduction under conscious sedation
- Sling and swathe for 4 weeks
- ROM exercises
- Surgical repair for nonreducible dislocations

Gamekeeper's Thumb

DEFINITION

- Avulsion of ulnar collateral ligament of first metacarpophalangeal (MCP) joint (Figure 14-3)

ETIOLOGY

- Forced abduction of the thumb
- Can be associated with an avulsion fracture of the metacarpal base

SIGNS AND SYMPTOMS

Inability to pinch

DIAGNOSIS

Application of valgus stress to thumb while MCP joint is flexed will demonstrate laxity of ulnar collateral ligament.

TREATMENT

- Rest, ice, elevation, analgesia
- Thumb spica cast for 3 to 6 weeks for partial tears
- Surgical repair for complete tears

Carpal Tunnel Syndrome

DEFINITION

Compression of the median nerve, resulting in pain along the distribution of the nerve

FIGURE 14-3. Gamekeeper's thumb.

(Reproduced, with permission, from Scaletta TA, et al. *Emergent Management of Trauma.* New York: McGraw-Hill, 1996: 220.)

ETIOLOGY

- Tumor (fibroma, lipoma)
- Ganglion cyst
- Tenosynovitis of flexor tendons due to rheumatoid arthritis (RA) or trauma
- Edema due to pregnancy or thyroid or amyloid disease
- Trauma to carpal bones
- Gout

RISK FACTORS

Repetitive hand movements

EPIDEMIOLOGY

More common in women 3:1

SIGNS AND SYMPTOMS

- Pain and paresthesia of volar aspect of thumb, digits 2 and 3, and half of digit 4
- Activity and palmar flexion aggravate symptoms.
- Thenar atrophy: Uncommon, but irreversible and indicates severe long-standing compression
- Sensory deficit (two-point discrimination > 5 mm)

DIAGNOSIS

- Tinel's sign: Tapping over median nerve at wrist produces pain and paresthesia. (See Figure 14-4.)
- Phalen's test: One minute of maximal palmar flexion produces pain and paresthesia. (See Figure 14-4.)
- Consider erythrocyte sedimentation rate (ESR), thyroid function tests, serum glucose, and uric acid level to look for underlying cause.

Typical scenario:
A 37-year-old woman presents with pain in her right wrist and fingers, accompanied by a tingling sensation. The pain awakens her from sleep, and she is unable to perform her duties as a word processor. *Think: Carpal tunnel syndrome*

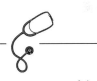

Twenty to 50% of the population normally have a positive Phalen's test and Tinel's sign.

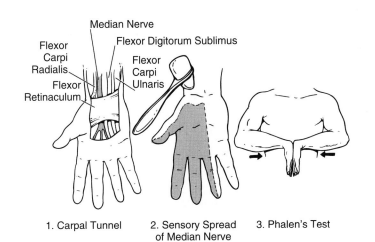

1. Carpal Tunnel   2. Sensory Spread of Median Nerve   3. Phalen's Test

FIGURE 14-4. Carpal tunnel syndrome. **1.** The flexor retinaculum in the wrist compresses the median nerve to produce hyperesthesia in the radial 3.5 digits. **2.** Tinel's sign: Percussion on the radial side of the palmaris longus tendon produces tingling in the 3.5 digit region. **3.** Phalen's test: Hyperflexion of the wrist for 60 seconds may produce pain in the median nerve distribution, which is relieved by extension of the wrist.

(Reproduced, with permission, from DeGowin RL, Brown DD. *DeGowin's Diagnostic Examination,* 7th ed. New York: McGraw-Hill, 2000: 720.)

TREATMENT

- Treat underlying condition.
- Rest and splint.
- NSAIDs for analgesia
- Surgery for crippling pain, thenar atrophy, and failure of nonoperative management

Ganglion Cyst

DEFINITION

A synovial cyst, usually present on radial aspect of wrist

ETIOLOGY

Idiopathic

SIGNS AND SYMPTOMS

- Presence of mass that patient cannot account for
- May or may not be painful
- Pain aggravated by extreme flexion or extension
- Size of ganglia increases with increased use of wrist.
- Compression of median or ulnar nerve may occur (not common).

DIAGNOSIS

Radiographs to ascertain diagnosis; since a ganglion cyst is a soft-tissue problem only, no radiographic changes should be noted.

TREATMENT

- Reassurance for most cases
- Wrist immobilization for moderate pain
- Aspiration of cyst for severe pain
- Surgical excision for cases involving median nerve compression and cosmetically unacceptable ganglia

> Differential diagnosis includes bone tumor, arthritis, and intraosseous ganglion.

Mallet Finger

DEFINITION

Rupture of extensor tendon at its insertion into base of distal phalanx (Figure 14-5)

ETIOLOGY

- Avulsion fracture of distal phalanx
- Other trauma

SIGNS AND SYMPTOMS

Inability to extend distal interphalangeal (DIP) joint

TREATMENT

- Splint finger in extension for 6 to 8 weeks.
- Surgery may be required for large avulsions of distal phalanx and for injuries that were not splinted early.

> If left untreated, mallet finger results in permanent boutonniere deformity.

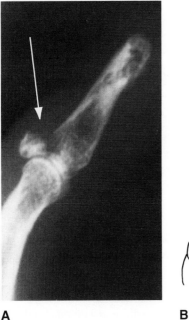

A   **B**

FIGURE 14-5. Mallet finger. **A.** Radiograph of an avulsion fracture of the base of the distal phalanx (arrow), which is often associated with mallet finger. **B.** Avulsion of the extensor tendon.

(Reproduced, with permission, from Schwartz DT, Reisdorff EJ. *Emergency Radiology.* New York: McGraw-Hill, 2000: 40.)

Trigger Finger

DEFINITION

Stenosis of tendon sheath flexor digitorum leading to nodule formation within the sheath

RISK FACTORS

- RA
- Middle-aged women
- Congenital

SIGNS AND SYMPTOMS

Snapping sensation or click when flexing and extending the digit (Figure 14-6)

FIGURE 14-6. Trigger finger. Usually involves third or fourth digit. Flexion is normal, but extension involves a painful "snap."

(Reproduced, with permission, from DeGowin RL, Brown DD. *DeGowin's Diagnostic Examination,* 7th ed. New York: McGraw-Hill, 2000: 701.)

TREATMENT

- Splinting of MCP joint in extension
- Injection of corticosteroid into tendon sheath
- Surgical repair if above fail

See Table 14-1 for more upper extremity problems.

TABLE 14-1. Common Hand and Wrist Injuries

Injury	Description	Treatment

Boxer's fracture	Fracture of neck of fifth metacarpal sustained in a closed fist injury	■ Thumb spica cast for 3–6 weeks for partial tears
		■ Surgical repair for:
		  ■ Any rotational deformity
		  ■ Angulation of fourth/fifth metacarpal > 40°
		  ■ Angulation of second/third metacarpal > 10°–15°

Bennett's fracture	Fracture–dislocation of base of thumb	■ Initially immobilization in thumb spica cast ■ Definitive treatment is with surgical fixation.
Rolando's fracture	Comminuted fracture of the base of the thumb	■ Initially immobilization in thumb spica cast ■ Definitive treatment is with surgical fixation.
Scaphoid fracture	■ Most commonly caused by fall on outstretched hand ■ Snuffbox tenderness is classic.	■ Immobilization in thumb spica cast with wrist in neutral position for 12 weeks ■ May take up to 2 weeks to be seen on radiographs

Colles' fracture	■ Distal radius fracture with dorsal angulation
	■ Most commonly caused by fall on outstretched hand
	■ "Dinner fork deformity" is classic.
		■ Short arm cast 4–6 weeks with volar flexion and ulnar deviation
		■ Surgical repair for:
		  ■ Open fracture
		  ■ Comminuted fracture
		  ■ Intra-articular displaced fracture > 5 mm

Smith's fracture	■ Distal radius fracture with volar angulation ■ Most commonly caused by direct trauma to dorsal forearm	■ Surgical repair needed for most cases
Galeazzi's fracture	■ Distal one third radial fracture with dislocation of distal radioulnar joint ■ Commonly caused by fall on outstretched hand with forearm in forced pronation or direct blow to back of wrist	■ Surgical repair needed for most cases
Monteggia's fracture	■ Proximal one third ulnar fracture with dislocation of the radial head ■ Commonly caused by fall on outstretched hand with forearm in forced pronation or direct blow to posterior ulna ■ May note injury of radial nerve	■ Surgical repair for adults ■ Closed reduction for children (children can tolerate a greater degree of displacement)

Nightstick fracture	■ Isolated fracture of the ulnar shaft	■ Long arm cast for 3–6 weeks
		■ Surgical repair for:
		  ■ Angulation > 10°
		  ■ Displacement > 50%

See Table 14-2 for lower extremity problems.

TABLE 14-2. Common Lower Extremity Injuries

Injury	Description	Treatment
Lisfranc fracture	▪ Fracture through base of second metatarsal ▪ The second metatarsal is the stabilizing force of the tarsometatarsal joint.	▪ Surgical fixation (can be open or closed)

Maisonneuve fracture	▪ Malleolar (ankle) and proximal fibula fracture with disruption of the medial deltoid ligament	▪ Long leg cast for 6–12 weeks
		▪ Surgical fixation for:
		  ▪ Medial malleolar fracture
		  ▪ Widened medial joint space

Baker's cyst	▪ Cyst in the medial popliteal fossa ▪ Associated with arthritis and joint trauma ▪ Rupture of cyst can mimic symptoms of deep vein thrombosis.	▪ Treat underlying cause (adults). ▪ Symptomatic relief with NSAIDs
Calcaneal fracture	▪ Most frequently injured foot bone ▪ Usually occurs due to fall from a height with patient landing on his feet	▪ Posterior splint for nondisplaced fractures ▪ Surgical repair for displaced fractures
Jones fracture	▪ Fracture of diaphysis of fifth metatarsal ▪ Usually occurs due to force applied to ball of foot, as in pivoting or dancing	▪ Short leg cast for nondisplaced fractures ▪ Surgical repair for displaced fractures

INFECTIONS

Felon

DEFINITION

Infection of the pulp space of any of the distal phalanges (Figure 14-7)

ETIOLOGY

Caused by minor trauma to the dermis over the finger pad

COMPLICATIONS

Results in increased pressure within the septal compartments and may lead to cellulitis, flexor tendon sheath infection, or osteomyelitis if not effectively treated

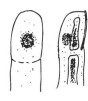

FIGURE 14-7. Felon (infection of pulp space).
(Reproduced, with permission, from DeGowin RL, Brown DD. *DeGowin's Diagnostic Examination.* 7th ed. New York: McGraw-Hill, 2000: 703.)

TREATMENT

- Using a digital block, perform incision and drainage with longitudinal incision over the area of greatest induration but not over the flexor crease of the DIP.
- A drain may be placed and the wound checked in 2 days.
- 7- to 10-day course of antibiotics: Usually first-generation cephalosporin or anti-*Staphylococcus* penicillin

Paronychia

DEFINITION

Infection of the lateral nail fold (Figure 14-8)

ETIOLOGY

Caused by minor trauma such as nail biting or manicures

TREATMENT

- Without fluctuance, this may be treated with a 7-day course of antibiotics, warm soaks, and retraction of the skin edges from the nail margin.
- For more extensive infections, unroll the skin at the base of the nail and at the lateral nail or incise and drain at area of most fluctuance using a digital block.
- Pus below the nailbed may require partial or total removal of the nail.
- Advise patient to do warm soaks and return for wound check in 2 days.
- Antibiotics are usually not necessary unless area is cellulitic.

Tenosynovitis

DEFINITION

- This is a surgical emergency requiring prompt identification.
- Infection of the flexor tendon and sheath is caused by penetrating trauma and dirty wounds (i.e., dog bite).
- Infection spreads along the tendon sheath, allowing involvement of other digits and even the entire hand, causing significant disability.

ETIOLOGY

- Polymicrobial
- *Staphylococcus* most common
- *Neisseria gonorrhoeae* with history of sexually transmitted disease

FIGURE 14-8. Paronychia.

(Reproduced, with permission, from DeGowin RL, Brown DD. *DeGowin's Diagnostic Examination,* 7th ed. New York: McGraw-Hill, 2000: 703.)

SIGNS AND SYMPTOMS

Kanavel criteria:
- Digit is flexed at rest.
- Passive extension produces pain.
- Symmetrical swelling of finger
- Tenderness over flexor tendon sheath

TREATMENT

- Immobilize and elevate hand.
- Immediate consultation with hand surgeon
- Intravenous (IV) antibiotics

Cellulitis

DEFINITION

A local erythematous inflammatory reaction of the subcutaneous tissue following a cutaneous breach, which leads to infection

ETIOLOGY

- *Streptococcus pyogenes* (most common)
- *Staphylococcus*
- *Haemophilus influenzae* in unimmunized individuals
- Enterobacteriaceae in diabetics

SIGNS AND SYMPTOMS

- Localized tenderness and swelling
- Warmth
- Erythema
- If immunocompromised, may see fever and leukocytosis

TREATMENT

- For uncomplicated cellulitis in healthy individuals, cephalexin or dicloxacillin 500 mg qid × 10 days or azithromycin 500 mg × 1, then 250 mg qd × 4 days
- IV antibiotics for head and face involvement and the immunocompromised: Cefazolin 1 g IV qid and nafcillin or oxacillin 2 g IV q4h. Ceftriaxone or imipenem for severe cases.

Gas Gangrene

ETIOLOGY

A life- and limb-threatening soft-tissue infection caused by one of the spore-forming *Clostridium* spp., resulting in myonecrosis, gas production, and sepsis

ORGANISM

- *Clostridium perfringens* (80 to 90%)
- *Clostridium septicum*
- These are spore-forming G+ anaerobic bacilli found in soil, gastrointestinal tract, and female genitourinary tract.

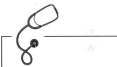

PATHOPHYSIOLOGY

- Dirty wounds with jagged edges become infected with the ubiquitous organism that produces exotoxins.
- These cause systemic toxicity and cellular destruction.
- Bacteremia is rare.

SIGNS AND SYMPTOMS

- 3-day incubation period
- Patient complains of **pain out of proportion** to physical findings.
- Limb feels heavy.
- Skin becomes discolored (brown).
- Crepitance
- Fever
- Tachycardia
- Diabetics are particularly susceptible due to immunocompromise (impaired white blood cell [WBC] chemotaxis), peripheral neuropathy (delaying detection of small wounds), and impaired peripheral perfusion.

DIAGNOSIS

- Metabolic acidosis
- Leukocytosis
- Myoglobinuria, myoglobinemia
- Coagulopathy
- Elevated creatine phosphokinase (CPK)
- Gas in soft-tissue planes on radiograph

TREATMENT

- Fluid resuscitation, may require transfusion
- Monitor intake and output.
- Antibiotics: Penicillin G or clindamycin; metronidazole or chloramphenicol if penicillin allergic
- Surgical debridement is definitive treatment.
- Hyperbaric O_2 has been shown to help.

Septic Arthritis

DEFINITION

Infection of joint space

ETIOLOGY

- Neonates: *Staphylococcus aureus*, group B strep
- Children and adolescents: *S. aureus*
- Adults < 50: *N. gonorrhea, S. aureus*
- Adults > 50: *S. aureus, E. coli*
- IV drug users: *Pseudomonas aeruginosa*

EPIDEMIOLOGY

- Two peaks: In children and the elderly
- Males affected twice as often

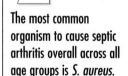

The most common organism to cause septic arthritis overall across all age groups is *S. aureus*.

RISK FACTORS

- RA
- OA
- Risky sexual behavior (*N. gonorrhoeae*)
- Immunocompromised states: Alcoholism, liver or kidney disease, diabetes, cancer

SIGNS AND SYMPTOMS

- Fever, chills
- Acute joint pain
- Joint stiffness
- Recent urethritis, salpingitis, or hemorrhagic vesicular skin lesions (*N. gonorrhoeae*)
- Maculopapular or vesicular rash (*N. gonorrhoeae*)
- Tenosynovitis → migratory polyarthritis → oligoarthritis (*N. gonorrhoeae*)
- Pain with passive motion of the involved joint
- Joint is warm, tender, and swollen, with evidence of effusion.

The most common joint involved is the knee, followed by hip, shoulder, and wrist.

DIAGNOSIS

- Via arthrocentesis (see Procedures chapter)
- A WBC count of 50,000 in the joint fluid with 75% granulocytosis is diagnostic.
- ESR and C-reactive protein often elevated, blood cultures usually positive
- Plain radiographs of joint should be obtained to look for underlying osteomyelitis or joint disease.
- If *N. gonorrhoeae* is suspected, culture the cervix, anus, and eye.

TREATMENT

- IV antibiotics
- Splinting of joint
- Analgesia
- Surgery recommended in children and for joints with loculated effusions
- Shoulder and hip septic arthritis are drained openly in the operating room due to risk of AVN.

Osteomyelitis

DEFINITION

Inflammation or infection of bone

ETIOLOGY

- *S. aureus*
- *Streptococcus* species
- *Pseudomonas aeruginosa* (especially in IV drug users and foot puncture wounds)

Patients with sickle cell disease and asplenism can get *Salmonella* osteomyelitis though *S. aureus* is still the most common cause.

EPIDEMIOLOGY

More common in males

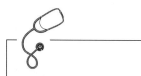

Typical scenario:
A 42-year-old male athlete steps on a nail through his sneaker. Two weeks later, he presents to the emergency department (ED) with pain and swelling of his left foot. *Think: Osteomyelitis due to Pseudomonas.*

It is important to differentiate osteomyelitis from septic joint, which is an emergency.

RISK FACTORS

- Trauma (including surgery)
- Immunocompromise (diabetes, sickle cell disease, alcoholism, etc.)
- Soft-tissue infection

SIGNS AND SYMPTOMS

- Pain, swelling, and warmth of bone or joint
- Decreased ROM
- Fever

DIAGNOSIS

- Bone scan will detect osteomyelitis within 48 hours.
- Radiograph will demonstrate periosteal elevation within 10 days. (See Figure 14-9.)
- Blood cultures will demonstrate causative organism in 50% of cases.

TREATMENT

- Antibiotics for 6 weeks (some bugs may need shorter courses)
- Splinting of joint

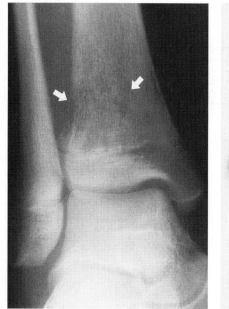
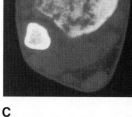

A   B   C

FIGURE 14-9. Osteomyelitis of the distal tibia. **A.** Plain film of tibia demonstrating slight lucency at arrow. **B.** Bone scan of the same tibia demonstrating increased uptake. **C.** Computed tomography scan (cross-section) demonstrating mottled appearance of the bony cortex.

(Reproduced, with premission, from Schwartz DT, Reisdorff EJ. *Emergency Radiology.* New York: McGraw-Hill, 2000: 23.)

Leading Causes of Lower Back Pain

- **F**racture
- **A**bdominal aortic aneurysm
- **C**auda equina syndrome
- **T**umor (cord compression)
- **O**ther (OA, severe musculoskeletal pain, other neurological syndromes)
- **I**nfection (e.g., epidural abscess)
- **D**isk herniation/rupture

Lumbar Disk Herniation

DEFINITION

- Disk herniation is a common cause of chronic lower back pain.
- L4–5 and L5–S1 are the most common sites affected.
- Herniation occurs when the nucleus pulposus prolapses through the annulus fibrosis.
- More common in men

SIGNS AND SYMPTOMS

- Limited spinal flexion
- Pain and paresthesia with a dermatomal distribution
- Specific signs depend on nerve root involved:
  - L4: Decreased knee jerk, weakness of anterior tibialis
  - L5: Weakness of extensor hallucis longus, decreased sensation over lateral aspect of calf and first web space
  - S1: Decreased ankle jerk, decreased plantar flexion, decreased sensation over lateral aspect of foot

Spondylolysis

DEFINITION

Defect or fracture of the pars interarticularis in the lumbar spine

ETIOLOGY

Possible etiology is a stress fracture that occurs during childhood that does not heal completely.

DIAGNOSIS

- Oblique view on radiograph will show a characteristic "Scotty dog with a collar" (Figure 14-10).
- Most often occurs at L4–5, L5–S1

TREATMENT

Rest, NSAIDs, possible bracing

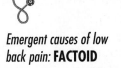

Emergent causes of low back pain: **FACTOID**

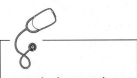

OA can lead to osteophytes and hypertrophy of spinal facets, which compress nerve roots.

The nucleus pulposus is a thick gel. Herniation of the nucleus pulposus is like toothpaste being squeezed out of the tube.

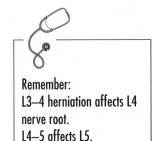

Remember:
L3–4 herniation affects L4 nerve root.
L4–5 affects L5.
L5–S1 affects S1.

HIGH-YIELD FACTS

Musculoskeletal Emergencies

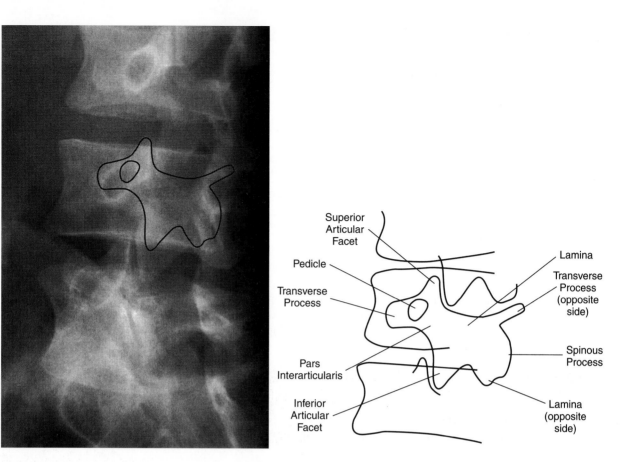

FIGURE 14-10. Normal lumbosacral spine with intact "Scotty dog."
(Reproduced, with permission, from Schwartz DT, Reisdorff EJ. *Emergency Radiology.* New York: McGraw-Hill, 2000: 344.)

Spondylolisthesis

Definition

- Forward displacement of one vertebra over another
- Usually occurs when spondylolysis is bilateral and becomes unstable

Diagnosis

- Oblique view on radiograph will show forward displacement of one vertebra with fracture at bilateral pars interarticularis or "Scotty dog decapitated."
- Felt as a stepoff when palpating the lumbar spine
- Most common at L4–5, L5–S1

Treatment

Orthopedic consultation, bracing

Vertebral Compression Fracture

- This is the most common manifestation of osteoporosis.
- It is also seen in patients on long-term steroids and in patients with lytic bony metastases.
- The thoracic spine is the most common site affected.

- Height loss
- Sudden back pain after mild trauma
- Local radiation of pain—the extremities are rarely affected (unlike a herniated disk)

DIAGNOSIS

Plain radiographs of lumbosacral spine will not show compression fracture until there is loss of 25 to 30% of bone height.

TREATMENT

- Symptomatic relief with NSAIDs
- Treatment of osteoporosis prevents compression fractures:
  - Recommend weight-bearing exercises
  - Estrogen replacement therapy
  - Calcium supplementation
  - Calcitonin (intramuscular) inhibits bone resorption.
  - Bisphosphonates increase bone mass by inhibiting osteoclast activity.

Epidural Abscess

- Spinal abscesses are most commonly found in the immunosuppressed, IV drug users, and the elderly.
- An abscess can form anywhere along the spinal cord, and as it expands, it compresses against the spinal cord and occludes the vasculature.

ETIOLOGY

- The infection is generally spread from the skin or other tissue.
- *Staphylococcus aureus,* gram-negative bacilli, and tuberculosis bacillus are the leading organisms involved.

SIGNS AND SYMPTOMS

- Triad of pain, fever, and progressive weakness
- The pain develops over the course of a week or two, and the fever is often accompanied by an elevated WBC count.

DIAGNOSIS AND TREATMENT

- Magnetic resonance imaging (MRI) can localize the lesion. Lumbar puncture is not required unless meningitis is suspected.
- Emergent decompressive laminectomy can prevent permanent sequelae. This should be followed up with long-term antibiotics.

Spinal Metastasis

- Metastatic lesions invade the spinal bone marrow, leading to compression of the spinal cord.
- Typically involves the thoracic spine
- The most common primary tumors involved include: Breast, lung, prostate, kidney, lymphoma, and multiple myeloma.

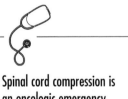

Bisphosphonates such as alendronate (Fosamax) irritate gastric mucosa, so advise patients to eat beforehand and stay upright for 30 minutes after taking it.

Spinal cord compression is an oncologic emergency. Missed diagnosis can lead to permanent paralysis.

SIGNS AND SYMPTOMS

- Pain is the primary symptom.
- Weakness and sensory loss follow.
- Upper motor neuron signs are seen:
  - Hyperreflexia
  - Upward Babinski sign

DIAGNOSIS

MRI is the preferred imaging technique.

TREATMENT

- Glucocorticoids are used to reduce inflammation and edema.
- Radiation therapy should be started as soon as possible.
- Surgery is indicated only if radiation fails to improve the symptoms.

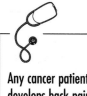

Any cancer patient who develops back pain should be investigated for spinal metastases.

Cauda Equina Syndrome

DEFINITION

Compression of the lumbar and sacral nerve roots that comprise the cauda equina

ETIOLOGY

- Tumor
- Midline disk herniations (rare)
- Congenital narrowing of the lumbar canal

SIGNS AND SYMPTOMS

- Typically present with *saddle anesthesia*
- Sensory and motor disturbances of the lower extremities can occur, as well as urinary and bladder incontinence.

Saddle anesthesia: Loss of sensation over the buttocks, perineum, and thighs. Frequently seen in cauda equina syndrome.

TREATMENT

- Bed rest on a hard surface and analgesia
- Neurosurgical evaluation for potential laminectomy

SYSTEMIC PROBLEMS

OA

DEFINITION

- OA is the result of mechanical and biological factors that destabilize articular cartilage and subchondral bone.
- There is softening, ulceration, and loss of articular cartilage, eburnation (sclerosis) of subchondral bone, osteophytes, and subchondral cysts.
- Cause is unclear but is probably multifactorial.

EPIDEMIOLOGY

- Most common form of arthritis
- Affects males and females equally

- Peak age is 45 to 55, but after 55 more common in women
- Fifty percent of people over 65 have radiographic changes in the knees.
- Obesity correlates with OA of the knees.
- Weight-bearing joints, including the lumbosacral spine, hips, knees, and feet, are most commonly involved.
- Cervical spine and proximal interphalangeal (PIP) and DIP joints are frequently involved.
- Elbows and shoulders are effected only when involved in trauma or overuse.

OA can cause morning stiffness but is usually short lived (in contrast to RA).

SIGNS AND SYMPTOMS

- Pain and stiffness in and around the joint
- Limitation of function
- Insidious onset
- Worse with activity, relieved by rest
- Worse in rainy, damp, and cool weather
- Gel phenomenon (stiffness after periods of rest) that resolves within several minutes
- Knee instability and buckling
- Hip-gait disturbance and pain in groin or radiation to anterior thigh and knee
- Hands: PIP (Bouchard's nodes) and DIP (Heberden's nodes) (Figure 14-11)
- Facet joints of cervical spine and lumbosacral spine cause neck and low back pain.

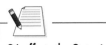

OA affects the Outer joints on the hand—the DIPs. RA affects the inner joints—MCPs and PIPs.

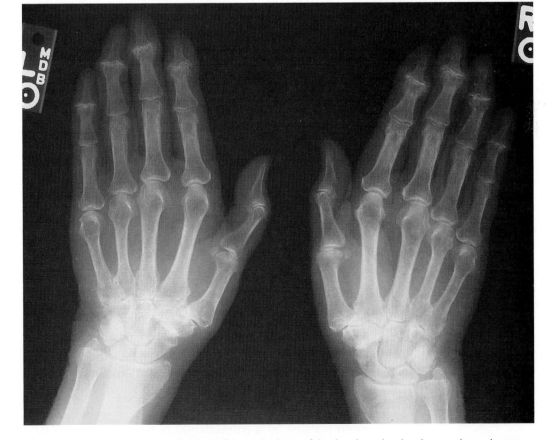

FIGURE 14-11. OA of the hands. Note the bony swelling at the base of the thumb and Heberden's nodes at the DIPs.

(Reproduced, with permission, from Simon RR, Koenigsknecht SJ. *Emergency Orthopedics: The Extremities,* 4th ed. New York: McGraw-Hill, 2001: 43.)

- Symptoms are localized, and limitation of function is secondary to osteophytes, cartilage loss, and muscle spasm.
- Locking of joint is secondary to loose bodies.
- Crepitation is present in 90%.

DIAGNOSIS

- Osteophytes and spurs at joint margin
- Asymmetric joint space narrowing
- Subchondral cysts and bone remodeling later on in the disease

TREATMENT

- Goals of treatment: Relieve symptoms, limit disability, improve function
- Physical and occupational therapy for ROM and strengthening exercises and providing assistive devices
- Weight loss
- Nonopioid analgesics (acetaminophen)
- NSAIDs
- Topical analgesics (capsaicin)
- Intra-articular steroid injections
- Surgical intervention: Arthroscopic debridement and lavage, osteotomy, and arthroplasty

RA

DEFINITION

- RA is a chronic, inflammatory, systemic disease that is manifested in the diarthrodial and peripheral joints.
- Etiology is still unknown; may be infectious.
- A combination of genetic and environmental factors control the progression.
- Disease process ranges from self-limited to progressively chronic with severe debilitation.

EPIDEMIOLOGY

- All ethnic groups affected; may be higher in Native Americans
- Worldwide distribution
- Affects all ages, prevalence increases with age, and peak incidence is between the fourth and sixth decades.
- Females affected more commonly than males
- Associated with HLA-DR4 and HLA-DRB1 genes

SIGNS AND SYMPTOMS

Common deformities:
- **Ulnar deviation** of the digits
- **Boutonniere's deformity**—hyperextension of the DIP and flexion of the PIP (Figure 14-2)
- **Swan's neck**—flexion of the DIP and extension of the PIP

DIAGNOSIS

- Diagnosis is based on a constellation of findings over several weeks to months or longer.
- Rheumatoid factor (RF) is present in 85% of patients.

- ESR correlates with the degree of inflammation and is useful in following the course of the disease.
- C-reactive protein can monitor inflammation.

CRITERIA FOR CLASSIFICATION OF RA

At least four of the following seven criteria must be present to diagnose RA; criteria 1 through 4 must have been present for ≥ 6 weeks.

1. Morning stiffness for ≥ 1 hour
2. Arthritis of ≥ three joint areas
3. Arthritis of hand joints (Figure 14-12)
4. Symmetric arthritis
5. Rheumatoid nodules
6. Positive serum RF
7. Radiographic changes: Erosions or bony decalcifications on posteroanterior hand and wrist

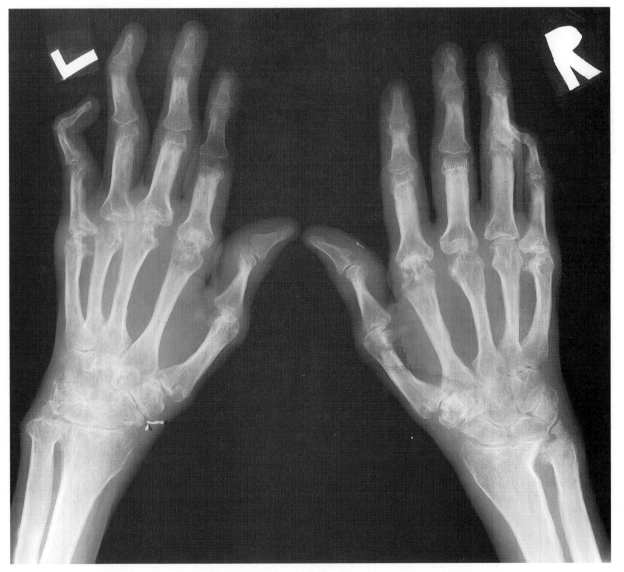

FIGURE 14-12. RA of the hands. Note inflammation and fusion of the PIP and metacarpointerphalangeal joints with relative sparing of the DIP joint, and the boutonniere deformities on the fifth digits.

(Reproduced, with permission, from Simon RR, Koenigsknecht SJ. *Emergency Orthopedics: The Extremities,* 4th ed. New York: McGraw-Hill, 2001: 50.)

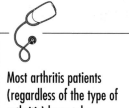

Most arthritis patients (regardless of the type of arthritis) have taken NSAIDs for long periods of time. This places them at high risk for ulcers.

TREATMENT

- Fifty percent of patients are refractory to treatment and display systemic disease.
- Physical and occupational therapy to maintain strength and flexibility and splinting of inflamed joints
- NSAIDs
- Corticosteroids
- Disease-modifying antirheumatic drugs: Gold compounds, hydroxychloroquine (Plaquenil) penicillamine, methotrexate, azathioprine (Imuran), sulfasalazine, cyclophosphamide (Cytoxan), cyclosporine

Gout

DEFINITION

A disorder in purine metabolism, resulting in the deposition of urate crystals in joint spaces, resulting in joint inflammation and exquisite pain

EPIDEMIOLOGY

Seen most commonly in middle-aged men

RISK FACTORS

- Age
- Hyperuricemia
- Alcohol consumption
- Drugs (e.g., thiazide diuretics)

The most common and frequent manifestation of gout is podagra.

SIGNS AND SYMPTOMS

- Acute onset of extreme pain in small joints, accompanied by redness and swelling
- **Tophi** are aggregates of gouty crystals and giant cells. They can erode away tissue.
- **Podagra** is inflammation of the first metatarsophalangeal joint, which presents in 50 to 75% of all patients as an exquisitely painful nodule on the medial aspect of the foot.

DIAGNOSIS

- Presence of **negatively birefringent crystals** in synovial fluid
- Elevated serum uric acid levels between attacks (may be low or normal during an acute attack)

TREATMENT

ED:
- Indomethacin to decrease inflammation is first line.
- Colchicine to inhibit chemotaxis is second line.

Outpatient:
- Allopurinol, a xanthine oxidase inhibitor, used as prophylaxis
- Uricosuric agents (probenecid)

Pseudogout

DEFINITION

Deposition of calcium pyrophosphate dihydrate (CPPD) crystals in joint spaces

ETIOLOGY

- Acute inflammatory reaction to the deposition of CPPD in joint spaces
- Changes related to age that make the synovial fluid environment more hospitable to CPPD growth

SIGNS AND SYMPTOMS

The most common presentation is erythema and swelling of the knee.

DIAGNOSIS

Presence of **positively birefringent crystals** in synovial fluid

TREATMENT

- Splint joint.
- Aspiration is both diagnostic and therapeutic.

Pseudogout:
Mostly large joints such as shoulder, wrist, and knee are involved.

Gout:
Small joints
Negative birefringence
Pseudogout:
Large joints
Positive birefringence

Polymyositis and Dermatomyositis

DEFINITIONS

Connective tissue diseases that result in proximal muscle weakness. Dermatomyositis differs only in that there is a rash, typically affecting the face, neck, and shoulders. There is also a significant risk of an occult malignancy associated with dermatomyositis.

ETIOLOGY

Etiology unknown. Many viruses including *Toxoplasma*, influenza, and coxsackie have been implicated. Family history of autoimmune disease or vasculitis is a risk factor.

SIGNS AND SYMPTOMS

- Symmetrical proximal muscle weakness
- Dysphagia
- Difficulty getting out of a chair, climbing or descending stairs, kneeling, raising arms

DIAGNOSIS

Look for the following four criteria:

1. Proximal muscle weakness
2. Elevated CPK (from necrotic muscle fibers)
3. Low-amplitude action potentials and fibrillations on electromyography (EMG)
4. Increased muscle fiber size on muscle biopsy

Polymyositis and dermatomyositis are both more common in women.

Polymyositis and dermatomyositis can be distinguished from myasthenia gravis by the lack of ocular involvement (ptosis).

LABORATORY

- Positive antinuclear antibody
- Elevated CPK, lactic dehydrogenase, serum glutamic oxaloacetic transaminase, aldolase
- ESR is elevated in only 50% of cases.
- Abnormal EMG
- Muscle biopsy shows inflammatory infiltrates.
- One fifth of patients have myositis-specific antibodies (Anti-Jo-1).
- Chest x-ray may show interstitial pulmonary disease.

PROGNOSIS

Presentation is usually insidious and progresses slowly, but disease can be fatal. Seventy-five percent survival at 5 years with long-term corticosteroid therapy.

TREATMENT

- ROM exercises
- Daily steroids
- If refractory to steroids, azathioprine or methotrexate is given.

PEDIATRIC MUSCULOSKELETAL PROBLEMS

Legg–Calvé–Perthes Disease

DEFINITION

- Also called coxa plana, juvenile osteochondrosis
- Childhood hip disorder that involves AVN of femoral head (Figure 14-13)
- Bilateral in 10 to 15% of patients

EPIDEMIOLOGY

- 1 in 1,200 children ages 3 to 10 years
- Peak incidence at age 6 years
- More common in males by factor of 4:1, but when it affects females, there is more extensive involvement of the epiphysis.

ETIOLOGY

Etiology is unknown but may be due to chronic synovitis, repeated trauma to hip in athletic children, infection, or congenital anomaly.

SIGNS AND SYMPTOMS

- Antalgic gait
- May or may not identify history of trauma or strenuous activity followed by sudden onset of limping and pain in the anterior groin, anterior thigh or knee, making diagnosis difficult
- Hip is held in external rotation and is limited in internal rotation. Muscle spasm may also be present.
- Buttock and thigh atrophy may be present on the affected side.

An antalgic gait is one that results from pain on weight bearing in which the stance phase of the gait is shortened on the affected side.

280

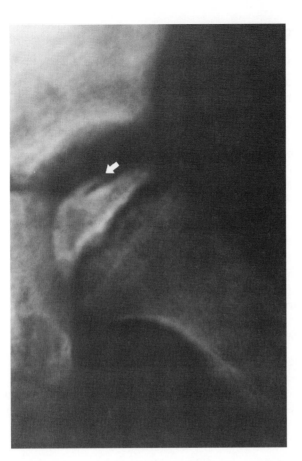

FIGURE 14-13. Anteroposterior (AP) view of pelvis demonstrating subchondral lucency of femoral head 2° to avascular necrosis. This is known as the "crescent sign" of Caffey.
(Reproduced, with permission, from Schwartz DT, Reisdorff EJ. *Emergency Radiology.* New York: McGraw-Hill, 2000: 238.)

DIAGNOSIS

- Stage 1: No findings to slight widening of the joint space and lateral displacement of the head
- Stage 2: Radiolucent and radiodense areas with epiphyseal fragmentation: This is the stage when most children present.
- Stage 3: Areas of radiolucency secondary to resorption of necrotic bone; this stage may last for several years in older children as new bone grows.
- Stage 4: Normal appearing radiograph; however, femoral neck and epiphysis may remain widened. This is the healed phase.

TREATMENT

- Depends on the severity of the disease
- Most cases are self-limited and no intervention is required.
- If ROM is limited, an abduction cast is applied. Traction may be used to relax adductor spasm and to maintain 45 degrees of abduction and slight internal rotation, which is the best position to center the femoral head to facilitate normal growth.
- The child may be mobilized using crutches and partial weight bearing with the cast. Cast should be removed periodically to mobilize the knee and ankle.
- Surgical intervention may be required for severe cases.

> **Typical scenario:**
> A 7-year-old boy presents with a limp and complains of groin and hip pain. Radiographs demonstrate a slight widening of the joint space. *Think: Legg–Calvé–Perthes disease.*

Slipped Capital Femoral Epiphysis (SCFE)

DEFINITION

- Condition in which the femoral head maintains its position in the acetabulum but the femoral neck is displaced anteriorly

EPIDEMIOLOGY

- Occurs between the ages of 10 and 15
- M:F = 2:1
- Bilateral in 15 to 20%

ETIOLOGY

Cause is unclear, may involve:

- History of trauma
- Weakened physis
- Obesity
- Endocrine disorder

SIGNS AND SYMPTOMS

- Antalgic gait that may have been present for months or may have occurred acutely
- Hip, medial thigh, or knee pain intermittently worsened with activity
- Hip may be held in external rotation, and internal rotation is limited.

DIAGNOSIS

AP radiograph of the pelvis (Figure 14-14) and lateral and frogleg views (if no acute slippage) to look for:

- Irregular widening of the epiphyseal plate
- Globular swelling of the joint capsule
- Posterior and inferior displacement of the femoral head (if slippage)

TREATMENT

Surgical stabilization

Osgood–Schlatter Disease

EPIDEMIOLOGY

- A cause of adolescent knee pain
- Cause is uncertain but may be due to:
  - Apophysitis at the insertion of the patellar tendon at the tibial tuberosity
  - Repeated quadriceps contraction resulting in tendonitis or partial avulsions at the tibial tubercle
- Seen at ages 9 to 15, when the apophysis is most prone to injury
- Males affected more commonly than females

SIGNS AND SYMPTOMS

- Pain at tibial tuberosity
- Symptoms worsened by palpation and knee extension against resistance

> **Typical scenario:**
> An 11-year-old obese boy presents with thigh and knee pain that worsens when he plays sports. He is walking with a limp and holds his hip in slight external rotation. *Think: SCFE.*

> **Typical scenario:**
> A 12-year-old boy presents complaining of knee pain for 2 weeks. Physical exam demonstrates a prominent tibial tubercle. *Think: Osgood–Schlatter disease.*

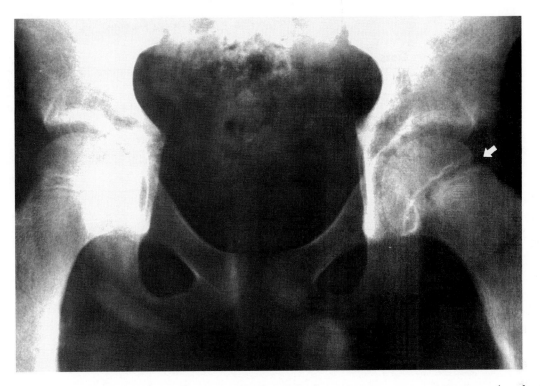

FIGURE 14-14. AP view of pelvis demonstrating widening of growth plate (arrow) as seen in SCFE. Note that if a line is drawn along the superior margin of the femoral neck, part of the femoral head will intersect it.
(Reproduced, with permission, from Schwartz DT, Reisdorff EJ. *Emergency Radiology.* New York: McGraw-Hill, 2000: 236.)

- Prominent tibial tubercle
- Soft-tissue swelling

DIAGNOSIS

Radiographs demonstrate:
- Prominence of the tibial tubercle
- Heterotopic ossification, which appears as irregularities

TREATMENT

- Self-limited and usually resolves with complete ossification of the tibial tuberosity by age 15
- NSAIDs
- Cryotherapy
- Stretching of the quadriceps
- Limit activity to pain tolerance.
- Avoid kneeling, running, and jumping.

Pediatric Fractures

See Table 14-3.

TABLE 14-3. Salter–Harris Fractures

Class	Definition	Treatment
I	■ Fracture through epiphyseal plate	Closed reduction
II	■ Fracture of metaphysis with extension into epiphyseal plate ■ Most common type of Salter–Harris fracture	Closed reduction
III	■ Intra-articular fracture of epiphysis with extension into epiphyseal plate	Open reduction
IV	■ Intra-articular fracture of epiphysis, metaphysis, and epiphyseal plate	Open reduction
V	■ Crush injury of epiphyseal plate	Open reduction

Musculoskeletal Emergencies

Endocrine Emergencies

ADRENAL CRISIS

DEFINITION

Acute life-threatening emergency that occurs secondary to cortisol and aldosterone insufficiency

ETIOLOGY

- Infections
- Withdrawal of steroid therapy
- Trauma
- Burns
- Pregnancy
- Drugs

SIGNS AND SYMPTOMS

- Acutely ill appearing
- Weakness, confusion, delirium
- Anorexia
- Nausea, vomiting, abdominal pain
- Fever
- Hypotension
- Increased motor activity, seizures
- Dehydration

TREATMENT

- Aggressive rehydration with 5% dextrose in normal saline (D_5NS)
- Steroid replacement with high-dose hydrocortisone
- Identification and treatment of precipitating cause

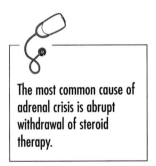

The most common cause of adrenal crisis is abrupt withdrawal of steroid therapy.

DIABETES MELLITUS

DEFINITION

- Most common endocrine disorder in the world (up to 3% of population)
- Type 1: Autoimmune disease with no insulin production
- Type 2: Hereditary disease with decreased insulin production

PATHOPHYSIOLOGY

- Insulin secreted in response to elevated blood glucose levels
- Inhibits ketogenesis, glycogenolysis, lipolysis, gluconeogenesis
- Counterregulatory hormones: Glucagon, epinephrine, cortisol, growth hormone (GH)

SIGNS AND SYMPTOMS

- Usually presents with symptomatic hyperglycemia or diabetic ketoacidosis (DKA) (discussed later)
- Polyuria
- Polydipsia
- Weight loss
- Dehydration
- Blurred vision
- Fatigue
- Foot ulcers
- Can get restrictive cardiomyopathy without coronary artery disease

TREATMENT

- Insulin for Type 1
- Oral hypoglycemic agents alone or in combination with insulin for Type 2

DAWN PHENOMENON

- The exaggeration of the normal tendency of the plasma glucose to rise in the early morning hours before breakfast, probably secondary to an increase in GH secretion

SOMOGYI EFFECT

Typical scenario:
A patient presents with persistent morning hyperglycemia, despite steadily increasing his nighttime neutral protamine Hagedorn insulin dose. Further, he complains of frequent nightmares. His wife brings him now because she witnessed him having a seizure in the middle of the night. *Think: Somogyi effect.*

- Characterized by nighttime hypoglycemia followed by a dramatic increase in fasting glucose levels and increased plasma ketones
- If Somogyi phenomenon is suspected, patients should get their blood glucose checked around 3 A.M. Hypoglycemia at this time confirms diagnosis.
- The morning hyperglycemia is a rebound effect.
- Intermediate-acting insulin administration at bedtime (rather than earlier in the evening) can prevent this effect (try to avoid peaking of insulin effect in the middle of the night).

DEFINITION

- Syndrome of relative insulin insufficiency with excess of counterregulatory hormones
- More common in Type 1 diabetics

ETIOLOGY

Most common causes:
- Infection
- Noncompliance with medications

PATHOPHYSIOLOGY

- Insulin deficiency causes hyperglycemia, which induces an osmotic diuresis.
- Profound dehydration, sodium loss, and potassium loss occurs.
- Ketosis occurs because of the loss of inhibition of free fatty acid oxidation in the liver.
- Metabolic acidosis resulting from the ketosis causes a profound respiratory compensation.
- Acetone is produced from spontaneous decarboxylation of acetoacetic acid. The acetone is disposed of by respiration, and its fruity odor is present on the patient's breath.
- Plasma ratio of beta-hydroxybutyric acid to acetoacetic acid is usually around 3:1 in DKA but can reach levels of 8:1.

SIGNS AND SYMPTOMS

- Polyuria, nausea, vomiting
- Lethargy and fatigue are later components.
- May progress to coma
- Signs of dehydration are present and patients may be hypotensive and tachycardic.
- Kussmaul's respirations (slow deep breaths) may be present.
- Acetone (fruity) odor may be present on the patient's breath.

DIAGNOSIS

- *Hyperglycemia*
- *Hyperketonemia*
- *Anion gap metabolic acidosis* (ketones are unmeasured ions)
- Usually, the diagnosis can be presumed at the bedside if patient's urine is strongly positive for ketones and the fingerstick glucose is high.
- Glucose is usually between 400 and 800 mg/dL.
- Initially, potassium is high due to acidosis but drops with treatment, so it is important to replace it.
- Blood urea nitrogen (BUN) may be increased because of prerenal azotemia.

TREATMENT

- Rapid administration of fluids (initially NS) should begin promptly (usual deficit is 5 to 10 L).
- Insulin to control hyperglycemia and reverse ketosis: Start with bolus 0.1 U/kg IV, then infuse at 0.1 U/kg/hr.

Typical scenario:
A 26-year-old man presents with vomiting. He reports several days of malaise and fatigue. He appears pale and diaphoretic. He is afebrile but tachycardic to 120 with a blood pressure (BP) of 105/70. His blood sugar is 550. *Think: DKA as a first presentation of diabetes mellitus.*

DKA treatment goals:
- Replacement of fluid losses
- Correction of metabolic derangements
- Reversal of ketosis
- Treatment of precipitating causes
- Restoration of normal diabetic regimen

- Continue until glucose is < 250 *and* ketosis is resolved (change intravenous (IV) fluid to D_5NS when glucose is < 250).
- Bicarbonate (to reverse acidosis) is controversial and not routinely recommended:
  - Side effects include lowering intracellular pH, hypokalemia, and shifting O_2 dissociation curve.
  - Use in small amounts in patients with pH < 6.9, severe hyperkalemia, or refractory hypotension.
- Frequent monitoring and replacement of serum potassium is essential.
- Replace other electrolytes as needed.
- Treatment of infection or other precipitating cause should begin as soon as possible.

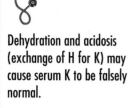

Dehydration and acidosis (exchange of H for K) may cause serum K to be falsely normal.

NONKETOTIC HYPEROSMOLAR CRISIS (NKHC)

DEFINITION

- Syndrome of hyperglycemia without ketoacidosis
- Small amounts of insulin protect against lipolysis and resultant ketoacidosis.
- Absence of ketosis leads to dramatic hyperglycemia (glucose > 800 to 1,000).
- More common in Type 2 diabetics (who produce small amounts of insulin) and the elderly

Typical scenario:
A 73-year-old woman who is a known diabetic is brought in due to altered mental status. The home health aide states the patient ran out of her medicines 4 days ago. Her fingerstick glucose is > 1,000. *Think: NKHC.*

CAUSES

- Infection
- Myocardial infarction (MI)
- Cerebrovascular accident (CVA)
- Gastrointestinal (GI) bleed
- Pancreatitis
- Uremia
- Drugs

SIGNS AND SYMPTOMS

- Osmotic diuresis is even more pronounced than in DKA, so patients are severely dehydrated.
- Water losses are greater than sodium losses, so patients become fluid depleted and hypertonic.
- Dehydration/stasis leads to hypercoagulability and vascular thrombosis.
- Hypertonicity leads to seizures (usually focal and resistant to anticonvulsants).
- Potassium, magnesium, and phosphate losses are also more pronounced than in DKA.

Rapid correction of hyperosmolar state may lead to cerebral edema (high mortality).

TREATMENT

- Replacement of fluid losses (usually 8 to 12 L) with NS solution
- Replacement and serial monitoring of electrolytes
- Insulin requirements usually less than in DKA (0.1 U/kg/hr)

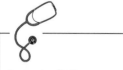

Aggressive fluid resuscitation in patients with heart failure may require invasive monitoring.

DEFINITION

Low serum glucose (< 70)

CAUSES

Multiple

SIGNS AND SYMPTOMS

- Decreased glucose causes central nervous system (CNS) dysfunction (confusion, lethargy).
- Release of counterregulatory hormones (epinephrine) causes sweating, tachycardia, and tremor.

TREATMENT

- Replacement of glucose is accomplished by the most clinically appropriate method.
- Oral replenishment (juice, soft drink, etc.) is appropriate for patients with intact mental status.
- Elderly or obtunded patients should receive IV dextrose.
- Patients with adrenal insufficiency may require hydrocortisone in addition to dextrose.
- Patients who require prolonged monitoring of blood sugar (overdose of long-acting insulin or oral hypoglycemics) or are unable to maintain adequate oral glucose intake should be admitted.

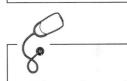

Causes of hypoglycemia:
I NEED SUGAR
Insulin/sulfonylurea excess

Neoplasms
Endocrine (Dawn, Somogyi)
Exercise
Dieting/starvation

Sepsis
Unreal (factitious)
GI (alimentary/postprandial)
Alcohol (inhibits gluconeogenesis)
Renal failure

Hypoglycemia due to oral hypoglycemic agents lasts approximately 24 hours, so it cannot be corrected quickly. Patients with oral hypoglycemia overdose should be admitted to the hospital for 24-hour monitoring and continuous glucose administration.

PARATHYROID DISORDERS

Parathyroid Physiology

- Parathyroid hormone (PTH), calcitonin (from thyroid), and vitamin D work in concert to regulate calcium.
- PTH increases serum calcium by three mechanisms:
  1. Increasing resorption of calcium (and phosphate) from bone
  2. Decreasing renal excretion of calcium (and increasing phosphate excretion)
  3. Increasing vitamin D levels in the intestine

Hyperparathyroidism

CAUSES

- Primary hyperparathyroidism is most common: Parathyroid adenoma, hyperplasia, carcinoma
- Multiple endocrine neoplasia types I and IIA both feature parathyroid neoplasms as part of the syndrome.

HIGH-YIELD FACTS

Endocrine Disorders

289

Signs of hyperparathyroidism: "Stones, bones, abdominal groans, and psychic moans"

SIGNS AND SYMPTOMS

- Renal stones (hypercalcemia)
- Bone pain (increased osteoclastic activity)
- Abdominal pain (ulcers, pancreatitis)
- Lethargy, confusion, stupor, coma

TREATMENT

Emergency management involves treatment of hypercalcemic crisis.

Hypoparathyroidism

DEFINITION

Syndrome of decreased calcium, increased phosphate, decreased PTH

CAUSES

- Most commonly seen as a complication of thyroid/parathyroid surgery (inadvertent excision)
- Less common causes: Autoimmune, congenital (DiGeorge's), infiltrative (Wilson's), hemochromatosis

SIGNS AND SYMPTOMS

- Perioral and digital paresthesias
- Decreased myocardial contractility
- Chvostek's and Trousseau's signs

TREATMENT

Treat hypocalcemia.

Pheochromocytoma

DEFINITION

Catecholamine-secreting tumor of neural crest cells, most often found in adrenal medulla

EPIDEMIOLOGY

- Equal incidence in men and women
- Tumors in women are three times as likely to be malignant.

CAUSES

Episodes precipitated by abdominal movement, trauma, drugs, or idiopathic

Rule of 10s:
10% are extra-adrenal.
10% are bilateral.
10% are malignant.
10% are familial.
10% are pediatric.
10% calcify.
10% recur after resection.

SIGNS AND SYMPTOMS

Clinical presentation is of catecholamine excess:
- Hypertensive crisis with headaches, chest pain, palpitations, shortness of breath, sweating
- Sequelae may include arrhythmias, MI, renal failure, lactic acidosis, CVA, and death.
- Hallmark of disease is marked hypertension (sustained or paroxysmal).

5 Hs:

- Headache
- Hypertension
- Hot (diaphoretic)
- Heart (palpitations)
- Hyperhidrosis

DIAGNOSIS

- Elevated urine vanillylmandelic acid (urine catecholamines)
- Hypercalcemia
- Hyperglycemia
- Computed tomography (CT) to look for adrenal mass

TREATMENT

- Control of hypertension with alpha blockade (phentolamine, labetalol) or nitroprusside
- Tachycardia may be controlled with beta blockers (propranolol, esmolol) after alpha blockade.
- Avoid use of beta blockers alone (unopposed alpha activity may lead to paradoxical increase in BP).

PITUITARY DISORDERS

Pituitary Physiology

- Pituitary gland sits in sella turcica (near optic chiasm and cavernous sinus).
- Anterior pituitary produces thyroid-stimulating hormone (TSH), adrenocorticotropic hormone (ACTH), GH, follicle-stimulating hormone (FSH), luteinizing hormone (LH), and prolactin.
- Posterior pituitary stores and releases oxytocin and vasopressin (antidiuretic hormone).
- Tumors of pituitary gland (most commonly prolactinoma) may present with visual field defects (most commonly bitemporal hemianopsia) or cranial nerve palsies (III, IV, V, VI) from local compression.

Pituitary Apoplexy

- Sudden enlargement of pituitary tumor secondary to infarct or hemorrhage, causing clinical signs/symptoms of local compression and intracranial bleeding
- Treatment is prompt neurosurgical decompression.

Sheehan's Syndrome

"Postpartum pituitary necrosis" seen after episode of hypotension during delivery (patients fail to lactate and resume menstruation after delivery)

Panhypopituitarism

Hormone loss follows typical sequence:
GH (first) $\rightarrow$ LH/FSH $\rightarrow$ TSH $\rightarrow$ ACTH $\rightarrow$ prolactin (last)

Thyroid Physiology

- Thyroid function controlled by hypothalamus (thyrotropin-releasing hormone) $\rightarrow$ pituitary (TSH) $\rightarrow$ thyroid (T_3, T_4)
- Peripheral conversion of T_4 to T_3 (active form) takes place in liver/kidney.

Causes of Hyperthyroidism

- Graves' disease (autoimmune stimulation of TSH receptors)
- Toxic multinodular goiter
- Toxic adenoma
- Thyroiditis (autoimmune or viral)

Thyroid Storm

DEFINITION

Exaggerated manifestation of hyperthyroidism

EPIDEMIOLOGY

Mortality is high (20 to 50%) even with the correct treatment.

ETIOLOGY

- Infection
- Trauma and major surgical procedures
- DKA
- MI, CVA, pulmonary embolism
- Withdrawal of antihyperthyroid medications, iodine administration, thyroid hormone ingestion
- Idiopathic

SIGNS AND SYMPTOMS

Overactivated sympathetic nervous system causes most of the signs and symptoms of this syndrome:
- Fever > 101°F
- Tachycardia (out of proportion to fever) with a wide pulse pressure
- High-output congestive heart failure and volume depletion
- Exhaustion
- GI manifestations: Diarrhea, abdominal pain
- Continuum of CNS alterations (from agitation to confusion when moderate, to stupor or coma with or without seizures when most severe)
- Jaundice is a late and ominous manifestation.

Typical scenario:
A 41-year-old woman with known hyperthyroidism is brought in by her family, who state that she has had days of diarrhea and has now started acting "crazy" with labile mood. She is febrile to 102°F, has a pulse of 140, and has rales on auscultation. *Think: Thyroid storm.*

HIGH-YIELD FACTS

Endocrine Disorders

- This is a clinical diagnosis, and since most patients present in need of emergent stabilization, treatment is initiated empirically.
- Patients may have improperly treated hyperthyroidism.
- May also occur in the setting of unintentional or intentional toxic ingestion of synthetic thyroid hormone in the hypothyroid patient

TREATMENT

Primary stabilization:

- Airway protection
- Oxygenation
- Assess circulation (pulse/BP) and continuous cardiac monitoring
- IV hydration
- Beta blocker therapy (e.g., propranolol) to block adrenergic effects
- Treat fever with acetaminophen (not aspirin, which would displace T_4 from thyroid-binding protein).
- Propylthiouracil (PTU) or methimazole to block synthesis of new thyroid hormone
- Iodine to decrease release of preformed thyroid hormone. Do not give iodine until the PTU has taken effect (1.5 hours) because more thyroid hormone will be produced.
- Treat any possible precipitating factors that may be present.

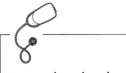

In initial stabilization, cooling blankets can be applied to treat hyperpyrexia, if present.

Never send any thyroid storm patient for a procedure involving iodine contrast before giving PTU.

Causes of Hypothyroidism

- Hashimoto's thyroiditis (most common cause)
- Iodine deficiency or excess
- Radiation therapy to neck (from other malignancy)
- Medications (lithium is most common)
- Secondary causes include pituitary tumor, tuberculosis, and Sheehan's syndrome.

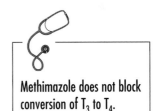

Methimazole does not block conversion of T_3 to T_4.

Myxedema Coma

DEFINITION

Life-threatening complication of hypothyroidism, with profound lethargy or coma usually accompanied by hypothermia: Mortality is 20 to 50% even if treated early.

ETIOLOGY

- Sepsis
- Prolonged exposure to cold weather
- CNS depressants (sedatives, narcotics)
- Trauma or surgery

SIGNS AND SYMPTOMS

- Profound lethargy or coma is obvious.
- Hypothermia: Rectal temperature < 35°C (95°F)
- Bradycardia or circulatory collapse
- Delayed relaxation phase of deep tendon reflexes, areflexia if severe (this can be a very important clue)

Hypothermia is often missed by regular thermometers. Use a rectal probe if profound hypothermia is present.

HIGH-YIELD FACTS

Endocrine Disorders

Differential diagnosis:
- Severe depression or primary psychosis
- Drug overdose or toxic exposure
- CVA
- Liver failure
- Hypoglycemia
- CO_2 narcosis
- CNS infection

DIAGNOSIS

Lab tests for the patient presenting with profound altered mental status:
- Complete blood count with differential
- Blood and urine cultures
- Serum electrolytes
- BUN and creatinine
- Blood glucose
- Urine toxicology screen
- Serum transaminases and lactic dehydrogenase
- Arterial blood gas to rule out hypoxemia and CO_2 retention
- Cortisol level
- Carboxyhemoglobin

CT scan and chest radiograph are also commonly ordered because myxedema coma is often a diagnosis of exclusion.

TREATMENT

- Airway management with mechanical ventilation is often necessary.
- Prevent further heat loss but do not initiate external rewarming unless cardiac dysrhythmias are present, as peripheral vasodilation can lead to hypotension.
- Monitor patient in an intensive setting.
- Pharmacologic therapy:
  - IV levothyroxine
  - Glucocorticoids (until coexisting adrenal insufficiency is excluded)
- IV hydration (D_5NS)
- Rule out and treat any precipitating causes (antibiotics for suspected infection).

Dermatologic Emergencies

Shapes

- Annular: Ring-shaped
- Arcuate: Arc-shaped
- Confluent: Coalescence of lesions
- Discoid: Coin- or disc-shaped
- Linear: Line-shaped
- Serpiginous: Wavy linear lesions
- Target: Concentric rings (like a target sign)

Definitions

Flat Lesions
- **Macule:** Nonpalpable, discrete area of change in color. Generally < 10 mm diameter (Figure 16-1)
- **Erythema:** Nonpalpable, diffuse redness
- **Patch:** Nonpalpable, discrete area of change in color > 10 mm diameter
- **Telangiectasia:** Blanchable, visibly dilated blood vessel at skin surface (Figure 16-2)
- **Petechiae:** Nonblanching purple spots < 2 mm
- **Purpura:** Nonblanching purple spots > 2 mm (can be palpable in some conditions)

Raised, Solid Lesions
- **Papule:** Solid, raised lesion < 5 mm diameter (Figure 16-3)
- **Nodule:** Solid, raised lesion > 5 mm diameter
- **Tumor:** Solid, palpable lesion > 10 mm
- **Induration:** Raised "hardening" of the skin
- **Wheal:** Transient localized skin edema (Figure 16-4)
- **Scale:** Flake of keratinized epidermal cells on top of skin surface (Figure 16-5)
- **Plaque:** Flat-topped lesion of induration (Figure 16-6)
- **Crust:** Dried serous/serosanguinous exudate (Figure 16-7)
- **Hyperkeratosis:** Thickened stratum corneum (Figure 16-8)
- **Lichenification:** Indurated and thickened skin caused by excessive scratching and chronic inflammation (Figure 16-9)

- **Filiform/Warty:** Flesh-colored, circumscribed hypertrophy of epidermal papillae (Figure 16-10)

Raised, Fluid-Filled Lesions
- **Vesicle:** Blister < 5 mm diameter
- **Bulla:** Blister > 5 mm diameter
- **Pustule:** Visible pus under the skin (yellow, white, or green in color)
- **Comedone:** Collection of sebum and keratin in a blocked, dilated sebaceous duct (Figure 16-11)
- **Cyst:** Sack of fluid-containing material
- **Abscess:** Tender, fluctuant pocket of pus with surrounding inflammation deep to skin

Depressed Lesions
- **Erosion:** Localized epidermal loss (Figure 16-12)
- **Atrophy:** Thinning of skin from layer loss (Figure 16-13)
- **Excoriation:** Abraded or scratched skin
- **Ulcer:** Localized dermal and epidermal loss (can be deeper) (Figure 16-14)
- **Fissure:** Cleft-shaped ulcer (Figure 16-15)

Color

Black, white, yellow, red, flesh, brown, hyper- or hypopigmented, blanchable, or nonblanchable

Distribution

Flexor/extensor surfaces, sun-exposed, dermatomal, clothing-covered, intertriginous, discrete/scattered/grouped.

Size (Does Matter)

- Planar dimensions: Circular—average diameter, oblong—length and width
- Height/depth: If raised or depth discernible, or if biopsied
- Large lesions: Estimate body surface area involved (see Environmental Emergencies chapter).

Use the "Rule of 9s" to estimate body surface area.

GENERAL DIAGNOSIS

History of Present Illness

- Signs and symptoms (painless, itching, burning, etc.)
- How long present?
- Where are lesions?
- Evolutionary changes?
- Systemic complaints?
- Exposures (chemicals, foods, animals, plants, medications, etc.)?
- Allergies?
- Ever have this before?
- Partially treated?

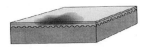

FIGURE 16-1. Macule.
(Reproduced, with permission, from Rycroft RJG, Robertson SL. *A Color Handbook of Dermatology.* London, England: Manson Publishing Ltd., 1999: 9.)

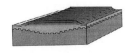

FIGURE 16-6. Plaque.
(Reproduced, with permission, from Rycroft RJG, Robertson SL. *A Color Handbook of Dermatology.* London, England: Manson Publishing Ltd., 1999: 9.)

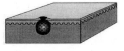

FIGURE 16-11. Comedone.
(Reproduced, with permission, from Rycroft RJG, Robertson SL. *A Color Handbook of Dermatology.* London, England: Manson Publishing Ltd., 1999: 11.)

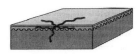

FIGURE 16-2. Telangiectasia.
(Reproduced, with permission, from Rycroft RJG, Robertson SL. *A Color Handbook of Dermatology.* London, England: Manson Publishing Ltd., 1999: 10.)

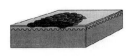

FIGURE 16-7. Crust.
(Reproduced, with permission, from Rycroft RJG, Robertson SL. *A Color Handbook of Dermatology.* London, England: Manson Publishing Ltd., 1999: 11.)

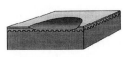

FIGURE 16-12. Erosion.
(Reproduced, with permission, from Rycroft RJG, Robertson SL. *A Color Handbook of Dermatology.* London, England: Manson Publishing Ltd., 1999: 10.)

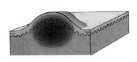

FIGURE 16-3. Papule.
(Reproduced, with permission, from Rycroft RJG, Robertson SL. *A Color Handbook of Dermatology.* London, England: Manson Publishing Ltd., 1999: 9.)

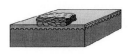

FIGURE 16-8. Hyperkeratosis.
(Reproduced, with permission, from Rycroft RJG, Robertson SL. *A Color Handbook of Dermatology.* London, England: Manson Publishing Ltd., 1999: 11.)

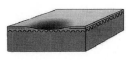

FIGURE 16-13. Atrophy.
(Reproduced, with permission, from Rycroft RJG, Robertson SL. *A Color Handbook of Dermatology.* London, England: Manson Publishing Ltd., 1999: 11.)

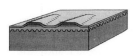

FIGURE 16-4. Wheal.
(Reproduced, with permission, from Rycroft RJG, Robertson SL. *A Color Handbook of Dermatology.* London, England: Manson Publishing Ltd., 1999: 9.)

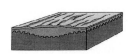

FIGURE 16-9. Lichenification.
(Reproduced, with permission, from Rycroft RJG, Robertson SL. *A Color Handbook of Dermatology.* London, England: Manson Publishing Ltd., 1999: 11.)

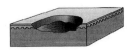

FIGURE 16-14. Ulcer.
(Reproduced, with permission, from Rycroft RJG, Robertson SL. *A Color Handbook of Dermatology.* London, England: Manson Publishing Ltd., 1999: 10.)

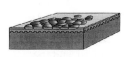

FIGURE 16-5. Scale.
(Reproduced, with permission, from Rycroft RJG, Robertson SL. *A Color Handbook of Dermatology.* London, England: Manson Publishing Ltd., 1999: 11.)

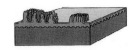

FIGURE 16-10. Warty.
(Reproduced, with permission, from Rycroft RJG, Robertson SL. *A Color Handbook of Dermatology.* London, England: Manson Publishing Ltd., 1999: 11.)

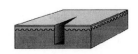

FIGURE 16-15. Fissure.
(Reproduced, with permission, from Rycroft RJG, Robertson SL. *A Color Handbook of Dermatology.* London, England: Manson Publishing Ltd., 1999: 10.)

Dermatologic Emergencies

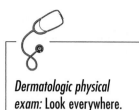

Dermatologic physical exam: Look everywhere.

These are the problems you'll most likely be tested on, not necessarily the ones you'll see most frequently in the emergency department.

Examination

See above.

Diagnostic Procedures

See Table 16-1.

Top Dermatologic Problems in Emergency Medicine

- Decubitus ulcer
- Abscess
- Cellulitis
- Erysipelas
- Necrotizing infection
- Herpes zoster
- Erythema multiforme (EM)
- Henoch–Schönlein purpura (HSP)
- Purpura
- Urticaria
- Pemphigus
- Staphylococcal scalded syndrome
- Stevens–Johnson syndrome (SJS)
- Toxic epidermal necrolysis (TEN)

TABLE 16-1. Diagnostic Procedures Used in Dermatology

	Definitions
Diascopy	Pressing of a glass slide firmly against a red lesion will determine if it is due to capillary dilatation (blanchable) or to extravasation of blood (nonblanchable).
KOH preparation	Used to identify fungus and yeast. Scrape scales from skin, hair, or nails. Treat with a 10% KOH solution to dissolve tissue material. Septated hyphae are revealed in fungal infections, and pseudohyphae and budding spores are revealed in yeast infections.
Tzanck preparation	Used to identify vesicular viral eruptions. Scrape the base of a vesicle and smear cells on a glass slide. Multinucleated giant cells will be identified in herpes simplex, herpes zoster, and varicella infections.
Scabies preparation	Scrape skin of a burrow between fingers, side of hands, axilla, or groin. Mites, eggs, or feces will be identified in scabies infection.
Wood's lamp	Certain conditions will fluoresce when examined under a long-wave ultraviolet light ("black" lamp). Tinea capitis will fluoresce green or yellow on hair shaft.
Patch testing	Detects type IV delayed hypersensitivity reactions (allergic contact dermatitis). Nonirritating concentrations of suspected allergen are applied under occlusion to the back. Development of erythema, edema, and vesicles at site of contact 48 hours later indicates an allergy to offending agent.
Biopsy	Type of biopsy performed depends on the site of lesion, the type of tissue removed, and the desired cosmetic result. Shave biopsy is used for superficial lesions. Punch biopsy (3 to 5 mm diameter) can remove all or part of a lesion and provides tissue sample for pathology. Elliptical excisions provide more tissue than a punch biopsy and are used for deeper lesions or when the entire lesion needs to be sent to pathology.

Top Causes of Rash with Fever

- Rubella
- Measles
- Staphylococcal scalded skin syndrome
- Toxic shock syndrome
- Scarlet fever
- Meningococcemia
- Disseminated gonococcal infection
- Bacterial endocarditis
- Rocky Mountain spotted fever (RMSF)
- Kawasaki's disease
- Erythema nodosum
- Hypersensitivity vasculitis

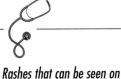

Rashes that can be seen on palms and soles: **Mrs. HE**
- **M**eningococcemia
- **R**MSF
- **S**yphilis

- **H**and–foot–mouth disease
- **E**M

GENERAL TREATMENTS

Initial Modalities

- Astringents (drying agents): Domeboro solution
- Emollients (moisturizers): Eucerin cream, lotion

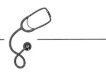

- If it's wet . . . dry it.
- If it's dry . . . wet it.
- If present, remove offending agent.

Antihistamines (Topical)

For pruritic (itchy) disorders:
- Diphenhydramine: Adult, 25 to 50 mg PO q6h; child, 4 to 6 mg/kg/24 hr ÷ q6 to 8 (max 200 mg)
- Hydroxyzine: Adult, 25 to 100 mg PO q8h; child, 2 to 4 mg/kg/24 hr ÷ q8 to 12 (max 200 mg)
- Cetirizine/loratadine/fexofenadine

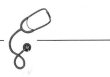

Absorption of topical antihistamines is unpredictable.

Antibacterials (Topical)

- Mupirocin: Used for impetigo
- Bacitracin: Used for burns and cuts
- Neomycin/polymixin B: Used for cuts
- Silver sulfadiazine: Used for burns

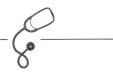

Warn patients about drowsiness associated with antihistamines.

Antifungals (Topical)

- Polyenes: Nystatin, amphotericin B 3%
- Imidazoles: Ketoconazole 1%, clotrimazole 1%, miconazole 2%, econazole 1%

Antiparasitics (Topical)

- Lindane (for age > 1 year):
  - Lice: 1% shampoo 30 mL for 4 minutes, then rinse thoroughly; again after 5 days
  - Scabies: Lotion 30 to 60 mL and wash after 8 hours

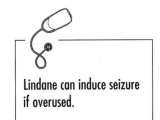

Lindane can induce seizure if overused.

Dermatologic Emergencies

- Permethrin (for age > 2 months):
  - Lice: 1% rinse—wash after 10 minutes, again after 5 days for next generation
  - Scabies: 5% cream all over and wash thoroughly after 8 to 12 hours

Antivirals (Topical)

- Acyclovir: 5% ointment q3h × 7 days
- Used for herpes (varicella, zoster, simplex, and genitalis)

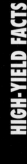
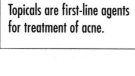

The thicker the skin, the more potent steroid needed.

Antivirals (Oral)

- Acyclovir:
  - Genitalis: 400 mg PO tid × 10 days
  - Zoster: 800 mg PO 5/day × 7 to 10 days
  - Varicella: 20 mg/kg PO qid × 5 days—max 800 mg
- Famciclovir:
  - Genitalis: 250 mg PO tid × 10 days
  - Zoster: 500 mg PO tid × 7 days
- Valacyclovir:
  - Genitalis: 1 g PO bid × 10 days
  - Zoster: 1 g PO tid × 7 days

Topicals are first-line agents for treatment of acne.

Corticosteroids (Topical)

- Potency graded on ability to vasoconstrict: High potency, group I; low potency, group VII
- Avoid using groups I, II, III, and IV in pregnancy, infancy, face, genitalia, flexure creases, and intertriginous areas.
- Bid–tid therapy for 1 to 2 weeks (potent), or 2 to 4 weeks (less potent)

Tretinoin and isotretinoin are teratogenic.

Acne (Topical Agents)

- Benzoyl peroxide: Many preparations
- Clindamycin: 10 mg/mL bid
- Tretinoin: Many preparations
- Erythromycin: 1.5 to 2% bid

Acne (Oral Agents)

Exposure to sun while on tetracycline or doxycycline can cause a rash.

- Tetracycline: 250 mg PO qid
- Doxycycline: 100 mg PO bid
- Isotretinoin: 0.5 mg/kg PO bid

CUTANEOUS BACTERIAL INFECTIONS

Abscess

- Location: Back, buttocks, axillae, groin, and anywhere pus can accumulate (acne, wounds)

- Definition: Pocket of pus from skin flora
- Signs and symptoms: Red, hot, swollen, and tender
- Treatment: Incise, drain, pack, wound check

Cellulitis

- Location: Commonly lower extremities (diabetics and peripheral vascular disease), but can be anywhere
- Definition: Superficial skin and subcutaneous tissue infection from skin flora (*Staphylococcus aureus, Streptococcus pyogenes*)
- Signs and symptoms: Red, hot, swollen, and tender
- Treatment: Outpatient oral antibiotics in the young and healthy (first-generation cephalosporin) or inpatient intravenous (IV) antibiotics in the frail/elderly

Impetigo

- Location: Face (usually), can be anywhere (Figure 16-16)
- Definition: Bacterial superinfection of epidermis from broken skin. Bullous (*S. aureus*) and nonbullous (group A beta-hemolytic strep [GAS])
- Signs and symptoms:
  - Initial lesion is a transient erythematous papule or thin-roofed vesicle that ruptures easily and forms a "honey-colored" crust.
  - Lesions can be discrete and scattered or become confluent, forming a superficial crusted plaque.
- Treatment:
  - Remove crusts by soaking in warm water.
  - Antibacterial washes (benzoyl peroxide)
  - Topical antibiotic if disease is limited (mupirocin)
  - Oral antibiotics (e.g., first-generation cephalosporin)

Erysipelas

- Location: Face (most often), extremities (Figure 16-17)
- Definition: An acute onset of superficial spreading cellulitis, arising in inconspicuous breaks in skin; involves dermis and epidermis. Pathogens include *S. aureus*, GAS, and occasionally *Haemophilus influenzae*.

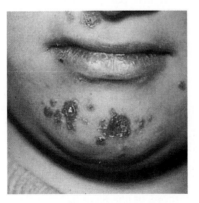

FIGURE 16-16. Impetigo.
(Reproduced, with permission, from Pantell R, et al. *The Common Symptom Guide,* 4th ed. New York: McGraw-Hill, 1996.)

Typical scenario:
A 55-year-old diabetic man presents with a right lower extremity that is red, warm, and tender to the touch. The rash has poorly demarcated borders and has been spreading over the last day. He is febrile to 101°F. *Think: Cellulitis.*

Erysipelas, erysipeloid, and necrotizing fasciitis are variants of cellulitis.

Complications of GAS impetigo include acute glomerulonephritis and guttate psoriasis. If untreated, patients can develop cellulitis, lymphangitis, and septicemia.

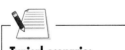

Typical scenario:
A 67-year-old woman presents with an erythematous, shiny area of warm and tender skin on her face with a well-demarcated and indurated advancing border. *Think: Erysipelas.*

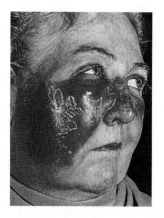

FIGURE 16-17. Erysipelas.

(Reproduced, with permission, from Fauci AS, et al. *Harrison's Principles of Internal Medicine,* 14th ed. New York: McGraw-Hill, 1997.)

- Signs and symptoms:
  - An erythematous, shiny area of warm and tender skin with a well-demarcated and indurated advancing border
- Less edematous than cellulitis, but margins are more sharply demarcated and elevated
- Face is most commonly involved, but can affect any area, especially sites of chronic edema
- Treatment: Same as for cellulitis of the face (IV antibiotics), with care taken if orbital involvement to consult ophthalmologist

Lyme Disease

- Location: Usually affects the trunk, proximal extremities, axilla, and inguinal area
- Definition: Chronic multisystem infection with spirochete *Borrelia burgdorferi* transmitted through *Ixodes* ticks in Atlantic and northeast states. Rash is erythema chronicum migrans (ECM), a spreading, annular, macular erythema seen 2 to 20 days from site of tick bite (Figure 16-18).
- Signs and symptoms: Mild–moderate itch, mild burn. If untreated, progresses with systemic illness (arthralgias, fever, adenopathy, flulike symptoms, facial nerve palsies, cranial neuritis, myocarditis, cardiac conduction abnormalities, encephalopathy, polyneuropathy, more rash)
- Treatment: Doxycycline 100 mg PO bid × 21 days (or clarithromycin, amoxicillin, cefuroxime)

RMSF

- Location: Wrists and ankles (acral rash), then spreads to trunk (Figure 15-19)
- Definition:
  - A potentially life-threatening disease due to a tick bite, with highest incidence in children aged 5 to 10 years old
  - Ninety-five percent of cases occur from April through September.
  - Occurs only in the western hemisphere, primarily in southeastern states and most often in Oklahoma, North and South Carolina, and Tennessee

Typical scenario:
A 39-year-old woman presents with a rash on her right leg that she initially thought was an insect bite. It is an erythematous annular plaque with a central clearing. *Think: ECM.*

Typical scenario:
A 7-year-old boy presents with a high fever, myalgias, and a rash of 2 days that consists of 2- to 6-mm pink, blanchable macules that first appear peripherally on wrists, forearms, ankles, palms, and soles, then spread to the trunk. *Think: RMSF.*

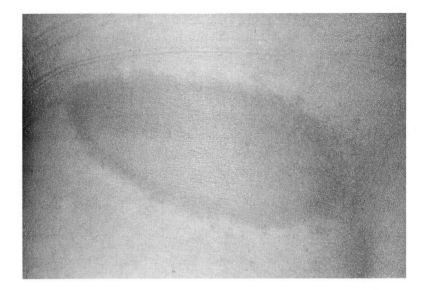

FIGURE 16-18. ECM rash of Lyme disease.

(Reproduced, with permission, from Fitzpatrick TB, et al. *Color Atlas and Synopsis of Clinical Dermatology: Common and Serious Diseases,* 4th ed. New York: McGraw-Hill, 2001: 675.)

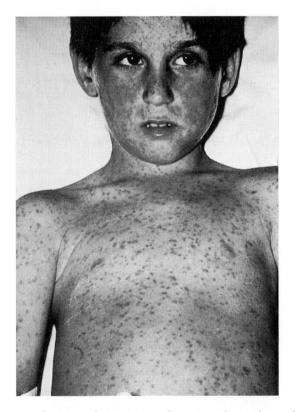

FIGURE 16-19. Late manifestation of RMSF. Note disseminated macules and papules. Initial lesions were noted on the palms and soles, wrists, and ankles and extended centripetally.

(Reproduced, with permission, from Fitzpatrick TB, et al. *Color Atlas and Synopsis of Clinical Dermatology: Common and Serious Diseases,* 4th ed. New York: McGraw-Hill, 2001: 753.)

- Rarely occurs in the Rocky Mountains
- Only 60% of patients report a history of a tick bite.
- Signs and symptoms:
  - *Rickettsia rickettsii* through tick bite invades bloodstream and causes blanching, maculopapular lesions that become petechial and can coalesce and become ecchymotic or gangrenous.
  - Sudden onset of high **fever,** myalgia, severe headache, rigors, nausea, and photophobia within first 2 days of tick bite
  - Fifty percent develop rash within 3 days. Another 30% develop the rash within 6 days.
  - Rash consists of 2- to 6-mm pink **blanchable macules** that first appear peripherally on wrists, forearms, ankles, palms, and soles.
  - Within 6 to 18 hours the exanthem spreads centrally to trunk, proximal extremities, and face.
  - Within 1 to 3 days, the macules evolve to deep red papules, and within 2 to 4 days, the exanthem is hemorrhagic and no longer blanchable.
  - Up to 15% have no rash.
  - Many patients have exquisite tenderness of the gastrocnemius muscle.
- Treatment: Doxycycline 100 mg PO bid × 14 days. Use chloramphenicol for pregnant patients and children under age 8.

Scarlet Fever

The sandpaper rash is typical of scarlet fever.

- Location: Diffuse
- Definition: A toxin-mediated disease caused by GAS
- Signs and symptoms:
  - Pain precedes rash and follows fever.
  - A finely punctate pink-scarlet exanthem first appears on upper trunk 12 to 48 hours after onset of fever.
  - As the exanthem spreads to extremities, it becomes confluent and feels like sandpaper and fades within 4 to 5 days, followed by desquamation.
  - Linear petechiae evident in body folds (Pastia's sign)
  - Pharynx is beefy red and tongue is initially white, but within 4 to 5 days, the white coating sloughs off and tongue becomes bright red ("strawberry tongue").
- Treatment: Oral penicillin or erythromycin, acetaminophen

Complications of untreated scarlet fever include:
- Acute rheumatic fever
- Acute glomerulonephritis
- Erythema nodosum

Gonococcemia

- Location: Anywhere
- Definition: Emboli of disseminated *Neisseria gonorrhoeae*, usually in menstruating or peripartum females. Looks like multiple papular, vesicular, and pustular petechial lesions with erythematous base that become hemorrhagic; associated fever and arthralgias
- Signs and symptoms: Painful
- Treatment: IV ceftriaxone or ciprofloxacin

Typical scenario:
A 20-year-old college student has a low-grade fever, chills, and migratory polyarthralgias accompanied by a tender rash. The rash initially consisted of erythematous macules that have now evolved into hemorrhagic pustules. *Think: Disseminated gonococcal infection.*

Meningococcemia

- Location: Extremities and trunk (anywhere) (Figure 16-20)
- Definition: Infectious vasculitis from emboli of disseminated *Neisseria meningitidis,* usually in age < 20, sometimes in epidemics

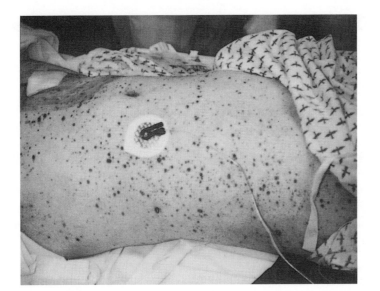

FIGURE 16-20. Meningococcemia.
(Reproduced, with permission, from Knoop KJ, Stack LB, and Storrow AB. *Atlas of Emergency Medicine.* New York: McGraw-Hill, 1997: 404.)

- Signs and symptoms:
  - Petechia, urticaria, hemorrhagic vesicles, macules, and papules with surrounding erythema
  - Associated with fever, altered mental status and vitals, headache, arthralgias, and stiff neck
- Treatment: IV ceftriaxone, add vancomycin for cephalosporin-resistant pneumococcus

> Complications of meningococcemia include meningitis and Waterhouse–Friderichsen syndrome (fulminant meningococcemia with adrenal hemorrhage).

Toxic Shock Syndrome

- Location: Diffuse or just extremities/trunk
- Definition: Severe, life-threatening, multisystem syndrome arising because of *S. aureus* toxic shock syndrome toxin (TSST-1) in menstruating women using tampons, or enterotoxins B and C also from *Staphylococcus* but unrelated to tampon use.
- Signs and symptoms:
  - Nonpruritic, tender erythroderma
  - Fever, hypotension, diffuse tender erythroderma, pharyngitis, mucosal hyperemia, diarrhea, and malaise
  - Erythema may resolve in 3 to 5 days with subsequent desquamation of hands and feet in 5 to 14 days.
- Treatment: Hospital admission, aggressive IV fluid resuscitation, IV oxacillin or cefazolin, vancomycin if penicillin allergic

Candida (Oral)

- Location: Can be on mucous membranes (palate, pharynx, tongue, vagina) or can be cutaneous (intertriginous, groin, under fat pannus)
- Definition: *Candida albicans*, normally a nonpathogenic colonizer of moist skin and mucosa, causes painful, raised, whitish plaques that detach and leave red erosions.
- Signs and symptoms: Painful, pruritic in vagina
- Treatment: Oral nystatin swish and swallow 5 mL tid for oral lesions; topical nystatin or clotrimazole cream for cutaneous and vaginal types. Fluconazole 150 mg PO single dose for both oral and vaginal types.

Tinea Infection

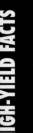

All tinea infections except tinea capitis are treated with a topical antifungal cream.

Tinea are fungal infections caused by *Trichophyton* and *Microsporum* species and are named according to the part of the body they are on:

- Tinea cruris: Groin, gluteal cleft
- Tinea pedis: Feet, in between toes (athlete's foot)
- Tinea versicolor: On trunk, multiple-colored lesions that do not tan with surrounding skin in sunlight
- Tinea capitis: Invade hair shafts and surrounding skin; causes red, circular patches with raised edges, sometimes swollen, boggy, and crusted, with loss of hair:
  - Treatment: Griseofulvin 7.5 mg/kg PO bid × 6 weeks
- Tinea corporis: See Figure 16-21.

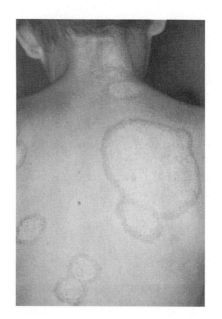

FIGURE 16-21. Tinea corporis.

(Reproduced, with permission, from Pantell R, et al. *The Common Symptom Guide,* 4th ed. New York: McGraw-Hill, 1996.)

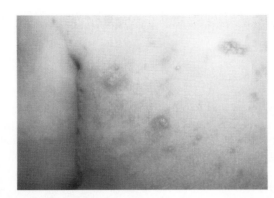

FIGURE 16-22. Scabies. Notice the papulovesicular nature of the rash, which tends to occur in places where mites can burrow, such as the web spaces of the digits and the axilla, as shown here.

(Reproduced, with permission, from Rudolph A, et al. *Rudolph's Pediatrics*, 20th ed. Stamford, CT: Appleton & Lange, 1997.)

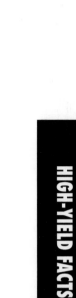
PARASITIC INFECTIONS

Pediculosis (Lice)

- Location: *Phthirus capitis* on scalp and neck. *Phthirus pubis* (crabs) in pubic hair
- Definition: *P. capitis* mite lives on scalp and lays eggs (nits) on hair shafts; lives on human blood
- Signs and symptoms: Severe itch
- Treatment: Permethrin, then lindane, fine-toothed comb to manually remove nits

Scabies

- Location: Flexural creases, hands, feet
- Definition: *Sarcoptes scabiei*, the "itch mite," burrows into the skin and lays its eggs.
- Signs and symptoms: Intense itch and mild burning; excoriations and pruritic red papules (Figure 16-22)
- Treatment: Lindane or permethrin

Typical scenario:
A 27-year-old human immunodeficiency virus (HIV)-positive patient presents due to an intensely painful erythematous rash that is over his right flank in a dermatomal distribution. *Think: Varicella-zoster.*

VIRAL INFECTIONS

Varicella Zoster: Shingles

- Location: Commonly thoracic and facial dermatomes
- Definition: An acute dermatomal viral infection caused by reactivation of latent varicella-zoster virus that has remained dormant in a sensory root ganglion. The virus travels down the sensory nerve, resulting initially in dermatomal pain, followed by skin lesions. Risk factors include age, malignancy, immunosuppression, and radiation.
- Signs and symptoms:
  - Prodrome of pain, burning, itching, and paresthesia in affected dermatome precedes eruption by 3 to 5 days.

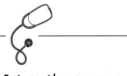

Patients with zoster can infect nonimmune contacts with chickenpox. Exposed nonimmune contacts should be treated with varicella-zoster immune globulin.

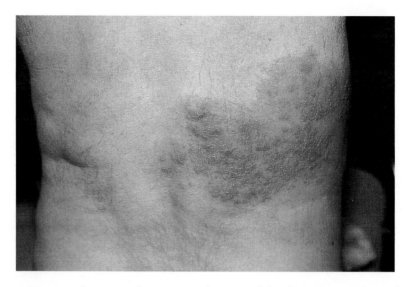

FIGURE 16-23. Varicella-zoster infection. Note dermatomal distribution (T8–T10) to rash.

(Reproduced, with permission, from Fitzpatrick TB, et al. *Color Atlas and Synopsis of Clinical Dermatology: Common and Serious Diseases*, 4th ed. New York: McGraw-Hill, 2001: 807.)

Dermatologic Emergencies

Varicella-zoster infection of cranial nerve VIII is called Ramsay Hunt syndrome and results in hearing loss, vertigo, and tinnitus.

Varicella-zoster infection of VI (ophthalmic branch of trigeminal nerve) can be vision threatening. Ophthalmic consultation should be obtained for these cases.

There is an increased incidence of verrucae in atopic and immunocompromised patients.

- Accompanied by fever, headache, and malaise, and heightened sensitivity to stimuli (allodynia)
- Grouped vesicles on an erythematous base distributed unilaterally along a dermatome (Figure 16-23)
- Crust formation within 5 to 10 days
- Some vesicles may occur outside of involved dermatome.
  - Treatment:
  - Moist and cool compresses to affected dermatome
  - Oral acyclovir, valacyclovir, or famciclovir (accelerate healing of lesions and decrease duration of pain if started within 3 days of infection)
  - Analgesics

Molluscum Contagiosum

- Location: Anywhere, typically head and neck
- Definition: A self-limited contagious poxvirus infection transmitted by direct contact and characterized by an umbilicated "pearly" papule; commonly seen with HIV
- Signs and symptoms:
  - Mild pruritus
  - Shiny, umbilicated, slightly translucent skin or flesh-colored papules (Figure 16-24); slow growing, < 10 mm diameter, sometimes grouped
- Treatment: Cryotherapy, surgical excision, or wait it out; resolves in 12 to 18 months

Verruca (Warts)

- Location: Anywhere, typically hands
- Definition: Human papillomavirus (common warts—hard, rough, skin-colored papules) and others (plantar warts—bottom of foot; plane warts, also called flat warts; mosaic warts) caused by different viruses
- Signs and symptoms:
  - Initial lesion is skin colored with a smooth surface.

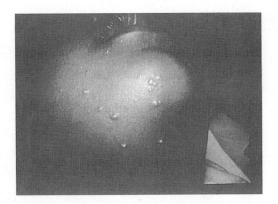

FIGURE 16-24. Molluscum contagiosum.

(Reproduced, with permission, from Seltzer V, Pearse WH. *Women's Primary Health Care: Office Practice and Procedures*, 2nd ed. New York: McGraw-Hill, 2000.)

- As lesion enlarges with time, the surface becomes roughened and papillomatous.
- Several types of warts exist and are named according to their location.
- Treatment:
    - Cryotherapy with liquid nitrogen or carbon dioxide (requires multiple treatments every 2 to 3 weeks and is painful)
    - Topical application of keratolytic agents (salicylic acid and lactic acid) and destructive agents (podophyllin or cantharidin)
    - Curettage and desiccation
    - Topical imiquimod (an immune response modifier that stimulates the immune system to fight the virus)
    - Or wait it out; resolves in 2 to 3 years

IMMUNOGENIC CUTANEOUS DISORDERS

Angioedema

- Location: Face (tongue, lips, larynx, more), anywhere (Figure 16-25)
- Definition:
    - Immunologic (associated with food, cold, insect venom, pollen) mechanism is immunoglobulin E (IgE)–antigen complex triggered massive histamine release.
    - Nonimmunologic (associated with angiotensin-converting enzyme [ACE] inhibitors, contrast dye) mechanism not well understood
- Signs and symptoms: Warm; itchy; difficulty breathing, talking, and swallowing due to airway edema
- Treatment:
    - ABCs
    - For stridor, wheezing, or low SaO_2:
        - Subcutaneous (SQ) epinephrine
        - Albuterol nebulizer
        - Consider early intubation (patient's airway can be rapidly lost due to significant airway edema).
    - IV methylprednisolone
    - IV diphenhydramine (H_1 blocker)
    - Some people give IV H_2 blocker (thought to provide some cross-reactive antihistamine benefit).
    - Admit for observation.

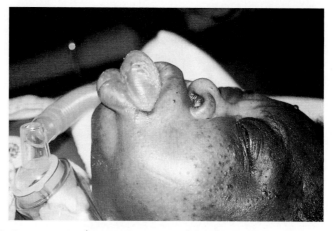

FIGURE 16-25. Severe angioedema requiring cricothyroidectomy.
(Reproduced, with permission, from Knoop K, Stack LB, and Storrow AB. *Atlas of Emergency Medicine.* New York: McGraw-Hill, 1997.)

Urticaria

- Location: Anywhere
- Definition: An immunologic reaction that results in mast-cell degranulation of histamine, causing localized capillary and postcapillary venule leak of proteinaceous fluid that is gradually resorbed. Histamine also causes vasodilation, giving localized erythema and classic wheal appearance. Types include immune type I (IgE) and type III immune-complex IgG and IgM (drugs, pollen, dust, animal dander) and non–immune mediated (cold, pressure, heat, cholinergic, dermatographism, strawberries)
- Signs and symptoms:
  - Characterized by **wheals:** An abrupt development of transient, edematous, pink papules and plaques that may be localized or generalized and are usually pruritic (Figure 16-26)
  - Wheals may develop after exposure to circulating antigens (drugs, food, insect venom, animal dander, pollen), hot and cold temperatures, exercise, and pressure or rubbing (dermatographism).

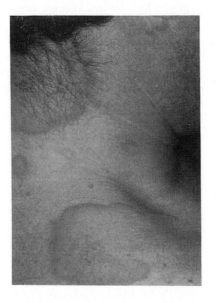

FIGURE 16-26. Urticaria.
(Reproduced, with permission, from Pantell R, et al. *The Common Symptom Guide,* 4th ed. New York: McGraw-Hill, 1996.)

- Wheals usually last < 24 hours and may recur on future exposure to the antigen.
- Treatment:
  - Antihistamines (H_1 and H_2 blockers)
  - SQ epinephrine if anaphylactic/impending associated airway compromise
  - PO or IV corticosteroids if severe
  - Observation
  - Supportive therapy

Bullous Pemphigoid

- Location: Anywhere (skin and mucosa—usually oral)
- Definition: Autoimmune disorder with IgG antibodies to the dermoepidermal junction giving vesicles and bullae that lyse and yield erosions
- Signs and symptoms:
  - Occasional pruritus and tenderness
  - Large, erythematous urticarial plaques may precede bullae by months.
  - Multiple, intact, tense bullae become crusted after rupturing.
  - Bullae can be localized or generalized, primarily distributed on flexural areas of axilla, groin, medial thighs, forearms, and lower legs (Figure 16-27).
  - Only one third of patients have oral involvement.
- Treatment: Oral/IV steroids; consult dermatologist for management

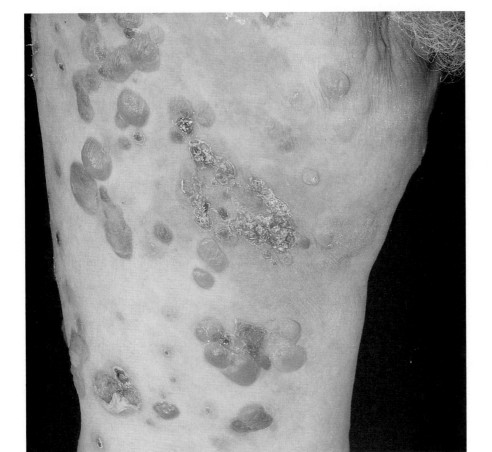

FIGURE 16-27. Bullous pemphigoid.
(Reproduced, with permission, from Fitzpatrick TB, et al. *Color Atlas and Synopsis of Clinical Dermatology: Common and Serious Diseases*, 4th ed. New York: McGraw-Hill, 2001: 100.)

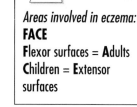

Areas involved in eczema:
FACE
Flexor surfaces = **A**dults
Children = **E**xtensor surfaces

Psoriasis is worse in winter.

Typical scenario:
A 35-year-old man has salmon-colored papules covered with silvery white scales on his scalp, elbows, and knees. *Think: Psoriasis.*

Eczema

- Location: Extremities (usually)
- Definition:
  - Also called dry skin; from loss of epidermal lipids by excessive washing or decrease in production (elderly), causing flaking and cracking
  - *Eczema* is a broad term used to describe several inflammatory skin reactions and is used synonymously with dermatitis. Eczema is an inherited skin condition with a discrete classification system (atopic, contact, allergic, stasis, or seborrheic).
- Signs and symptoms:
  - Lesions can be described as acute or chronic.
  - Acute lesions are red, blistery, and oozy.
  - Chronic lesions are thickened, lichenified, and pigmented.
- Treatment: Decrease frequency of washing or use moisturizer after each washing.

Psoriasis

- Location: Elbows, knees, scalp, gluteal cleft, nails, palms, soles
- Definition: Inherited disorder in which the keratinocyte life cycle is shortened (i.e., rapid cell turnover) looking like erythema, scaly silvery plaques, fissures, and nail plate separation from nail bed with pitting of nails. Variant exists with pustules on palms and soles, minimal scale.
- Signs and symptoms:
  - Well-demarcated, thick, "salmon-pink" **plaques** with an adherent silver-white scale (Figure 16-28)
  - Distributed bilaterally over **extensor surface** of extremities, often on elbows, knees, trunk, and scalp

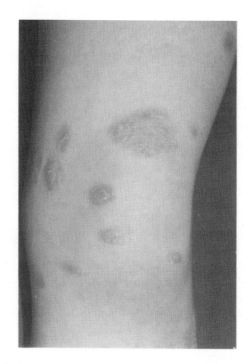

FIGURE 16-28. Psoriasis.
(Reproduced, with permission, from Rudolph A, et al. *Rudolph's Pediatrics,* 20th ed. Stamford, CT: Appleton & Lange, 1997.)

- Nails are commonly involved: Pitting of nails, oil spots (yellow-brown spots under nail plate), onycholysis (separation of distal nail plate from nail bed), subungual hyperkeratosis (thickening)
- Can occur at site of injury (Koebner phenomenon)
- Pinpoint capillary bleeding occurs if scale is removed (Auspitz sign).
- Treatment: Tar emulsion (1 tsp in quart of water) applied bid followed by group I topical steroid cream, moisturizer creams

EM

- Location: Palms, soles, extremities, anywhere
- Definition: Immune complex–mediated (IgM, C3) vasculitis of blood vessels at dermo-epidermal junction that give rise to multiple pink-red, target-shaped bullae and papules of varying sizes; most commonly due to drugs, infections, x-ray therapy, malignancy, and unknown etiology
- Signs and symptoms:
  - Viral-like prodrome may precede eruption.
  - Lesions itch and burn, may lyse yielding erosions
  - Although characterized by target lesions, multiforme refers to the wide variety of lesions that may be present, including papules, vesicles, and bullae (Figure 16-29).

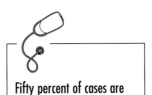

Fifty percent of cases are idiopathic, but herpes simplex virus accounts for most cases of recurrent EM.

FIGURE 16-29. EM. Note the many different-sized lesions.

(Reproduced, with permission, from Knoop KJ, Stack LB, and Storrow AB. *Atlas of Emergency Medicine*. New York: McGraw-Hill, 1997.)

- Treatment:
  - Cessation of medication (if possible)
  - Antihistamines for itch
  - Wet-to-dry dressings with topical bacitracin for erosions
  - Look for underlying cause.
  - Supportive care

SJS

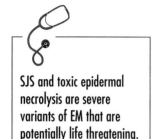

SJS and toxic epidermal necrolysis are severe variants of EM that are potentially life threatening.

- Location: Mucous membranes, conjunctiva, respiratory tract, various areas of skin
- Definition: Bullous variant of EM most often secondary to medication (sulfonamides, barbiturates, phenytoin, carbamazepine, thiazide diuretics, penicillins) or infection (upper respiratory infections, gastroenteritis, mycoplasma, herpes simplex virus).
- Signs and symptoms:
  - Viral-like prodrome precedes skin and mucosal lesions, which are itchy, burning, red-pink, target-shaped bullae, lysing to give erosions (Figure 16-30).
  - Bullous target lesions often less than 10% of epidermis
  - High morbidity and mortality
- Treatment:
  - Hospital admission may be required.
  - Antihistamines for the itch
  - Corticosteroid (IV/oral) use is controversial, with most favoring its use.

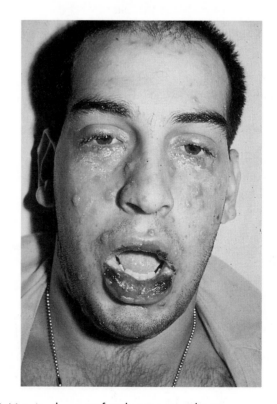

FIGURE 16-30. SJS. Note involvement of oral mucous membranes.

(Reproduced, with permission, from Knoop KJ, Stack LB, and Storrow AB. Atlas of Emergency Medicine. New York: McGraw-Hill, 1997: 343.)

314

- Removal of offending medication if possible
- Soft/liquid diet
- Eroded lesions treated with wet-to-dry dressings and topical bacitracin

TEN

- Location: Everywhere, with mucosal involvement
- Definition: EM variant that is a true emergency from lysis of 30 to 100% of epidermis at dermal junction caused by similar things that cause EM/SJS; mortality high
- Signs and symptoms:
  - Prodrome of fever and influenza-like symptoms
  - Pruritus, pain, tenderness, and burning
  - Classic target-like lesions symmetrically distributed on dorsum of hands, palms, soles, face, and knees
  - Initial **target lesions** can become confluent, erythematous, and tender, with bullous formation and subsequent loss of epidermis.
  - Epidermal sloughing may be generalized, resembling a second-degree burn, and is more pronounced over pressure points (Figure 16-31).
  - Positive Nikolsky's sign
  - Ninety percent of cases have mucosal lesions—painful, erythematous erosions on lips, buccal mucosa, conjunctiva, and anogenital region.
- Treatment:
  - Hospital admission (usually to burn unit)
  - Wounds treated as second-degree burns
  - Avoid steroid use.
  - Studies suggest that plasmapheresis or exchange, hyperbaric O_2, and cyclosporine can decrease extent of disease and facilitate healing.

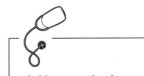

Nikolsky's sign: Sloughing of epidermis with light pressure over lesion.

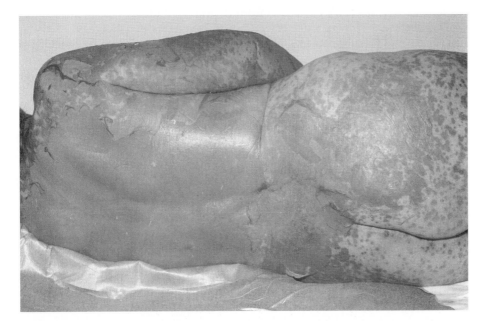

FIGURE 16-31. TEN. Note the generalized macular eruption and large denuded erosive area.

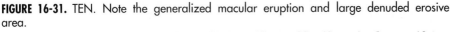

(Reproduced, with permission, from Fitzpatrick TB, et al. *Color Atlas and Synopsis of Clinical Dermatology: Common and Serious Diseases,* 4th ed. New York: McGraw-Hill, 2001: 141.)

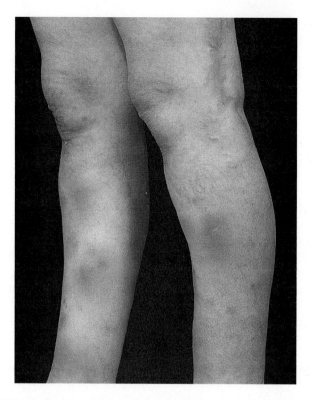

FIGURE 16-32. Erythema nodosum. Note indurated, very tender inflammatory nodules mostly over pretibial region. Palpable as deep nodules.

(Reproduced, with permission, from Fitzpatrick TB, et al. *Color Atlas and Synopsis of Clinical Dermatology: Common and Serious Diseases,* 4th ed. New York: McGraw-Hill, 2001: 145.)

Erythema Nodosum

- Location: Shins, lower extremities (Figure 16-32)
- Definition: Hypersensitivity vasculitis of venules in subcutaneous tissue from drugs (sulfonamides, oral contraceptives), infections (tuberculosis, *Streptococcus* spp., coccidioidomycosis), or systemic disease (sarcoidosis, inflammatory bowel disease, lymphoma, leukemia) and look like red subcutaneous nodules with surrounding erythema; can last 6 weeks
- Signs and symptoms:
  - Painful and tender lesions accompanied by fever, malaise, and arthralgias
  - ± Regional adenopathy
- Treatment: Cessation of medication (if possible), nonsteroidal anti-inflammatory drugs for pain, look for underlying etiology

HSP

- Location: Lower legs and buttocks
- Definition: IgA immune complex vasculitis involving arterioles and capillaries caused by drugs, infections, foods, immunizations, and insect bites; usually a childhood disorder
- Signs and symptoms:
  - Purplish raised papules and "palpable purpura" (Figure 16-33)
  - Arthralgias

Typical scenario:
A 5-year-old child presents with a palpable purpura over his buttocks and back of his legs and also complains of joint pains and nausea. *Think: HSP.*

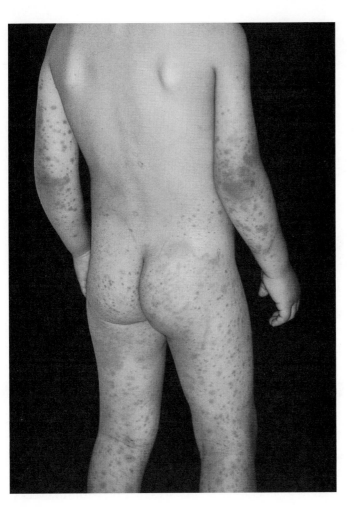

FIGURE 16-33. HSP.

(Reproduced, with permission, from Knoop KJ, Stack LB, Storrow AB. *Atlas of Emergency Medicine.* New York: McGraw-Hill, 1997: 345.)

- Gastrointestinal complaints (nausea, vomiting, diarrhea, abdominal pain—70%)
- Renal involvement (hematuria, red blood cell [RBC] casts—50%)
- Treatment:
    - Admit for IV steroids if renal involvement.
    - Otherwise, discharge home on PO prednisone 1 mg/kg/day, and remove the offending agent if possible.

Systemic Lupus Erythematosus (SLE)

- Location: Face (malar rash), widespread (discoid) (Figure 16-34)
- Definition: Multisystem anti–double-stranded DNA autoantibody-mediated inflammatory disorder.
- Signs and symptoms: Systemic symptoms include fever, arthralgia, pneumonitis, nephritis, pericarditis, and vasculitis.
- Treatment: Systemic steroids and immunosuppressive therapy for flare-ups

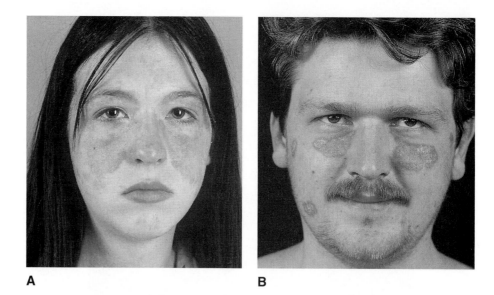

A   **B**

FIGURE 16-34. Malar (A) and discoid (B) rashes of SLE.

(Reproduced, with permission, from Fitzpatrick TB, et al. *Color Atlas and Synopsis of Clinical Dermatology: Common and Serious Diseases,* 4th ed. New York: McGraw-Hill, 2001: 363, 364.)

MISCELLANEOUS RASHES

Typical scenario:
A 21-year-old male presents with a pruritic, spotted rash on the trunk that began as one solitary larger patch. *Think: Pityriasis rosea.*

Pityriasis Rosea

- Location: Chest or back or both
- Definition: A common self-limiting eruption of a single herald patch followed by a generalized secondary eruption within 2 weeks; ages 10 to 35 commonly
- Signs and symptoms:
  - A 2- to 10-cm solitary, oval, erythematous "herald patch" with a collarette of scale precedes the generalized eruption in 80% of patients.
  - Within days, multiple, smaller, pink, oval, scaly patches appear over trunk and upper extremities.
  - Secondary eruption occurs in a Christmas tree distribution, oriented parallel to the ribs (Figure 16-35).
- Treatment: Antihistamines for itch

Seborrheic Dermatitis

- Location: Skin folds and hair-bearing areas of face, scalp, chest, groin
- Definition: Waxy, erythematous scale possibly related to yeast (*Pityrosporum ovale*); "cradle cap" in infancy
- Signs and symptoms: Mild itch
- Treatment: Zinc pyrethrin (Head and Shoulders), selenium sulfide (Selsun Blue), or tar (Neutrogena T-Gel) shampoo—lathered for 10 minutes, then rinsed, 3 times a week; 1 to 2.5% hydrocortisone cream for face

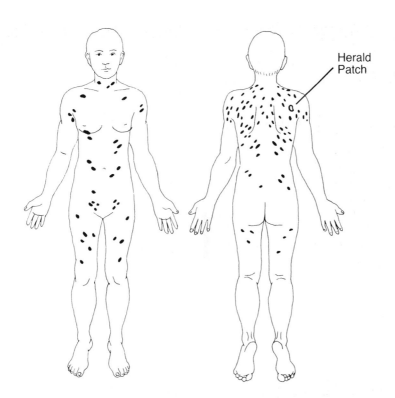

Herald Patch

FIGURE 16-35. Distribution of pityriasis rosea. Note "Christmas tree" pattern of rash and location of herald patch.

(Reproduced, with permission, from Fitzpatrick TB, et al. *Color Atlas and Synopsis of Clinical Dermatology: Common and Serious Diseases*, 4th ed. New York: McGraw-Hill, 2001: 107.)

Decubitus Ulcers

- Location: Over bony prominences (sacrum, ischial tuberosities, iliac crests, greater trochanters, heels, elbows, knees, occiput)
- Definition: Any pressure-induced ulcer that occurs secondary to external compression of the skin, resulting in ischemic tissue necrosis (i.e., bedsore, pressure ulcer). Early ulcers have irregular, ragged borders, but chronic ulcers have smooth, well-demarcated borders. Infection is usually polymicrobial: *S. aureus, Streptococcus, Pseudomonas, Enterococcus, Proteus, Clostridium,* and *Bacteroides.*
- Signs and symptoms: Painful, ulcerated
- Treatment:
  - *Prophylaxis:*
    - Mobilizing patients as soon as possible
    - Repositioning patients every 2 hours
    - Pressure-reducing devices (foam, air, or liquid mattresses)
    - Correction of nutritional status
  - *Local wound care:*
    - Proper cleansing with mild agents
    - Moisturizing to maintain hydration and promote healing
    - Polyurethane, hydrocolloid, or absorptive dressings, and topical antibiotics for wound
    - Necrotic tissue may require surgical debridement, flaps, and skin grafts.
    - Appropriate antibiotic therapy for infected ulcer

Risk factors for decubitus ulcers:
- Immobility, fracture
- Malnutrition
- Age > 70
- Hypoalbuminemia
- Spinal cord injury
- Fecal incontinence
- Diabetes mellitus
- Inadequate nursing care
- Decreased level of consciousness

HIGH-YIELD FACTS

Dermatologic Emergencies

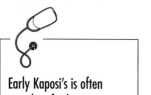

Stages of decubitus ulcers:
I—nonblanching erythema of intact skin
II—partial-thickness skin loss involving epidermis and/or dermis (superficial ulcer)
III—full-thickness skin loss involving epidermis and dermis (deep, crateriform ulcer); may involve damage to subcutaneous tissue, extending down to, but not through, fascia
IV—full-thickness skin loss with extensive damage to muscle, bone, or other supporting structures

Early Kaposi's is often mistaken for bruising.

Basal Cell Carcinoma (Rodent Ulcer)

- Location: Sun-exposed areas (forehead, nose)
- Definition: Slow-growing proliferation of basal keratinocytes
- Signs and symptoms:
  - Asymptomatic, rarely painful
  - Flesh-colored or hyperpigmented nodule with surface telangiectasia that expands outward leaving central ulcer and "rolled" raised edge (Figure 16-36)
- Treatment: Surgical excision

Kaposi's Sarcoma

- Location: Anywhere (skin and mucosa)
- Definition: Multisystem vascular neoplasm characterized by mucocutaneous violaceous lesions, commonly seen in acquired immune deficiency syndrome patients
- Signs and symptoms: Cutaneous, nonblanching, reddish-purple macules, plaques, and nodules made of vasoformative tissue (spindle cells, vascular spaces, hemosiderin-stained macrophages, extravasated RBCs) (Figure 16-37)
- Treatment: Radiation therapy (if limited disease), chemotherapy, and radiation (if disseminated—palliative)

Melanoma

- Location: Anywhere
- Definition: A malignant proliferation of melanocytes (> 10 mm diameter, crusting or inflammation, change in size, color, contour, texture, or sensation) (Figure 16-38)
- Signs and symptoms: May itch or lose sensation
- Treatment: Wide surgical excision

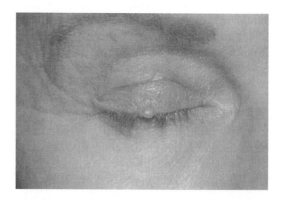

FIGURE 16-36. Basal cell carcinoma. Note the translucent nature of the lesion.

(Reproduced, with permission, from Seltzer V, Pearse WH. *Women's Primary Health Care: Office Practice and Procedures*, 2nd ed. New York: McGraw-Hill, 2000.)

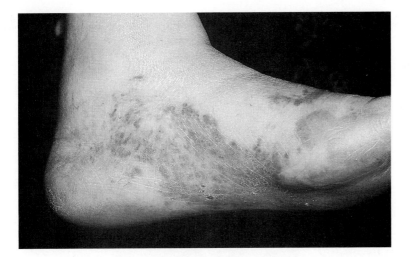

FIGURE 16-37. Kaposi's sarcoma. Note multiple purplish confluent papules, often mistaken for bruising.

(Reproduced, with permission, from Fitzpatrick TB, et al. *Color Atlas and Synopsis of Clinical Dermatology: Common and Serious Diseases,* 4th ed. New York: McGraw-Hill, 2001: 527.)

Squamous Cell Carcinoma

- Location: Sun-exposed areas (face, neck, forearms)
- Definition: Malignant proliferation of epidermal keratinocytes, sometimes locally invasive; expanding nodular plaque, with indurated base and central ulcer with crust/scale (Figure 16-39)
- Signs and symptoms: A cut that won't heal, bleeds easily
- Treatment: Surgical excision

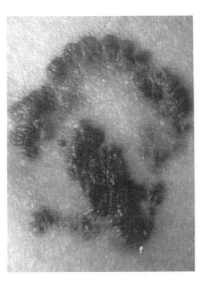

FIGURE 16-38. Melanoma.

(Reproduced, with permission, from Pantell R, et al. *The Common Symptom Guide,* 4th ed. New York: McGraw-Hill, 1996.)

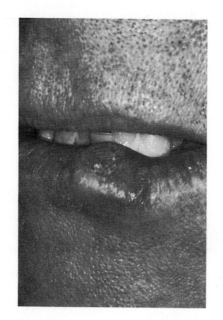

FIGURE 16-39. Squamous cell cancer.
(Reproduced, with permission, from Pantell R, et al. *The Common Symptom Guide,* 4th ed. New York: McGraw-Hill, 1996.)

Procedures

TUBE THORACOSTOMY

DEFINITION

Tube thoracostomy, commonly called a chest tube, is used to remove air or fluid from the pleural space.

INDICATIONS

- Pneumothorax
- Hemothorax
- Hemopneumothorax
- Open pneumothorax (sucking chest wound)
- Drainage of recurrent pleural effusion
- Empyema
- Chylothorax

RELATIVE CONTRAINDICATIONS

- Multiple adhesions
- Need for thoracotomy
- Recurrent pneumothorax requiring definitive treatment
- Severe coagulopathy

PROCEDURE (MIDAXILLARY LINE PLACEMENT)

1. Elevate the head of the bed at least 30 degrees to reduce the chances of injury to abdominal organs.
2. Identify the fourth intercostal space in the midaxillary line.
3. Prep and sterilize the area (Figure 17-1A).
4. Anesthetize the skin, muscle, periosteum, and parietal pleura through which the tube will pass by utilizing a local anesthetic such as lidocaine. If time permits, do intercostal blocks above and below to provide better anesthesia.
5. Estimate the distance from incision to apex of the lung on the chest tube, ensuring that the distance is enough to allow the last drainage hole of the chest tube to fit inside the pleura. Place a clamp at this point of the chest tube.
6. Make a 2- to 4-cm skin incision over the rib below the one the tube will pass over. The incision should be big enough for the tube and

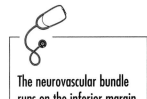

The neurovascular bundle runs on the inferior margin of each rib.

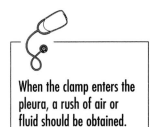

When the clamp enters the pleura, a rush of air or fluid should be obtained.

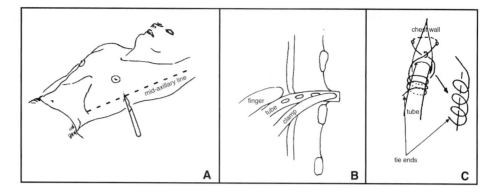

FIGURE 17-1. Procedure for tube thoracostomy. **A.** An incision is made in the fourth or fifth intercostal space in the midaxillary line. **B.** Following finger exploration to confirm space, the tube is advanced, guided by the curved clamp. **C.** The tube is secured in place.
(Modified, with permission, from Scaletta TA, Schaider JJ. *Emergent Management of Trauma.* New York: McGraw-Hill, 1996: 359–361.)

Size of chest tube to use:
For adult large hemothorax: 36–40 French
For adult pneumothorax: 24 French
For children: Four times the size of appropriate endotracheal tube

one finger to fit through at the same time. Use blunt dissection to penetrate down to the fascia overlying the intercostal muscles.

7. Insert a closed, heavy clamp over the rib and push through the muscles and parietal pleura. Spread the tips of the clamp to enlarge the opening.

8. Close the clamps and insert one finger next to the clamp into the pleural space. Sweep the finger around to ensure that you are in the pleural space and there are no adhesions. While leaving your finger in, remove the clamp and insert the chest tube by clamping the tip with a curved clamp and following the path of your finger (Figure 17-1B).

9. Remove the clamp and guide the chest tube in a superior and posterior direction.

10. Insert the tube until your previously placed marker clamp is against the skin.

11. Attach the tube to a water seal.

12. Secure the tube by using suture material to close the skin and then wrapping it around the chest tube tightly enough to prevent slipping (the two ends of the suture are wrapped in opposite directions [Figure 17-1C]). A purse string stitch also works nicely.

13. Place an occlusive dressing over the area.

14. Chest tube placement should be confirmed by chest x-ray.

COMPLICATIONS

- Subcutaneous (SQ) (versus intrathoracic) placement
- Bleeding from intercostal vessels
- Injury to intercostal nerves
- Infection
- Lung laceration
- Diaphragm injury
- Liver injury

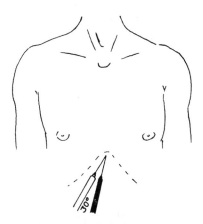

FIGURE 17-2. Pericardiocentesis via subxiphoid approach.

(Reproduced, with permission, from Scaletta TA, Schaider JJ. *Emergent Management of Trauma*, 2nd ed. New York: McGraw-Hill, 2001: 450.)

PERICARDIOCENTESIS

DEFINITION

The drainage of fluid from the pericardium, which relieves tamponade (Figure 17-2)

PROCEDURE

1. If possible, electrocardiographic (ECG) monitoring should be utilized by clamping one of the precordial leads to the needle.
2. After prepping the area, insert a 16- or 18G needle at a 30-degree angle into the left xiphocostal angle about 0.5 cm below the costal margin.
3. Advance the needle to the inner aspect of the rib cage.
4. Depress the needle to get under the ribs and point it toward the left shoulder.
5. Advance the needle as you aspirate until fluid is reached; this should not be much more than 1 cm.

COMPLICATIONS

- Dry tap
- Dysrhythmias
- Air embolism
- Cardiac, vessel, or lung injury

LOCAL ANESTHESIA

- Local anesthesia is done by local infiltration into and around the wound or by regional block.
- Anesthetic is slowly injected adjacent to the wound edge in a sequential fashion or directly into the dermis and SQ tissue through the open wound edge using a small-gauge (25G) needle.
- Epinephrine may be added to provide vasoconstriction and prolong the action of the anesthetic.
- Commonly used local anesthetic agents are listed in Table 17-1.

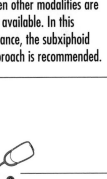

Pericardiocentesis is usually performed with ultrasound guidance or under fluoroscopy. Blind pericardiocentesis should be performed only in the unstable patient or as part of cardiac arrest protocols when other modalities are not available. In this instance, the subxiphoid approach is recommended.

Places you should not use epinephrine: **SPF-10**
Scrotum
Penis
Fingers

Toes
Ears
Nose

TABLE 17-1. Commonly Used Local Anesthetic Agents

Agent	Concentration	Onset of Action	Maximum Dosage
Lidocaine (Xylocaine)	1% or 2%	Immediate: 4–10 min Duration: 1–2 hr	4.5 mg/kg = 30 mL of 1% solution
Mepivacaine (Carbocaine)	1% or 2%	Immediate: 6–10 min Duration: 1.5–2.5 hr	5 mg/kg = 35 mL of 1% solution
Bupivacaine (Marcaine)	0.25%	Slower: 8–12 min Duration: 6–8 hr	3 mg/kg = 80 mL of 0.25% solution

ARTHROCENTESIS

- Indications:
  - Diagnose acute, painful nontraumatic or traumatic joint disease by synovial fluid analysis.
  - Therapeutic intervention to drain an effusion or hemarthrosis
- Contraindications: Infection (i.e., cellulitis or abscess) overlying affected joint

PROCEDURE

- Under sterile conditions, use povidone–iodine solution to prep skin, then wipe off with alcohol to prevent introduction of iodine into the joint space.
- Apply sterile drape and anesthetize skin and overlying SQ tissue down to the joint capsule.
- When joint space is entered, there will be an abrupt decrease in resistance.
- Remove anesthetizing needle and syringe and follow same track using an 18G needle, or catheter for large joints, with a 30-mL syringe so as to completely drain the joint space.
- Once in joint space, gently aspirate. Then send fluid for analysis, which should include: Gram stain and culture, microscopy for crystals, complete blood count with differential, glucose, and protein.
- Cover area with sterile dressing.

JOINT FLUID ANALYSIS

Septic	White blood cell (WBC) > 50,000 Polymorphonuclear neutrophil (PMN) 　> 85% Glucose < 50 mg/dL Gram stain positive in 65% Culture positive
Gout/pseudogout	WBC 2,500–50,000 PMN 40–90% Urate crystals (gout) Ca^{2+} pyrophosphate crystals (pseudogout)
Inflammatory	WBC 10,000–50,000 PMN 65–85%
Degenerative joint disease	WBC < 5,000 PMN < 25%

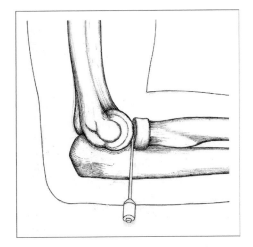

FIGURE 17-3. Elbow arthrocentesis.
(Reproduced, with permission, from Wilson FC, Lin PP. *General Orthopaedics.* New York: McGraw-Hill, 1997: 121.)

Traumatic	Bloody
	WBC < 1,000
	Fat droplets (with fracture)

ASPIRATION SITES

Shoulder	Patient sits upright with arm held in neutral position. Enter joint space anteriorly and inferiorly to the coracoid process.
Elbow	Place elbow at 90 degrees of flexion with hand prone. Locate the radial head, lateral epicondyle, and lateral aspect of the olecranon tip (anconeus triangle). Needle enters at center of triangle, perpendicular to radius (Figure 17-3).
Knee	With knee held in extension and slight flexion, enter joint space medially and inferior to the patella at its midpoint (Figure 17-4).
Ankle	With the foot in plantar flexion, place needle just medial to the anterior tibial tendon at the anterior edge of the medial malleolus.
Fingers/toes	With the digit flexed 15 to 20 degrees and traction applied, enter joint from the dorsal aspect medially or laterally to extensor tendon.
Wrist	With the wrist held at 20 to 30 degrees of flexion and traction applied, place needle dorsal and ulnar to the extensor pollicis longus tendon.
Thumb	With the thumb opposed, place the needle at the base of the first metacarpal on the palmar side of the abductor pollicis longus.

INTRAOSSEOUS ACCESS

INDICATIONS

- When vascular access cannot be obtained through other means
- In children up to age 6 with difficult peripheral or central access. After age 6, red marrow is replaced by yellow marrow, making infusion more difficult.

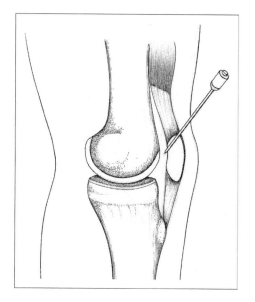

FIGURE 17-4. Knee arthrocentesis. Viewing the patella as the face of a clock, the needle is inserted just behind the patella at either 10 or 2 o'clock (medially or laterally).

(Reproduced, with permission, from Wilson FC, Lin PP. *General Orthopaedics.* New York: McGraw-Hill, 1997: 123.)

SITES

- Proximal tibia (most common in children) puncture site is 1 to 3 cm below the tibial tuberosity, midline on the medial flat surface of the anterior tibia. Direct needle 15 degrees off the perpendicular away from the epiphysis (Figure 17-5).
- Distal tibia (common in adults) puncture site is the medial surface of the of ankle proximal to the medial malleolus.
- Distal femur puncture site is on the dorsal surface where the condyle meets the shaft of bone.
- Sternum (high complication rate)

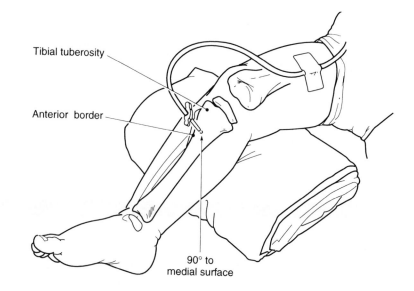

FIGURE 17-5. Intraosseous access.

(Reproduced, with permission, from *Textbook of Pediatric Life Support,* ©1997 American Heart Association.)

PROCEDURE

- Using sterile technique, a bone marrow aspiration needle, intraosseous infusion needle, or spinal needle is grasped in the palm of the hand and using a twisting motion is bored into the periosteum until the resistance decreases.
- Proper placement is confirmed by bone marrow aspiration or successful infusion of several milliliters of normal saline (NS).
- Local anesthesia is optional.

COMPLICATIONS

- Cellulitis
- Osteomyelitis (< 1%)
- Fracture
- Fat embolism (rare)
- Growth plate injury

CONSCIOUS SEDATION

INDICATIONS

- Painful procedures done in the emergency department (ED) (incision and drainage [I&D], reduction of bone)
- Anxious patient
- Uncooperative/anxious child who needs procedure or diagnostic test performed

GOALS

- To provide an adequate state of sedation and analgesia while allowing patient to maintain an independent airway, reflexes, and response to verbal stimulation
- To allow patient to be discharged quickly and safely

PATIENT SELECTION

- Healthy individuals with mild or no systemic disease
- No history of neurologic impairment
- Fasting at least 4 hours from solid food or 2 hours from liquids (non-emergent cases only)

MONITORING

- Cardiac monitor and pulse oximetry
- O_2, intubation equipment, and medical reversal agents should be readily available.
- Peripheral access should be obtained.
- Initial set of vitals, vitals 10 minutes after administration, and every 15 minutes thereafter until patient is alert and oriented × 3 and can sit up (if previously able to sit up)

MEDICATIONS

- Two agents are usually used, one for sedation (benzodiazepine) and another for analgesia (opiate).

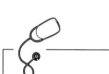

An emergence reaction is the occurrence of hallucinations and nightmares during the wearing off of ketamine. Occurs in about half of all adults and in about 10% of children. Allowing the patient to recover in a dark, quiet room minimizes this phenomenon.

Naloxone is an opiate antagonist. Flumazenil is a benzodiazepine antagonist. Have these on hand when doing conscious sedation in case quick reversal becomes necessary.

- Although medications may be given IV, IM, PO, or PR, the IV route is preferred because of ease of titration of medications and quicker action.
- **Midazolam** (Versed):
  - Benzodiazepine
  - 0.05 to 0.1 mg/kg IV, incremental dose at 2-minute intervals to desired effect
  - Duration 30 to 45 minutes
- **Diazepam** (Valium):
  - Benzodiazepine
  - 0.1 to 0.2 mg/kg IV (max 10 mg)
  - Duration 2 to 6 hours, do not give IM (erratic absorption)
- **Fentanyl:**
  - Opioid
  - 50 to 400 μg IV, incremental dose at 2-minute intervals to desired effect
  - Onset 1 to 3 minutes
  - Duration 30 to 60 minutes
- **Ketamine** (Ketalar):
  - Dissociative hypnotic
  - 1 to 3 mg/kg
  - Onset 30 to 60 seconds
  - Duration 15 minutes
  - Contraindications: Age < 3 months, increased intracranial pressure, seizure, glaucoma, psychosis, thyroid disorder, porphyria
  - May see emergence reaction after age 10
- **Pentobarbital:**
  - Barbiturate
  - 4 to 6 mg/kg IV
  - Onset 30 to 60 seconds
  - Duration 2 to 4 hours
- **Nitrous Oxide** (N_2O):
  - 50% N_2O/50% O_2 via inhalation
  - Onset 2 to 5 minutes
  - Duration 2 to 5 minutes
  - Must administer continuously
- **Flumazenil:**
  - Benzodiazepine antagonist
  - 0.2 mg q1min to max of 1 mg in 5 minutes
  - Onset 30 to 60 seconds
  - Duration 20 minutes
- **Naloxone:**
  - Opiate receptor antagonist
  - 0.2 to 2.0 mg IV
  - Onset 30 to 90 seconds
  - Duration 2 to 3 hours

SPLINTING

INDICATIONS

- Fractures to be seen by orthopedics at a later date
- Dislocations that have been reduced

- Fiberglass or plaster

PREPARATION

Plaster
- Measure the length of the affected extremity with the plaster, then place the plaster roll on a flat surface and unroll the plaster back and forth on itself to a total of 12 layers.
- Measure several layers of padding to be both longer and wider than the plaster.
- Submerge the plaster in water and hold until the bubbling stops.
- Strip excess water from plaster by holding plaster up in one hand and stressing plaster between thumb and index finger with the other from top to bottom.
- Place plaster on flat surface and massage layers together.
- Place padding on top, then apply to extremity with padding against skin and mold with palms, not fingers, to avoid creating pressure points.
- Wrap with Ace bandage (over gauze) for compression.

Fiberglass
- Cut material to desired length.
- Do not submerge in water. Put one strip of water down center of splint then curl up splint in a towel to remove excess moisture.
- Stretch outer padding over the ends of the fiberglass to avoid sharp edges and apply to extremity and Ace wrap.
- Fiberglass will harden within 10 minutes, much more quickly than plaster.

Upper Extremity Splints
- Reverse sugar tong (Figure 17-6):
  - Indications: Forearm or Colles' fracture
  - Use 3″ to 4″ adult; cut splint in center, leaving small piece to overlie thumb.

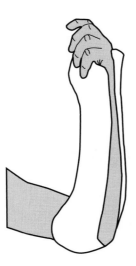

FIGURE 17-6. Reverse sugar tong splint.

331

Procedures

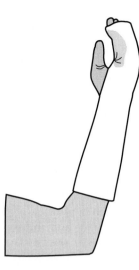

FIGURE 17-7. Boxer splint.

- Boxer splint (Figure 17-7):
  - Indications: Fourth and fifth metacarpal fracture
- Long arm ulnar gutter (elbow) splint (Figure 17-8):
- Indications: Supracondylar fracture, elbow sprain, radial head fracture
  - Elbow is held at 90 degrees. Splint extends from metacarpal heads to upper arm below axillary crease along ulnar surface.
- Cock-up splint:
  - Indications: Wrist sprain, carpal tunnel syndrome
  - Wrist is in extension, splint extends from midforearm to metacarpophalangeal (MCP) on volar surface of hand.
- Thumb spica (Figure 17-9):
  - Indications: Navicular or scaphoid fracture, thumb dislocation, ulnar collateral ligament sprain, thumb proximal phalanx fracture, MCP fracture

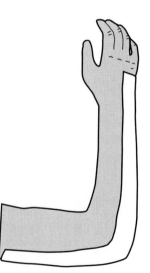

FIGURE 17-8. Elbow splint.

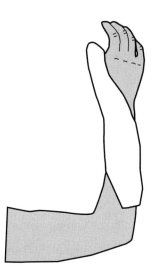

FIGURE 17-9. Thumb spica splint.

- The wrist is in neutral position and the thumb in abduction; the splint extends from the ulnar aspect of forearm and comes radially over dorsum of wrist and hand to encompass thumb.

Lower Extremity Splints

- Posterior leg (ankle) splint (Figure 17-10):
    - Indications: Distal tibia and fibula fracture, ankle sprain, Achilles' tendon tear, metatarsal fracture
    - The ankle is in neutral position, except for Achilles' tears in which the patient should be immobilized in plantar flexion. The splint extends from 2″ posterior to knee to metatarsophalangeal heads.
- Ankle stirrup (Figure 17-11):
    - Indications: Ankle strain/sprain, shin splint, hairline fracture

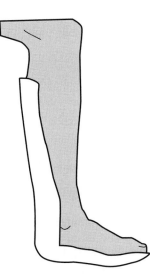

FIGURE 17-10. Posterior ankle splint.

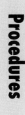

Procedures

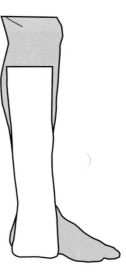

FIGURE 17-11. Ankle stirrup splint.

- The splint extends from medial to lateral aspect of lower leg at mid-calf to encompass the calcaneus. This prevents inversion/eversion.
- Long leg splint:
  - Indications: Femoral fracture
  - Apply like posterior leg splint, but superior aspect of splint extends to 3″ below buttock.
- Knee immobilizer:
  - Indications: Knee sprain, postop knee surgery
  - Usually ready-made device that wraps around posterior and sides of the lower extremities from upper thigh to lower leg above the ankle. It is held in place by anterior Velcro straps.

SUTURES

Types of Closure

- Primary:
  - Closure within 6 to 8 hours of any wound on body
  - Face and scalp may be closed primarily up to 24 hours because of good vascular supply.
- Secondary: Wound heals by granulation alone ("2 degree intention").
- Delayed primary closure: Closure of a wound 3 to 5 days following injury

Tetanus

- If unknown history or fewer than three doses, give Td (tetanus and diptheria) toxoid.
- If three doses given and within 7 years, no immunization necessary
- If tetanus-prone wound (> 6 hours, avulsion, crush, > 1 cm depth, abrasion, contusion, contamination, devitalized tissue, or frostbite) and unknown tetanus history, give Td and tetanus immune globulin.

Give tetanus prophylaxis to anything that is **CUT:**
Contaminated wounds
Unknown tetanus history
Tetanus status expired

Prevent Infection

- Irrigation is the most important procedure required to clean a wound.
- Use NS, a 8G needle, and 30-cc syringe to irrigate wound with 8 to 10 psi.
- Antibiotics are not proven to be of prophylactic benefit. Do give for grossly contaminated wounds.

*Prevent infection with **PSI:***
Pressure 8 to 10 psi
Sterile saline
Irrigate with 500 to 1,000 mL

Suture Equipment

- Needles:
  - Cutting: Has two cutting edges for shallow bites
  - Reverse cutting: Has three cutting edges for deeper bites
- Needle holder:
  - Place at 90-degree angle
  - One third from swage
  - Needle at tip of needle holder
- Dissecting forceps: To gently evert skin edges
- Skin hooks
- Scissors
- Local anesthetic
- Suture material: See Tables 17-2 and 17-3. See Table 17-4 for closure recommendations by wound site.

TABLE 17-2. Suture Materials: Absorbable

Material	Half-Life	Type	Comments
Gut	5–7 days	Natural	Stiff, rapidly absorbed, used for mucosal closure only
Chromic gut	10–14 days	Natural	Used for intraoral lacerations
Polyglycolic acid (Dexon)	10–15 days	Synthetic multifilament	Used for SQ sutures, difficult to tie
Polyglactin 910 (Vicryl)	14–21 days	Synthetic multifilament	Use clear variety on face, easy workability, SQ
Polydioxanone (PDS II)	28 days	Synthetic monofilament	Very strong, low reactivity, large knot mass

TABLE 17-3. Suture Materials: Nonabsorbable

Material	Type	Comments
Silk	Natural multifilament	Easiest to handle but poses greatest risk of infection, not used on face
Nylon (Ethilon and Dermalon)	Synthetic mono- or multifilament	Low tissue reactivity, most often used for cutaneous closure
Polypropylene (Prolene)	Synthetic monofilament	Stiffest sutures, requires five to six knots, tends to untie
Polyester (Mersilene)	Synthetic multifilament	Easy handling with excellent security, often used for vascular or facial wounds
Polybutester (Norafil)	Synthetic monofilament	Slight elasticity allows wound swelling

TABLE 17-4. Closure Recommendations by Wound Sites

Location	Material	Technique
Scalp	3-0 or 4-0 nylon or polypropylene	Interrupted in galea, single tight layer in scalp, horizontal mattress if bleeding not well controlled
Pinna	5-0 Vicryl/Dexon in perichondrium	Close perichondrium with interrupted Vicryl and close skin with interrupted nylon.
Eyebrow	4-0 or 5-0 Vicryl (SQ) 6-0 nylon	Layered closure
Eyelid	6-0 nylon	Single-layer horizontal mattress or simple interrupted
Lip	4-0 Vicryl (mucosa) 5-0 Vicryl (SQ or muscle) 6-0 nylon (skin)	If wound through lip, close three layers (mucosa, muscle, skin); otherwise do two-layer closure.
Oral cavity	4-0 Vicryl	Simple interrupted or horizontal mattress if muscularis of tongue involved
Face	6-0 nylon (skin) 5-0 Vicryl (SQ)	Simple interrupted for single layer, layered closure for full-thickness laceration
Trunk	4-0 Vicryl (SQ, fat) 4-0 or 5-0 nylon (skin)	Single or layered closure
Extremity	3-0 or 4-0 Vicryl (SQ, fat, muscle) 4-0 or 5-0 nylon (skin)	Single-layer interrupted or vertical mattress; apply splint if over a joint
Hands and feet	4-0 or 5-0 nylon	Single-layer closure with simple interrupted or horizontal mattress; apply splint if over a joint
Nail bed	5-0 Vicryl	Meticulous placement to obtain even edges, allow to dissolve

Suturing Techniques

- Simple interrupted (Figure 17-12):
  - To close most simple wounds
  - Edges should always be everted to prevent depression of scar. Do this by entering needle at 90 degrees to skin surface and follow curve of needle through skin.
  - Entrance and exit point of needle should be equidistant from laceration.
  - Do not place suture too shallow, as this will cause dead space.
  - Use instrument tie or surgeons knot and place knot to one side of laceration not directly over laceration.
- Running suture (Figure 17-13):
  - Not commonly used in the ED
  - Disadvantage: One nicked stitch or knot means the entire suture is out.
  - Advantage: Done well with sturdy knots, it provides even tension across wound.
- Vertical mattress (Figure 17-14):
  - This suture helps in reducing dead space and in eversion of wound edges.

336

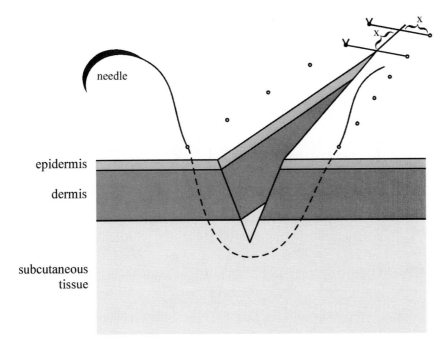

FIGURE 17-12. Simple interrupted suture.

- It does not significantly reduce tension on wound.
- The needle enters the skin farther away (more lateral) from the laceration than the simple interrupted and also exits further away on the opposite side.
- It then enters again on the same side that it just exited from but more proximal to the laceration and exits on the opposite side (where it originally entered) proximally.

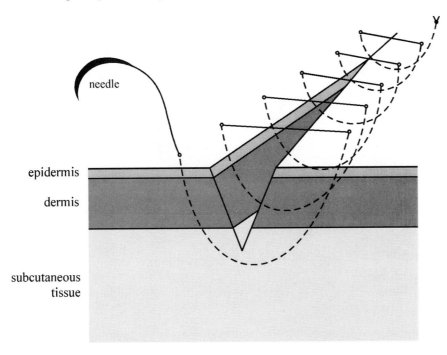

FIGURE 17-13. Running suture.

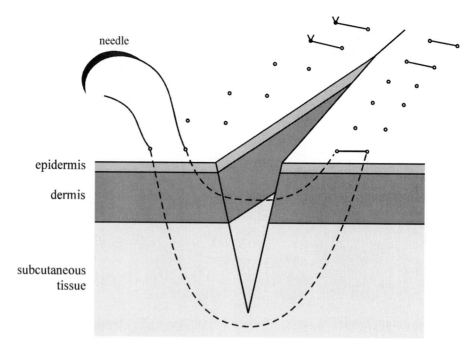

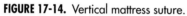

FIGURE 17-14. Vertical mattress suture.

- Horizontal mattress (Figure 17-15):
  - This suture also assists in wound edge eversion and helps to spread tension over a greater area.
  - This stitch starts out like a simple interrupted suture; however, after the needle exits, it then enters again on the same side that it exited from only a few millimeters lateral to the stitch and equidistant from the wound edge and exits on the opposite side.

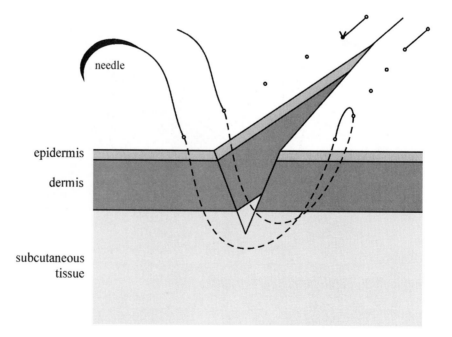

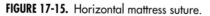

FIGURE 17-15. Horizontal mattress suture.

- Deep sutures (absorbable):
  - Used for multilayered closure
  - Deep sutures are absorbable because you will not be removing them.
  - Use your forceps (pickups) to hold the skin from the inside of the wound.
  - The first stitch is placed deep inside wound and exits superficially in dermal layer on same side of wound.
  - Then it enters in the superficial dermal layer on the opposite side and exits deep.
  - Tie a square knot and cut the tail of the suture close to the knot, which is called a *buried knot.*
  - Now proceed with your superficial closure of the skin with nonabsorbable sutures.
- Corner stitch (Figure 17-16):
  - This is used to repair stellate lacerations and help to preserve the blood supply to the tips of the skin.
  - The needle enters the epidermis of the nonflap or nontip portion of the wound.
  - It then enters the dermal layer of the skin tip on one side and proceeds through the dermal layer to exit the dermis on the other side of the tip (this portion will be buried).
  - It then enters and exits the other side of the stellate wound. It will appear as a simple interrupted suture.

Dressing

- Bacitracin ointment may be used over the repair.
- Cover the laceration with a single layer of nonadherent dressing, then cover that with gauze.
- For an extremity, wrap with gauze bandage (Kerlix) and take care not to tape circumferentially.

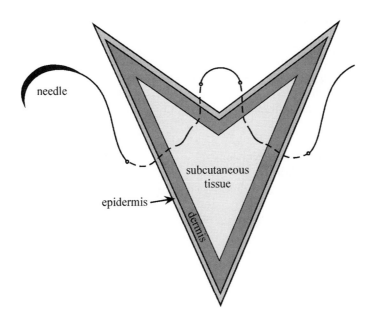

FIGURE 17-16. Corner stitch.

- The patient should come back for a wound check in 2 to 3 days for contaminated or deep wounds.
- The dressing should be changed every day and replaced with a Band-Aid or gauze.
- Keep area dry and look for signs of infection: Increased warmth, swelling, increasing erythema, streaking, dehiscence, more-than-normal discharge from wound, and fever.

See Table 17-5 for when to remove sutures.

TABLE 17-5. Suture Removal Times

Site	Days
Face, eyelid, ear, nose	3–5
Neck	5–7
Scalp, trunk	7–12
Arm, hand	8–12
Leg, foot, extensor surface of joints	10–14

CENTRAL VENOUS ACCESS

Subclavian vein cannulation can be infraclavicular (IC) or supraclavicular (SC).

Relative Indications

- Patient undergoing cardiopulmonary resuscitation: Internal jugular (IJ), SC subclavian, femoral
- Patient unable to lie flat: SC subclavian
- Coagulopathy: Femoral because more readily compressible

Relative Contraindications

General (applies to all routes)
- Distorted anatomy
- Overlying cellulitis or severe dermatitis
- Prior scarring of vein
- Significant coagulopathy

Subclavian
- Contralateral pneumothorax
- Chest wall deformity
- Chronic obstructive pulmonary disease

IJ
- Carotid artery stenosis (dislodging of plaque may occur due to inadvertent carotid artery cannulation)

Femoral
- Ambulatory patient
- Groin trauma

Procedure of Central Venous Cannulation

1. Use aseptic technique.
2. Place patient in Trendelenburg position.
3. Local anesthesia at point of needle entry
4. Insert and aim needle on syringe as appropriate for approach with gentle negative pressure to the syringe.
5. Nonpulsatile free flow flashback of blood indicates good position. Pulsatile flow may indicate inappropriate arterial placement.
6. Once within the vein, advancing of the guidewire depends on the commercial set you use. Some models will allow catheter insertion through the needle; others are over-the-needle.
7. Use scalpel to make small stab incision adjacent to guidewire (enlarges opening for catheter).
8. Pass catheter over guidewire. In most sets, removing the guidewire from the distal end of the catheter requires removal of the brown port.
9. NEVER let go of the guidewire.
10. Catheter should pass easily, without any forcing.
11. Once catheter is in to desired length, remove guidewire.
12. Check blood flow from catheter.
13. If not a triple lumen, connect catheter to IV tubing.
14. Suture catheter in place.
15. Place occlusive dressing over site.
16. Obtain chest x-ray for neck lines to confirm placement and to be certain no pneumothorax was caused by the procedure.

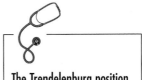

The Trendelenburg position is thought to prevent air embolism.

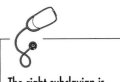

The right subclavian is preferred over the left in order to avoid thoracic duct (on left) or lung injury (dome of right lung is lower).

Landmarks for IC Subclavian

- Insert needle at junction of middle and proximal thirds of clavicle (Figure 17-17).
- Aim needle toward suprasternal notch.
- Vein entry at 4 cm

Landmarks for SC Subclavian

- Insert needle behind the clavicle, lateral to the clavicular head of the sternocleidomastoid (SCM) (Figure 17-18).

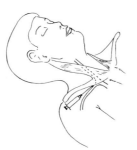

FIGURE 17-17. IC approach to subclavian vein cannulation.

(Reproduced, with permission, from Scaletta TA, Schaider JJ. *Emergent Management of Trauma,* 2nd ed. New York: McGraw-Hill, 2001: 441.)

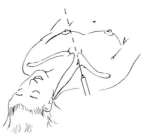

FIGURE 17-18. Supraclavicular (SC) approach to subclavian vein cannulation.
(Reproduced, with permission, from Scaletta TA, Schaider JJ. *Emergent Management of Trauma,* 2nd ed. New York: McGraw-Hill, 2001: 442.)

- Aim needle toward contralateral nipple.
- Vein entry at 3 cm

Landmarks for IJ Cannulation, Central Approach

- Insert needle at junction of the two heads of the SCM.
- Aim needle toward ipsilateral nipple.
- Maintain needle at 30- to 45-degree angle.
- Vein entry at 1 to 1.5 cm

Landmarks for IJ Cannulation, Anterior Approach

- Insert needle at medial edge of sternal head of SCM halfway up (Figure 17-19).
- Maintain needle at 30- to 45-degree angle.
- Aim needle toward ipsilateral nipple.
- Vein entry at 1.5 cm

Landmarks for IJ Cannulation, Posterior Approach

- Insert needle at lateral edge of clavicular head of SCM, a third of the way up between the clavicle and the mastoid (Figure 17-20).

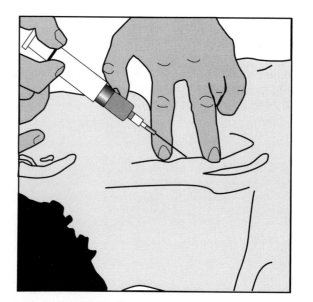

FIGURE 17-19. Anterior IJ cannulation.

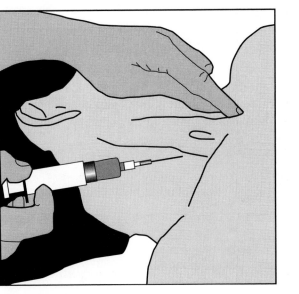

FIGURE 17-20. Posterior IJ cannulation.

- Aim needle toward sternal notch.
- Vein entry at 5 cm

Landmarks for Femoral Vein Cannulation

- Insert needle medial to pulsation of femoral artery.
- Maintain needle at 45-degree angle.
- Aim needle toward the head.
- Vein entry at 3 cm

Complications

- Infection
- Thrombosis
- Pneumothorax (not with femoral)
- SQ emphysema

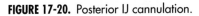

Remember the **VAN** *going from medial to lateral:*
Vein, Artery, Nerve

ABSCESS I&D

The I&D of abscesses is a very common procedure performed in the ED. Most skin abscesses are uncomplicated and can be drained easily with local anesthetic. Larger abscesses or ones in exquisitely sensitive areas may require conscious sedation or, occasionally, drainage in the operating room under general anesthesia.

Most Common Sites

- Axilla—25%
- Buttock/perirectal—25%
- Head/neck—20%

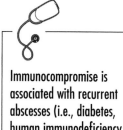

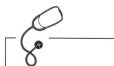

It is very difficult to completely anesthetize the abscess locally due to the acidic environment of abscesses. Use a regional block if possible.

While this is not a sterile procedure, it should be a clean procedure. Care should be taken not to infect areas not involved with the abscess.

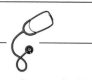

Antibiotics in healthy individuals are unnecessary. Consider antibiotics in immunocompromised individuals and in patients with valvular disease to prevent seeding due to transient bacteremia.

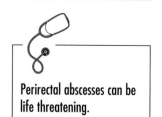

Perirectal abscesses can be life threatening.

- Extremities—18%
- Inguinal area—15%

Pathogens

Variety of aerobic and anaerobic. Most common:
- *Staphylococcus aureus*
- *Bacteroides fragilis*
- *Streptococcus viridans*

Equipment Needed

- Scalpel
- Hemostats
- Scissors
- Iodine solution
- Gauze
- Packing material—most commonly 1″ or 2″ plain or iodoform
- Dressing material
- Chucks
- Personal protective equipment
- Gloves
- Gown
- Eye protection
- Mask

Procedure

After explaining the procedure and placing the patient in a comfortable position with adequate exposure and lighting with chucks to minimize the mess:

1. Clean the area and prepare it with iodine solution.
2. Anesthetize the skin with the lidocaine preparation.
3. Make an incision large enough to ensure adequate exposure.
4. Care must be taken with the incision in the face and breast due to cosmetic considerations.
5. In these areas, cut along the natural wrinkle or crease lines to minimize scarring.
6. Explore the cavity with the hemostats to break up any loculations and express remaining pus.
7. If the abscess is large enough, pack it as much as possible, leaving some packing outside of the cavity.
8. Dress the area appropriately.
9. Patients should return in 24 hours for packing removal and wound check.

Special Considerations

- Perirectal abscesses require careful evaluation because they can extend deep into the perineum.
- Sebaceous cyst/abscesses can be excised with the shell intact, thus preventing recurrences.
- Cultures are generally unnecessary in first-time abscesses.

See Table 17-6 for procedures covered in other chapters.

TABLE 17-6. Procedures Covered in Other Chapters

Procedure	Chapter
Intubation, cricothyroidotomy (needle and surgical), laryngeal mask airway, Heimlich maneuver	Resuscitation
Interpretation of ECGs and imaging studies	Diagnostics
Reading a C-spine film, focused assessment with sonography for trauma, diagnostic peritoneal lavage, retrograde urethrogram, and cystogram	Trauma
Lumbar puncture	Neurologic Emergencies
Nasal packing	Head and Neck Emergencies
Testicular detorsion	Renal and Genitourinary Emergencies
Vaginal wet prep	Gynecologic Emergencies
Gastric lavage	Emergency Toxicology

Emergency Toxicology

OVERVIEW

Initial management of poisoned patient should emphasize supportive care:
- Stabilize ABCs and abnormal vital signs.
- Search to identify toxidromes.
- Perform a focused diagnostic workup.
- Decontamination, elimination, and antidotes as indicated
- Continuous reassessment is critical (patients may deteriorate rapidly).

Clinical pictures of symptoms and physical findings that correlate with a specific toxin recognize that "classic" toxidromes may be obscured in the setting of a multiple overdose (in which each toxin may cause competing signs/symptoms).

TOXIDROMES

Cholinergic

- Commonly seen with organophosphates and carbamates
- Symptoms are due to excessive stimulation of nicotinic/muscarinic acetylcholine (ACh) receptors.
- Muscarinic effects: Bronchorrhea, miosis, bradycardia
- Nicotinic effects: Fasciculations, cramping, hyperreflexia
- Use atropine and/or pralidoxime to reverse cholinergic excess.

Anticholinergic

- Many potential agents: Scopolamine, amanita muscaria, monoamine oxidase inhibitors (MAOIs)
- Think of the following four "anti" groups of drugs: Antidepressants, antihistamines, antipsychotics, antiparkinsons
- Clinical picture caused by antagonism/inhibition of ACh
- Other findings: Seizures, dysrhythmias, rhabdomyolysis
- Treatment is supportive: Benzodiazepines, cooling measures

Cholinergic toxidrome:
BAD SLUDGE
Bradycardia
Anxiety
Delirium

Salivation
Lacrimation
Urination
Defecation
Gastrointestinal (GI) upset
Emesis

Anticholinergic toxidrome:
- Mad as a hatter: *Altered mental status*
- Blind as a bat: *Mydriasis*
- Red as a beet: *Flushed skin*
- Hot as a hare: *Hyperthermia (can't sweat)*
- Dry as a bone: *Dry mucous membranes*

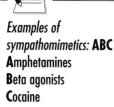

Toxins associated with mydriasis: **AAAAS**
Antihistamines
Antidepressants
Anticholinergics
Atropine
Sympathomimetics

Examples of sympathomimetics: **ABC**
Amphetamines
Beta agonists
Cocaine

Toxins associated with tachycardia: **FAST**
Free base (cocaine)
Anticholinergics/antihistamines/amphetamines
Sympathomimetics
Theophylline

Opiate toxidrome:
- **Coma**
- **Respiratory depression**
- **Pinpoint pupils**

Toxins associated with hypotension: **CRASH**
Clonidine
Reserpine
(antihypertensives)
Antidepressants
Sedative–hypnotics
Heroin

- Physostigmine:
  - Binds to acetylcholinesterase, increases ACh
  - Indicated only for unstable/refractory cases (seizures and dysrhythmias are common)
  - Avoid in tricyclic antidepressant (TCA) ingestions (asystole)

Sympathomimetic

- Agitation, mydriasis, tachycardia, hypertension, hyperthermia
- Sympathomimetic toxidrome resembles anticholinergic except for diaphoresis (sympathetic-mediated ACh stimulation of sweat glands causes diaphoresis).
- Bowel sounds (hyperactive in sympathomimetics)
- Multiple mechanisms of action of sympathomimetics:
  - Direct stimulation of alpha/beta-adrenergic receptors
  - Amphetamines stimulate release of norepinephrine (NE) into synapse.
  - Cocaine/TCAs prevent reuptake of NE from synapse.
  - MAOIs inhibit breakdown of NE.
- Treatment is supportive: Benzodiazepines, hydration, cooling

Opioid

- Heroin, morphine, propoxyphene, meperidine, codeine, fentanyl
- Hypothermia, bradycardia, hypotension, pulmonary edema
- Opiate receptors:
  - Euphoria, respiratory depression, miosis
  - Analgesia, dysphoria
  - Unknown
- Naloxone (Narcan): Competitive opiate receptor antagonist
- Dose depends on sensitivity of receptors to particular opiate.
- Caution: May precipitate seizures, agitation, withdrawal

Sedative–Hypnotic

- Mainly benzodiazepines and barbiturates both work by potentiating gamma-aminobutyric acid (GABA) (inhibitory neurotransmitter).
- Dose-dependent central nervous system (CNS) and respiratory depression (distinguish from ethanol [EtOH] intoxication by lack of vasodilation)
- Co-ingestion of alcohol, tranquilizers, or other depressants may potentiate these effects and lead to coma and/or apnea.
- Flumazenil: Competitive benzodiazepine receptor antagonist (caution—withdrawal seizures are common)
- Benzodiazepine overdoses usually low morbidity, flumazenil rarely used

DIAGNOSTIC ADJUNCTS

A variety of diagnostic studies and interventions are available to guide management.

"Coma Cocktail"

Serves as both a diagnostic and therapeutic intervention (hypoglycemia, hypoxia, opiates are common and easily reversible causes of CNS depression)

Acid–Base

- Arterial blood gas (ABG) evaluation should be obtained if indicated clinically:
  - Respiratory acidosis in comatose patients suggests opiates/sedatives.
  - Respiratory alkalosis may be seen in sympathomimetic overdoses.
  - Respiratory alkalosis with metabolic acidosis is suggestive of acetylsalicylic acid (ASA).
- Serial ABG may be indicated in patients who require mechanical ventilation.
- Alkalinization of serum (TCA) and urine (ASA)

Electrolytes

- Metabolic acidosis should be classified as anion gap versus nonanion gap using serum electrolytes (anion gap metabolic acidosis may be seen in certain toxic ingestions—CAT MUDPILES).
- STAT electrolytes may be sent with ABG for potassium (useful in management of digoxin overdoses).
- May be used in conjunction with serum osmolarity to detect toxic alcohol ingestion (with elevated osmole gap)

Spot Tests

- Classic example is ferric chloride test for salicylates (ferric chloride drops turn urine purple in presence of ASA).
- Spot tests also exist for acetaminophen, phenothiazines, barbiturates, ethanol, and certain types of mushrooms (most require high drug concentrations and have low sensitivity).

Immunoassays

- Most popular screening tool in emergency setting
- Antibodies generated to representative antigen in each class (i.e., amitriptyline for TCA, morphine for opiates, etc.)
- Tests have varying sensitivities and low specificity (negative test does not rule out all types of TCA, opiates, etc.).

Quantitative Tests

Useful for determining concentrations of specific toxins:
- May be useful in guiding management (acetaminophen)
- Serial levels (assess adequacy of decontamination/elimination)
- Predicting clinical outcome

Radiography

Certain toxins appear radiopaque on plain films.

Coma cocktail: **DON'T**
Dextrose (1 amp D$_{50}$)
Oxygen (supplemental)
Narcan (usually 0.4 mg titrated slowly)
Thiamine (to prevent Wernicke's)

Causes of anion gap metabolic acidosis: **CAT MUDPILES**
Carbon monoxide (CO), cyanide
Alcoholic ketoacidosis
Toluene

Methanol
Uremia
Diabetic ketoacidosis
Phenothiazines (Haldol)
Isoniazid (INH)
Lactic acidosis
Ethanol, ethylene glycol
Salicylates

Radiopaque substances: **CHIPS**
Chlorinated substances (pesticides)
Heavy metals (lead, mercury, arsenic)
Iodine/iron
Phenothiazines
Sustained-release preparations/salicylates (enteric coated)

METHODS OF DECONTAMINATION

Forced Emesis

- Syrup of ipecac:
  - Plant derivative containing alkaloids (emetine and cephaeline)
  - Direct emetic effect on stomach
  - Central effect on chemotactic trigger zone
  - Produces emesis in over 90% of patients after single dose
- Limit ipecac use to:
  - Prehospital (when access to emergency services may be significantly delayed)
  - Pediatric (where large-bore orogastric lavage may be contraindicated)
- Complications of ipecac include intractable vomiting, myocardial toxicity, and aspiration.

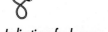

Contraindication: Ipecac should never be used when more controlled decontamination is possible. *Avoid in:*
- Patients without gag reflex
- Nontoxic ingestions
- Caustic ingestions
- Hydrocarbon ingestions
- Patients in whom charcoal administration is efficacious

Gastric Lavage

- Technique for orogastric lavage:
  - Use large-bore tubes for intact pills (size 36 to 40 in adults, 22 to 24 in children).
  - Place patient in left lateral decubitus position (to minimize aspiration risk).
  - Have suction ready, measure length of tube, insert, and confirm position in stomach.
  - Lavage with fluid until aspirate is clear.
- Usually must be performed within 1 hour to be of clinical utility except:
  - Diabetics (with impaired gastric motility)
  - Toxic ingestions that delay gastric emptying (i.e., anticholinergics)
  - Drugs that form concretions (aspirin) take longer to clear stomach.
- Complications include aspiration, esophageal/gastric perforation, and hypoxia during procedure.

Indications for lavage:
- Acute toxic ingestion
- Patient's condition may deteriorate rapidly.
- Toxin doesn't bind to charcoal.

Activated Charcoal

- Directly binds to toxin in gut lumen
- Decreases concentration of toxin in stomach, creating a gradient favoring flow of toxin from blood into stomach
- Binds to toxin in bile (interrupts enterohepatic circulation)
- Multiple-dose charcoal:
  - Proven benefit with certain toxins (digoxin, phenytoin, etc.)
  - Given empirically for ingestions of sustained-release products and drugs that form concretions
  - Avoid repeat doses of cathartics with charcoal.

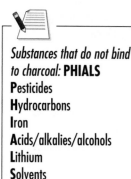

Substances that do not bind to charcoal: **PHIALS**
Pesticides
Hydrocarbons
Iron
Acids/alkalies/alcohols
Lithium
Solvents

Cathartics

- Limited role in toxic ingestions:
  - May relieve constipating effects of charcoal
  - May prevent "desorption" of toxin from charcoal over time
  - By decreasing transit time through gut

- Concerns about cathartics:
  - May cause significant fluid and electrolyte shifts
  - Decreased transit time gives charcoal less time to bind.
- Current recommendations are to routinely give single dose of cathartic with charcoal.

Whole Bowel Irrigation (WBI)

- WBI is a technique of flushing out the entire GI system with large volumes of fluid.
- Polyethylene glycol (Go-Lytely) is an isotonic fluid that does not cause significant bowel edema or fluid and electrolyte shifts.
- Sorbitol causes catharsis in < 2 hours; may cause abdominal cramping
- Magnesium citrate causes catharsis in 4 to 6 hours; contraindicated in patients with renal failure
- WBI minimally requires adults to drink 2 L/hr of polyethylene glycol (0.5 L/hr in children).
- Usually requires nasogastric tube and/or antiemetics to administer large volumes of fluid
- End point of therapy is clear rectal effluent.
- Concerns with WBI:
  - Vomiting, bloating, and rectal irritation are common.
  - Polyethylene glycol may occupy charcoal binding sites.
  - It is time consuming, labor intensive, and messy.

Urinary Alkalinization

- If pH of urine is raised to 7.5 to 8.0, "ion trapping" mechanism eliminates certain toxins.
- Hypokalemia impairs alkalinization by dumping H^+ ions in urine in exchange for K^+ (supplemental K^+ should be given intravenously (IV) with bicarbonate for alkalinization).

Hemodialysis and Hemoperfusion

- Hemoperfusion: Charcoal filter in series with dialysis:
  - Most useful for theophylline
- Toxins that can be dialyzed: STUMBLE

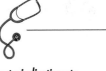

Contraindications to cathartic use:
- Patients with impaired gag
- Intestinal obstruction
- Caustics

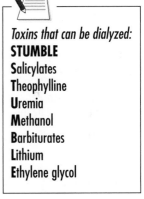

Toxins that can be dialyzed:
STUMBLE
Salicylates
Theophylline
Uremia
Methanol
Barbiturates
Lithium
Ethylene glycol

OVER-THE-COUNTER MEDICATIONS

Acetaminophen

- Chemical name is N-acetyl-para-aminophenol (commonly abbreviated as APAP)
- Most commonly reported potentially toxic ingestion, highest number of fatalities
- Frequent co-ingestant

EXPOSURE

- Tylenol
- Cold and flu preparations
- Percocet

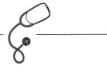

Indications for WBI:
- Toxins that do not bind to charcoal
- Ingestions of sustained-release products
- Body-packers (smuggling illicit drugs in GI tract)

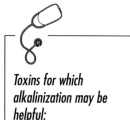

Toxins for which
alkalinization may be
helpful:
- Aspirin
- Phenobarbital
- Chlorpropamide

MECHANISM OF TOXICITY

- Metabolism of acetaminophen (therapeutic doses):
  - Over 90% is metabolized by liver into nontoxic sulfate and glucuronide conjugates.
  - Less than 5% is directly excreted in urine.
  - Less than 5% is processed by cytochrome P450 system in liver to form N-acetyl-para-benzoquinoneimine (NAPQI).
- Metabolism of acetaminophen (in overdoses):
  - Sulfation and glucuronidation pathways become saturated.
  - P450 processes more APAP, generating more NAPQI.
  - NAPQI is a toxic intermediate of APAP.
  - NAPQI depletes glutathione stores and starts to accumulate.
  - Glutathione reduces NAPQI into nontoxic mercaptate conjugate.
  - NAPQI binds nonspecifically to intracellular proteins, causing cell dysfunction.

CLINICAL SIGNS OF TOXICITY

- Acetaminophen (APAP) overdose is usually marked by a lack of clinical signs or symptoms in the first 24 hours.
- Toxic level of APAP at 4 hours is 150 mg/mL.
- 24 to 48 hours, begin to have right upper quadrant pain with elevation of liver function tests and prothrombin time/international normalized ratio
- 48 to 96 hours, severe liver dysfunction with coagulopathy, renal failure, death
- Survivors will recover hepatic function over next 2 weeks.

MANAGEMENT

- Decontamination:
  - Activated charcoal
  - Avoid emesis (this delays N-acetylcysteine [NAC] administration)
  - Lavage only for co-ingestants
- Administration of NAC:
  - Acts as glutathione precursor or substitute
  - Acts as a sulfate precursor
  - Directly reduces NAPQI back to APAP
  - After 24 hours, acts as a hepatocellular protectant

Factors that accelerate
acetaminophen toxicity:
- Prior induction of P450
  (smokers, alcoholics,
  certain drugs)
- Malnutrition (decreased
  glutathione stores)

Aspirin

ASA

EXPOSURE

- Present in over 200 oral and topical preparations (aspirin, Pepto-Bismol, Alka-Seltzer, Dristan, Ben-Gay, Tiger Balm, etc.)
- Present in oil of wintergreen

MECHANISM OF TOXICITY

- Absorption:
  - Normally 1 to 2 hours
  - 4 to 6 hours in overdose (delayed gastric emptying, concretion formation)

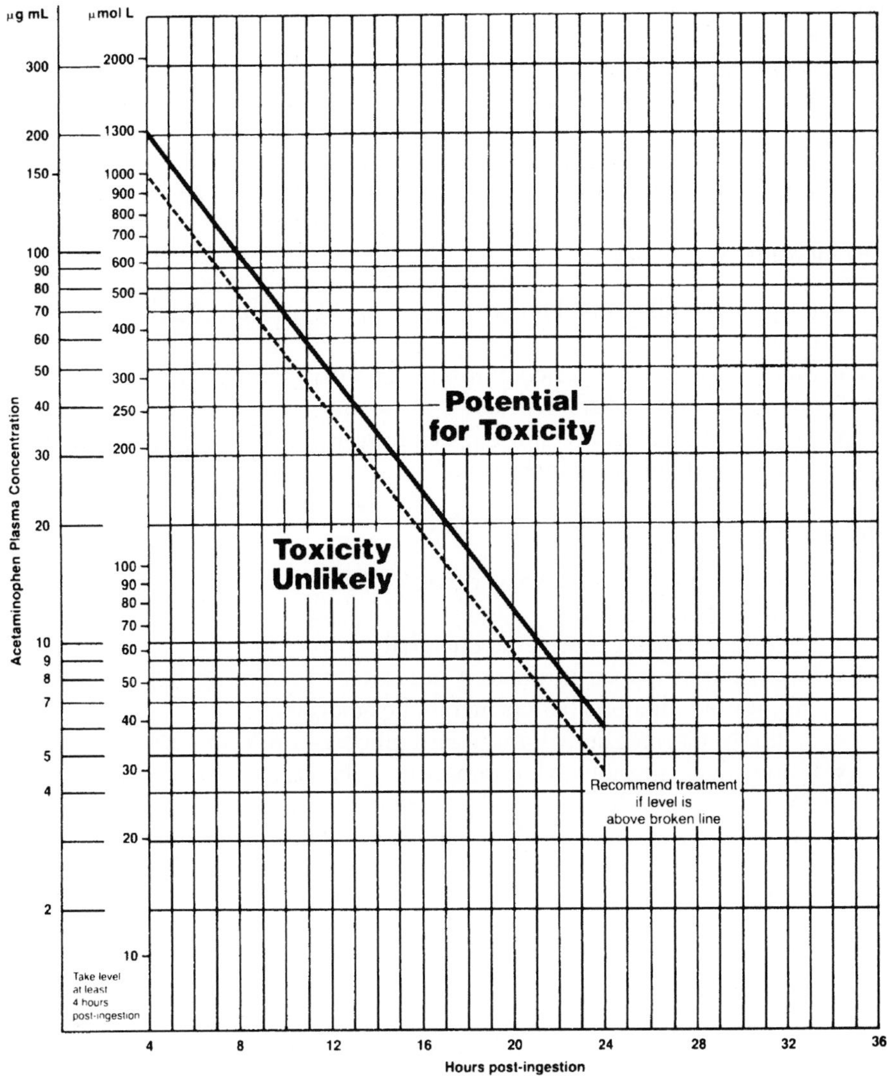

FIGURE 18-1. Rumack–Matthew nomogram.
(Reproduced, with permission, from *Management of Acetaminophen Overdose.* McNeil Consumer Products Co., 1986.)

How to administer NAC:
- Identify patients with a toxic level of APAP within 8 hours of ingestion (use Rumak–Matthew nomogram) (Figure 18-1). *Note:* Nomogram was designed for use with single APAP level.
- Give loading dose of 140 mg/kg PO, followed by 70 mg/kg q4h for 17 more doses.

- Distribution:
  - Normally weak acid that remains ionized
  - Acidosis in overdose makes it easier for ASA to penetrate tissues.
- Metabolism:
  - Conjugated in liver via first-order kinetics
  - Liver enzymes saturated in overdose, zero-order kinetics
- Elimination:
  - Small amount of free salicylate excreted in urine
  - Maximizing urinary excretion becomes critical in overdose.

Causes of noncardiogenic pulmonary edema: **MOPS**
Meprobamate/Mountain Sickness
Opioids
Phenobarbital
Salicylates

Clinical Signs of Toxicity

- Respiratory:
  - Tachypnea/hyperpnea
  - Noncardiogenic pulmonary edema

Typical scenario:
A 67-year-old woman presents with 6 days of headache and 2 days of "ringing in the ears" and fever. She is breathing deeply at a rate of 22/min. *Think: Aspirin toxicity.*

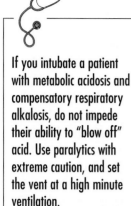

If you intubate a patient with metabolic acidosis and compensatory respiratory alkalosis, do not impede their ability to "blow off" acid. Use paralytics with extreme caution, and set the vent at a high minute ventilation.

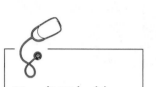

"Normal" ASA level does not rule out toxicity—repeat every 1 to 2 hours until levels decline and clinical status improves.

- CNS:
  - Tinnitus
  - Headache
  - Cerebral edema/coma
- Other:
  - Platelet dysfunction
  - Hyperthermia

ACID–BASE DISTURBANCES

- Respiratory alkalosis: Direct stimulation of medulla (tachypnea/hyperpnea)
- Metabolic acidosis: Uncoupling of oxidative phosphorylation leads to anaerobic metabolism with lactic acidosis.
- Metabolic alkalosis: Vomiting, diaphoresis, and tachypnea cause dehydration and volume contraction.

MANAGEMENT

- Check for presence of ASA: Ferric chloride—spot test turns urine purple if ASA is present.
- Decontamination: Activated charcoal
- Respiratory support: Intubate if necessary to maintain hyperventilation (respiratory alkalosis buffers metabolic acidosis).
- IV fluids: Correct dehydration with glucose-containing crystalloid fluid.
- Urine alkalinization: Maintain urine pH around 8.0 to trap ionized ASA in urine. Alkalinize with bicarbonate drip.
- Extracorporeal removal: Hemoperfusion is better at removing ASA; hemodialysis is better for correcting acid–base and electrolytes (consider for ASA level > 100 mg/dL or as indicated clinically).

Iron

Iron is an essential component of human red blood cells (RBCs), hemoglobin (Hgb), myoglobin, and cytochromes.

EXPOSURE

Accidental or intentional ingestion of iron-containing tablets

MECHANISM OF TOXICITY

- Less than 10% of ingested iron is bioavailable:
  - Iron absorbed by intestinal mucosa, stored as ferritin
  - Transported throughout body, complexed with transferrin
  - Elimination is primarily via sloughing of intestinal mucosa (ferritin).
- Overdose:
  - Ingested iron overwhelms protein carriers, enters via passive diffusion
  - Iron is corrosive to GI mucosa, enters circulation directly
- Free iron in circulation leads to toxicity:
  - Direct corrosive effect on GI tract
  - Causes vasodilation and myocardial depression
  - Disrupts oxidative phosphorylation, which leads to buildup of lactic acid (metabolic acidosis)
  - Delayed hepatotoxicity

CLINICAL SIGNS OF TOXICITY

Stage I: 1 to 6 Hours
- GI symptoms:
  - Abdominal pain
  - Nausea, vomiting, diarrhea
  - Hematemesis

Stage II: 6 to 24 Hours
- Resolution of GI symptoms
- Early shock

Stage III: Variable Time Course
- Shock
- Metabolic acidosis
- Coagulopathy
- Multiorgan failure may occur.

Stage IV: 2 to 5 Days
- Hepatic insufficiency, may progress to failure

Stage V: 4 to 6 Weeks After Ingestion
- Gastric outlet obstruction

MANAGEMENT

- Supportive care
- Decontamination:
  - WBI effective at clearing large GI loads
  - No ipecac (iron already induces emesis)
  - Lavage usually ineffective (large iron pills)
  - Charcoal does not adsorb well to iron.
- Deferoxamine:
  - Chelates free iron to form ferrioxamine (water soluble, excreted in urine)
  - Ferrioxamine turns urine "vin rosé" (or rusty brown) color.
  - Dose: 90 mg/kg IM up to 1 g in children and 2 g in adults, or 5 mg/kg/hr IV up to 15 mg/kg/hr for severe toxicity

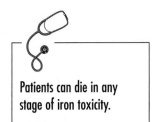

Patients can die in any stage of iron toxicity.

Toxic dose of iron:
< 20 mg/kg nontoxic
> 60 mg/kg severe toxicity
Calculate on basis of amount of elemental iron ingested.
Toxic level of iron:
< 300 µg/dL nontoxic
> 500 µg/dL severe toxicity

CARDIOVASCULAR DRUGS

Beta Blockers

EXPOSURE

Commonly prescribed for hypertension, hyperthyroidism

MECHANISM OF TOXICITY

- Stimulation of beta-adrenergic receptor causes an increase in intracellular cAMP → phosphorylation of calcium channels (opens channels).
- Increased calcium influx triggers release of intracellular calcium stores → excitation–contraction coupling.

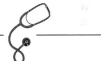

Beta-adrenergic receptors:
Beta-1:
- Myocardium (↑ inotropy)
- Eye (↑ aqueous humor)
- Kidney (↑ plasma renin)
Beta-2:
- Smooth muscle relaxation
- Liver (glycogenolysis, gluconeogenesis)
Beta-3:
- Adipose tissue (lipolysis)

- Pharmacologic differences among beta blockers:
  - Selectivity: Agents may have beta-1 or beta-2 selectivity, which is lost in overdose.
  - Solubility: More lipid-soluble agents are more likely to penetrate CNS.
  - Agents with intrinsic sympathomimetic activity may present atypically.
  - Membrane stabilizing: These agents may cause sodium channel blockade.

CLINICAL SIGNS OF TOXICITY

Hallmark of beta blocker toxicity: Bradycardia with hypotension

- Bradycardia
- Hypotension
- Sinus node suppression
- Slowed atrioventricular (AV) nodal conduction
- QRS widening with agents that block Na channels
- Decreased myocardial contractility
- Decreased cardiac output
- Smooth muscle relaxation, peripheral vasodilation
- Lipophilic agents may cause sedation and/or seizures (penetrate CNS).
- Beta-2 receptor blockade may lead to bronchospasm.

MANAGEMENT

- Supportive treatment
- Fluid resuscitation
- Decontamination: Gastric lavage (if within 1 to 2 hours) and activated charcoal
- Glucagon bypasses beta receptor to increase intracellular cyclic adenosine monophosphate (cAMP).
- Catecholamines (dopamine/NE) for pressor support
- Phosphodiesterase inhibitors (amrinone) block cAMP breakdown.
- Transcutaneous/transvenous pacing, intra-aortic balloon pump (IABP), bypass as indicated

Calcium Channel Blockers

EXPOSURE

Commonly prescribed for hypertension

MECHANISM OF TOXICITY

- Blockade of calcium channels in cell membranes
- Decreased calcium influx disrupts excitation–contraction coupling.
- Different classes of calcium channel blockers:
  - Phenylalkylamines (verapamil) and benzothiazepines (diltiazem) both cause decreased myocardial contractility and conduction, as well as vasodilation.
  - Dihydropyridines (nifedipine, amlodipine) cause mostly peripheral vasodilation.

CLINICAL SIGNS OF TOXICITY

- Hypotension
- Bradycardia
- Decreased conduction/automaticity

356

- Hypoperfusion
- Lactic acidosis
- Insulin resistance, hyperglycemia/hyperkalemia

MANAGEMENT

- Supportive care (including endotracheal intubation as indicated)
- Fluid resuscitation
- Decontamination with lavage (if early) and charcoal
- Consider WBI for sustained release.
- Correct acidosis.
- IV calcium
- Increases gradient across calcium channel
- Stabilizes membranes in presence of hyperkalemia
- Glucagon acts to increase cAMP and phosphorylate calcium channels.
- Electrical pacing and/or pressors (dopamine) as indicated
- Refractory cases: Consider amrinone (inhibits cAMP breakdown), insulin (inotrope/chronotrope), IABP, or dialysis.

Cardiac Glycosides (Digoxin)

Commonly used in the treatment of congestive heart failure (CHF) and supraventricular tachycardias

EXPOSURE

- Digoxin
- Foxglove plant
- Oleander plant

MECHANISM OF TOXICITY

- Inhibits Na^+-K^+ ATPase pump:
  - Increases intracellular Na^+, extracellular K^+
  - Less Ca^{2+} is pumped out in exchange for Na^+ (increased intracellular $Ca^{2+} \rightarrow$ increased inotropy).
  - Membrane resting potential becomes less negative (as Na^+ and Ca^{2+} accumulate inside cell), leads to increased automaticity (tachydysrhythmias)
- Increases vagal tone (leads to bradydysrhythmias)
  - Decreases conduction through AV node
  - Also leads to sinus bradycardia

CLINICAL SIGNS OF TOXICITY

- Cardiac toxicity (wide range of rhythm disturbances):
  - Sinus bradycardia/block
  - Atrial fibrillation/flutter
  - AV node blocks (junctional rhythms)
  - Premature ventricular contractions, ventricular tachycardia/fibrillation
- Hyperkalemia (inhibition of Na^+-K^+ pump)
- Nausea, vomiting, and headaches are common in acute overdose.
- Visual disturbances:
  - Amblyopia
  - Photophobia
  - Yellow-green halos around light

Causes of bradycardia:
PACED
Propranolol (beta blockers)
Anticholinesterase drugs
Clonidine/calcium channel blockers
Ethanol, other alcohols
Digoxin/Darvon (opiates)

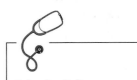

Toxicity from chronic digoxin use may be seen with normal levels.

Salvador Dali mustache: Scooped ST segments are seen with digoxin use at therapeutic levels *(not an indicator of toxicity).*

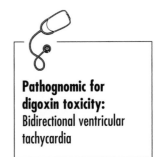

Pathognomic for digoxin toxicity: Bidirectional ventricular tachycardia

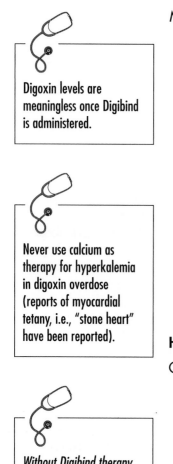

Digoxin levels are meaningless once Digibind is administered.

Never use calcium as therapy for hyperkalemia in digoxin overdose (reports of myocardial tetany, i.e., "stone heart" have been reported).

Without Digibind therapy, mortality in digoxin overdose is:
- 100% for K > 5.5
- 50% for K = 5.0–5.5
- 0% for K < 5.0

MANAGEMENT

- Decontamination with activated charcoal for acute overdose (avoid lavage, as it may increase vagal tone)
- Treat bradydysrhythmias—atropine and/or pacing
- Treat tachydysrhythmias—lidocaine, phenytoin
- Treat hyperkalemia—indicator for digoxin toxicity as above; severe hyperkalemia: Insulin/glucose and bicarbonate
- Treat hypokalemia—may potentiate digoxin toxicity, replace as indicated (may see toxic effects with normal digoxin levels)
- Digibind: Digoxin-specific antibody fragments bind to digoxin in serum, eliminated by kidneys. Use for:
  - Ventricular dysrhythmias
  - Hemodynamically significant bradydysrhythmias
  - Hyperkalemia > 5.0 in setting of overdose
- Digibind dosing:
  - Unknown ingestion (empiric): 5 to 10 vials
  - Known ingestion: 1.6 × amount ingested
  - Known digoxin level: [wt(kg) × level (ng/mL)/100]

Hypoglycemics

GLUCOSE METABOLISM

- Serum levels maintained by balance between three mechanisms:
  - Gut absorption of ingested glucose
  - Glycogenolysis—mobilization of liver stores
  - Gluconeogenesis—major mechanism for glucose control in hypoglycemic states
- Physiologic response to hypoglycemia:
  - CNS: Confusion, lethargy, seizures, coma, focal neurologic deficits
  - Autonomic response
  - Release of counterregulatory hormones (epinephrine, glucagon, etc.)
  - Diaphoresis, tremors, palpitations, anxiety

Insulin

EXPOSURE

Immediate- (Lispro), short- (regular), intermediate- (NPH), and long- (Ultralente) acting formulations

MECHANISM OF TOXICITY

- Secreted by beta-islet cells of pancreas
- Stimulates uptake/utilization of glucose in body
- Insulin absorption variable in overdose

CLINICAL SIGNS OF TOXICITY

- Hypoglycemia
- Hypothermia
- Delirium, coma, seizure, or focal neurologic deficit

MANAGEMENT

- IV dextrose
- Glucagon not recommended, as it may deplete glycogen stores

Sulfonylureas

Oral hypoglycemics

EXPOSURE

Commonly prescribed for type 2 diabetes

MECHANISM OF TOXICITY

Increases endogenous insulin secretion and sensitivity to insulin in peripheral tissues

CLINICAL SIGNS OF TOXICITY

- Long duration of hypoglycemia
- Hypothermia, hyponatremia, and disulfiram-like reactions have been reported.
- Delirium, coma, seizure, or focal neurologic deficit

MANAGEMENT

- IV dextrose
- Decontamination with charcoal for overdose
- Octreotide (somatostatin analog) inhibits glucose-stimulated insulin release.
- Diazoxide inhibits beta-islet cell insulin release.
- Chlorpropamide: Alkalinizing urine speeds elimination.

Biguanides

Oral hypoglycemics

EXPOSURE

- Phenformin (removed from market)
- Metformin (Glucophage)

MECHANISM OF TOXICITY

- Increases peripheral sensitivity to insulin
- Suppresses gluconeogenesis

CLINICAL SIGNS OF TOXICITY

- Hypoglycemia
- Hypothermia
- Delirium, coma, seizure, or focal neurologic deficit
- Lactic acidosis

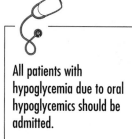
MANAGEMENT

- IV dextrose
- Decontaminate with charcoal for overdose.
- Consider bicarbonate for management of significant acidosis.
- Consider dialysis for correcting large fluid and electrolyte shifts.

ANTIDEPRESSANTS

TCAs

TCAs are responsible for more drug-related deaths than any other prescription medication.

EXPOSURE

Commonly prescribed for depression, chronic pain

MECHANISM OF TOXICITY

- Blocks reuptake of dopamine, serotonin, NE
- Binds to GABA receptor, lowering seizure threshold
- Sodium channel blockade: Wide QRS
- Alpha-adrenergic blockade: Orthostatic hypotension
- Antihistamine effect: Sedation
- Anticholinergic effect

CLINICAL SIGNS OF TOXICITY

- Hyperthermia, tachycardia, lethargy/coma, seizures/myoclonus
- Anticholinergic (dry skin/membranes, mydriasis, urinary retention, etc.)
- Abnormal electrocardiogram (ECG) (Figure 18-2):
  - Sinus tachycardia, right axis deviation (RAD), and prolongation of PR, QRS, and QT intervals

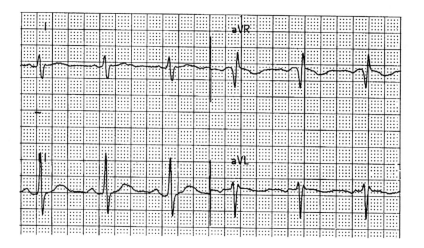

FIGURE 18-2. ECG of TCA toxicity.

(Reproduced, with permission, from Goldfrank LR et al. *Goldfrank's Toxicology*, 6th ed. Stamford, CT: Appleton & Lange, 1998: 112.)

- QRS widening secondary to sodium channel blockade:
  - QRS < 100, no significant toxicity
  - QRS > 100, seizures in one third of patients
  - QRS > 160, ventricular dysrhythmias in one half of patients
- RAD is most apparent in aVR → 40 msec positive R wave (this finding is sensitive but not specific for presence of TCA).

MANAGEMENT

- Decontamination:
  - Charcoal is effective at binding TCA.
  - Lavage only effective early in course
  - Ipecac contraindicated
- Treat hypotension:
  - Treat initially with IV crystalloid.
  - NE as pressor (if necessary)
  - Bicarbonate for refractory hypotension
- Treat seizures:
  - Treat with benzodiazepines/barbiturates.
  - Consider general anesthesia and paralytics for refractory seizures.
  - Avoid phenytoin (risk of dysrhythmia).
- Treat dysrhythmias:
  - Sodium bicarbonate is first-line intervention.
  - Lidocaine/bretylium as indicated
  - Cardioversion for unstable dysrhythmias
- Sodium bicarbonate:
  - Shown to improve conduction/contractility and decrease ectopy
  - Indications for sodium bicarbonate:
    - Refractory hypotension
    - QRS widening > 100 msec
    - Ventricular dysrhythmias
  - Goal of therapy is to maintain narrow QRS. Avoid excessive alkalemia (pH > 7.55).

Action of sodium bicarbonate in heart in TCA overdose is due to the *sodium* component; it alters the interaction between the drug and sodium channels.

Selective Serotonin Reuptake Inhibitors (SSRIs)

EXPOSURE

Commonly prescribed for depression, premenstrual syndrome

MECHANISM OF TOXICITY

- Selectively inhibit reuptake of serotonin without affecting dopamine/NE
- No direct effect on presynaptic/postsynaptic receptors (fewer side effects than TCAs)
- High toxic-to-therapeutic drug ratio (lower incidence of toxicity from overdose)

CLINICAL SIGNS OF TOXICITY

- Serotonin syndrome:
  - Hyperthermia
  - Tachycardia
  - Rigidity
  - Hyperreflexia
  - Confusion/agitation

Serotonin syndrome:
Usually results from combination of SSRI with:
- MAOI
- Cocaine
- Methylene dioxy metamphetamine (MDMA) (ecstasy)
- Lithium/tryptophan

- Extrapyramidal symptoms (EPS): Dystonic reactions, parkinsonism, etc.
- Hyponatremia secondary to syndrome of inappropriate antidiuretic hormone
- Seizures, QT prolongation: Rare, mostly with citalopram (Celexa)

MANAGEMENT

- Decontamination with activated charcoal
- Benzodiazepines/barbiturates for seizures
- Sodium bicarbonate for wide QRS
- For serotonin syndrome:
  - Supportive care, cooling
  - Consider cyproheptadine (antihistamine with antiserotonin properties).
  - Benzodiazepines, dantrolene, paralytics as needed

MAOIs

EXPOSURE

Commonly prescribed for depression

MECHANISM OF TOXICITY

- MAO: Enzyme found in nerve terminals; degrades epinephrine, NE, dopamine, and serotonin
- MAOIs: Form an irreversible covalent bond with MAO in nerve terminals
- Increase the amount of biogenic amines available at nerve terminals:
  - Increase catecholamines
  - Synergy with SSRIs may lead to serotonin syndrome.
  - Tyramine-containing foods may cause sympathomimetic crisis.
  - Other drugs (cocaine, amphetamines) may contribute to sympathomimetic crisis.

CLINICAL SIGNS OF TOXICITY

- Tachycardia, hyperthermia, hypertension, mydriasis, agitation
- Eventual catecholamine depletion can cause sympatholytic crisis (hypotension, bradycardia, CNS depression).
- Serum levels of MAOI correlate poorly with toxicity.
- Onset of toxicity may be delayed up to 24 hours.

MANAGEMENT

- Supportive care
- Gastric lavage, if acute
- Discontinue drugs that may interact with MAOI.
- Control hypertension (phentolamine, nitroprusside).
- Treat seizures, hyperthermia, and rigidity with benzodiazepines.
- Treat ventricular dysrhythmias with lidocaine or procainamide.
- Treat hypotension with fluids and NE.

Do not use the following agents in patients on MAOIs (partial list—check all agents given to patients on MAOIs):

- Other MAOIs
- Amphetamines
- Dopamine
- Epinephrine, NE
- Meperidine
- Buspirone
- Dextromethorphan
- SSRIs
- Tyramine-containing foods
- Cocaine

Lithium

EXPOSURE

Commonly prescribed for bipolar disorder

MECHANISM OF TOXICITY

- Increases synthesis and turnover of serotonin
- Downregulates number of adrenergic receptors (beta and alpha-2)
- Inhibits adenylate cyclase (decreases cAMP)
- Inhibits inositol monophosphatase
- Deposits in bone and other tissues, forming a reservoir of lithium
- Competes with other molecules of similar size
- 95% excreted in urine (glomerular filtration rate dependent)

CLINICAL SIGNS OF TOXICITY

- Acute toxicity:
  - Nausea, vomiting, abdominal pain
  - Serum lithium levels correlate poorly with symptoms/prognosis.
  - Acute ingestions can tolerate higher Li+ levels without toxicity.
- Chronic toxicity:
  - Resting tremor, hyperreflexia, seizure, coma, EPS
  - Serum lithium levels correlate well with symptoms/prognosis.
- Acute or chronic:
  - Prolonged QT, flipped T waves (hypokalemia)
  - Nephrogenic diabetes insipidus

MANAGEMENT

- Decontaminate with WBI for acute ingestions.
- Fluid resuscitation
- Kayexalate is effective at binding lithium.
- Hemodialysis for:
  - Lithium level > 4 (acute) or > 2.5 (chronic)
  - Significant CNS or cardiovascular toxicity
  - Renal failure
  - Heart failure

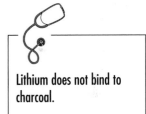

Lithium does not bind to charcoal.

Antipsychotics

EXPOSURE

- Older "typical" agents:
  - Haloperidol, chlorpromazine
  - More effective in controlling positive symptoms (hallucinations, delusions)
- Newer "atypical" agents:
  - Olanzapine, risperidone
  - More effective at controlling negative symptoms (apathy, blunted affect)

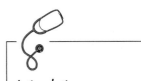

Antipsychotics:
Toxicity can occur with overdose or therapeutic dose.

MECHANISM OF TOXICITY

- Older agents block D_2 (dopaminergic) receptor, possess antihistamine, anticholinergic
- Newer agents block $5\text{-}HT_2$ (serotonergic) receptor
- Neuroleptic malignant syndrome (NMS) caused by central dopaminergic blockade

CLINICAL SIGNS OF TOXICITY

- EPS
- NMS
- Orthostatic hypotension with tachycardia
- Sedation

MANAGEMENT

- Decontamination
- Supportive care
- Treat EPS symptoms with IV diphenhydramine and discontinue agent if possible.
- Treat NMS with discontinuation of agent, cooling, benzodiazepines, and dantrolene. Consider carbidopa/levodopa to increase dopamine activity.

NMS:
- Hyperthermia
- Altered mental status
- Autonomic instability
- Muscular rigidity

ANTICONVULSANTS

Phenytoin

- First-line agent useful for all types of seizures except absence
- Blocks voltage-sensitive and frequency-dependent sodium channels in neurons
- Suppresses ability of neurons to fire action potentials at high frequency
- Fosphenytoin (Cerebyx):
  - Phenytoin prodrug, soluble in aqueous solution with pH ~8.8
  - Converted to phenytoin in blood and peripheral tissues
  - Well tolerated both IV and IM routes (fewer side effects—faster administration possible)

Toxicologic causes of hyperthermia: **NASA**
NMS/nicotine
Antihistamines
Salicylates/ sympathomimetics
Anticholinergics/ antidepressants (MAOIs)

EXPOSURE

Commonly prescribed for seizure disorder

MECHANISM OF TOXICITY

In overdose, kinetics change from first-order to zero-order.

CLINICAL SIGNS OF TOXICITY

- CNS toxicity: Nystagmus, lethargy, ataxia, seizures, coma
- Local effects (IM): Crystallization, abscess, tissue necrosis
- Hypersensitivity: Systemic lupus erythematosus, toxic epidermal necrolysis, Stevens–Johnson syndrome (1 to 6 weeks after initiating therapy)
- Gingival hyperplasia
- Cardiovascular toxicity:
  - Almost always seen as infusion rate–related complication of IV therapy due to diluent

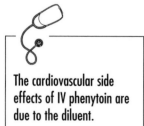

The cardiovascular side effects of IV phenytoin are due to the diluent.

- Phenytoin diluent: Propylene glycol, ethanol solution (pH ~12)
- Hypotension, bradycardia, AV blocks, asystole
- ECG: Prolonged PR and QRS, nonspecific ST-T wave changes

MANAGEMENT

- Use multiple-dose charcoal for oral overdose.
- Hemodialysis and hemoperfusion are ineffective.
- Supportive care; discontinue infusion for signs of toxicity.

Carbamazepine (Tegretol)

- First-line agent useful for all types of seizures except absence
- Also used in the management of trigeminal neuralgia and bipolar disorder
- Available only in oral formulation (no parenteral forms)

CLINICAL SIGNS OF TOXICITY

- CNS: Nystagmus, ataxia, dystonia, seizures, coma
- Cardiac: QRS widening, prolonged QT, AV blocks

MANAGEMENT

- Decontamination with multiple-dose charcoal
- Hemodialysis ineffective
- Hemoperfusion with charcoal is effective.
- Bicarbonate for QRS widening > 100 msec
- Benzodiazepines for seizures

Valproic Acid

- Used for the treatment of absence, myoclonic, and tonic–clonic seizures
- Also used as mood stabilizer for treatment of bipolar disorder
- Metabolized extensively in liver, with several biologically active metabolites (2-n-valproic acid is active and accumulates in CNS and other tissues)

CLINICAL SIGNS OF TOXICITY

- Nausea/vomiting and abdominal pain
- Cerebral edema from accumulation of metabolites
- Respiratory depression, cardiac arrest
- Metabolic derangements:
  - Hyperammonemia ± hypocarnitinemia
  - Metabolic acidosis
  - Hypernatremia
  - Hypocalcemia
- Hepatotoxicity up to fulminant hepatitis

MANAGEMENT

- Supportive care (including intubation as required)
- Decontamination with multiple-dose activated charcoal
- Hemodialysis improves clearance; reserve for most toxic patients.
- Carnitine supplementation in hyperammonemic patients

General Principals

- Group of structurally similar molecules with common R–OH group
- Level of inebriation after consumption is related to number of carbons in R group (methanol < ethanol < ethylene glycol < isopropyl alcohol).
- Calculated serum osmolarity: $2 (Na^+) + (BUN/2.8) + (Glucose/18)$
- Osmol gap: Difference between measured and calculated serum osmolarity
- Estimate toxic alcohol level as follows: Osmol gap = alcohol level/N (where N = molecular weight/10, i.e., N = 3.2 for methanol, 4.6 for ethanol, etc.)
- "Normal" osmol gap is between −14 and +10; baseline gap is usually unknown.
- Patients with "normal" gap may in fact be elevated from their baseline.
- Elevated gap of 10 corresponds to methanol level of 32, ethanol level 46, etc.
- Bottom line: Elevated gap is useful; normal gap does not rule out toxic ingestion.

Ethanol

Most commonly used and abused intoxicant in the United States

EXPOSURE

- Ethanol frequently consumed with other intoxicants (most common is cocaine)
- Ethanol + cocaine → cocaethylene (40 times more potent than regular cocaine)

MECHANISM OF TOXICITY

- CNS depressant that cross-reacts with other depressants (benzodiazepines, barbiturates)
- Majority of ethanol is absorbed in proximal small bowel.
- Up to 10% is eliminated by lungs, urine, and sweat.
- Remainder is metabolized by liver as follows:
  - Catalyzed by alcohol dehydrogenase and aldehyde dehydrogenase (inhibited by disulfiram)
  - Microsomal alcohol oxidizing system
- Elimination follows zero-order kinetics:
  - Approximately 15 to 20 mg/dL/hr in normal individuals
  - Approximately 30 mg/dL/hr in chronic alcoholics

CLINICAL SIGNS OF TOXICITY

- Slurred speech
- Nystagmus
- Disinhibition
- CNS depression
- Degree of intoxication clinically correlates poorly with blood alcohol level (BAL).

BAL:
- One drink equals ~25 to 35 mg/dL BAL.
- Average person metabolizes 15 to 20 mg/dL/hr.
- Chronic drinkers metabolize ~30 mg/dL/hr.

MANAGEMENT

Management of acute intoxication is supportive:

- Thiamine, folate, IV fluids
- "Banana bag" consists of 1 L of D₅NS with 100 mg thiamine, 1 mg folate, and 1 amp of multivitamin (which turns bag yellow).

ALCOHOLIC KETOACIDOSIS (AKA)

- Anion gap acidosis in heavy alcohol user who has temporarily stopped drinking and eating
- Acid–base: Frequently metabolic acidosis with respiratory alkalosis (compensatory) and metabolic alkalosis (vomiting). pH may be normal.
- Treat with IV fluid replacement, IV glucose, and thiamine.

Methanol

EXPOSURE

Product of wood distillation, found in:

- Antifreeze
- Automotive fluids
- Paint thinners

MECHANISM OF TOXICITY

Toxicity is secondary to metabolites: Formaldehyde and formic acid (Figure 18-3):

- Formic acid causes a lactic acidosis by inhibiting mitochondrial respiration.
- Formaldehyde accumulates in retina causing "snowfield vision."
- Onset of symptoms is usually delayed ~12 to 18 hours until metabolites form (delay is even longer if ethanol is co-ingested).

CLINICAL SIGNS OF TOXICITY

- CNS depression
- Visual changes
- Abdominal pain (direct GI mucosal irritation)
- High anion gap metabolic acidosis
- Severity of acidosis is better predictor of outcome than methanol level.

MANAGEMENT

- Charcoal:
    - Binds poorly to all alcohols
    - Rapid GI absorption of alcohols limits utility of charcoal.

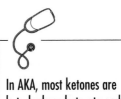

Causes of elevated osmol gap: **E-MEDIA**
Ethylene glycol

Methanol
Ethanol
Diuretics (mannitol)
Isopropyl alcohol
Acetone

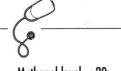

In AKA, most ketones are beta-hydroxybutyrate and are poorly detected by lab.

- Methanol level < 20: Patients are usually asymptomatic.
- Methanol level > 50: Patients usually have significant toxicity.

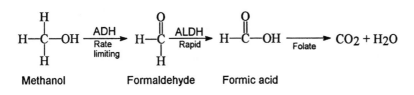

FIGURE 18-3. Methanol metabolism.

(Reproduced, with permission, from Goldfrank LR et al. *Goldfrank's Toxicology*, 6th ed. Stamford, CT: Appleton & Lange, 1998: 1054.)

- Fomepizole:
  - Competitive inhibitor of alcohol dehydrogenase
  - Blocks metabolism of methanol to toxic metabolites
- Ethanol:
  - Affinity for alcohol dehydrogenase 10 times greater than methanol
  - BAL of ethanol should be maintained ~100 to 150 mg/dL.
  - Methanol is cleared renally (slow) while on ethanol drip.
- Dialysis:
  - Indicated for large ingestions or with severe acidosis
  - Indicated when methanol level > 25 mg/dL

Ethylene Glycol

Colorless, odorless, and sweet-tasting liquid

EXPOSURE

- Coolant/antifreeze
- Commercial solvents
- Detergents
- Polishes
- De-icers

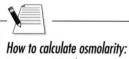

Ethylene glycol is often consumed as an ethanol substitute or in suicide attempts.

MECHANISM OF TOXICITY

Toxicity is secondary to toxic metabolites:
- Ethylene glycol → glycoaldehyde causes lactate formation.
- Glyoxylic acid broken down to glycine and ketoadipate (nontoxic)
- When above pathways are saturated, formic acid and oxalic acid are formed.
- Formic acid contributes to metabolic acidosis as with methanol.
- Oxalic acid crystallizes (calcium oxalate) causing renal stones and hypocalcemia.

CLINICAL SIGNS OF TOXICITY

- Early phase (1 to 12 hours): CNS depression, slurred speech, ataxia
- Cardiopulmonary phase (12 to 24 hours): Tachycardia, tachypnea, CHF, adult respiratory distress syndrome (ARDS)
- Nephrotoxic phase (24 to 72 hours): Oliguric renal failure, acute tubular necrosis, hypocalcemia

Hallmark of ethylene glycol toxicity: Calcium oxalate crystals in urine (50% present)

MANAGEMENT

- Quickly absorbed by gut and only 50% adsorbed to charcoal; charcoal has limited benefit
- Obtain blood levels of ethanol, methanol, and ethylene glycol.
- Ethanol infusion or fomepizole to competitively inhibit toxic pathways
- Calcium supplementation as indicated for hypocalcemia
- Pyridoxine and thiamine supplementation to preserve nontoxic pathways
- Dialysis as indicated clinically or for ethylene glycol level > 25 mg/dL

How to calculate osmolarity:
$2 \times Na + BUN/2 + Glucose/18 + ETOH/4.6$
If there is a difference between the measured (lab) and calculated osmolarity, consider toxic alcohols.

Isopropanol

Clear liquid with bitter burning taste and characteristic odor

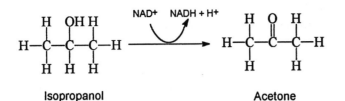

FIGURE 18-4. Isopropanol metabolism.
(Reproduced, with permission, from Goldfrank LR et al. *Goldfrank's Toxicology*, 6th ed. Stamford, CT: Appleton & Lange, 1998: 1058.)

EXPOSURE

- Rubbing alcohol
- Disinfectants
- Skin and hair products

MECHANISM OF TOXICITY

- Twice as potent as ethanol in causing CNS depression, with longer half-life
- Metabolism of isopropanol follows first-order (concentration dependent) kinetics (Figure 18-4).

CLINICAL SIGNS OF TOXICITY

- Hallmark of isopropanol ingestion is ketosis without significant acidosis:
  - Acetic acid and formic acid formation contribute to mild acidosis.
  - Acetone formation causes ketonemia/ketonuria in absence of hyperglycemia.
- Marked CNS depression (greater than ethanol)
- Hypotension secondary to peripheral vasodilatation
- Hemorrhagic gastritis from direct mucosal irritation

MANAGEMENT

- Rapidly absorbed and binds poorly to charcoal
- Supportive treatment for coma/respiratory depression
- IV fluids (pressors if necessary) for hypotension
- H_2 blockers and nasogastric tube as indicated for gastritis
- Dialysis for refractory hypotension or peak level > 400 mg/dL

> The hallmark of isopropanol ingestion is ketosis without significant acidosis.

DRUGS OF ABUSE

Cocaine

Naturally occurring alkaloid extract of *Erythroxylon coca* (South American plant)

EXPOSURE

- Cocaine hydrochloride: Absorbed across all membranes (usually snorted or injected)

- Cocaine alkaloid (crack): Stable to pyrolysis (may be inhaled), rapid onset/short duration

MECHANISM OF TOXICITY

- Mechanisms of action:
  - Blocks presynaptic reuptake of biogenic amine transmitters: Dopamine, serotonin, NE
  - Local anesthetic effect by blocking fast sodium channels
- Initial euphoria secondary to release of biogenic amines, subsequent dysphoria secondary to depletion of neurotransmitters (dopamine)

CLINICAL SIGNS OF TOXICITY

- Euphoria followed by dysphoria
- Hypertension
- Tachycardia, dysrhythmias
- Chest pain (coronary vasoconstriction)
- Seizures, infarction, hemorrhage (cerebral vasoconstriction)
- Cocaine psychosis
- Rhabdomyolysis
- Hyperthermia
- QRS widening and QT prolongation (sodium channel blockade)
- Adulterants and direct toxicity cause pulmonary edema, hemorrhage, and barotrauma (patients try Valsalva to increase drug effect).
- Mesenteric vasospasm (common in body-packers, body-stuffers)
- Uterine vasospasm causes abortions, abruption, prematurity, intrauterine growth retardation
- Cocaine wash-out syndrome

MANAGEMENT

- Initial supportive therapy includes sedation and cooling measures.
- Decontamination (charcoal and/or WBI) for ingestions (body-packers) (endoscopy contraindicated due to high incidence of bags rupturing)
- Benzodiazepines are effective in controlling tachycardia, hypertension, and seizures.
- Aggressive fluid resuscitation to maintain urine output
- Aspirin/nitrates/morphine for myocardial ischemia
- Bicarbonate for patients with widened QRS
- Nitroprusside or phentolamine for control of severe hypertension (beta blockers contraindicated, unopposed alpha stimulation may increase blood pressure)

Opioids

EXPOSURE

Naturally occurring or synthetic derivatives of poppy plant:
- Morphine
- Codeine
- Fentanyl
- Heroin
- Methadone
- Others

Causes of toxin-induced seizures:
OTIS CAMPBELL
Organophosphates/oral hypoglycemics
Tricyclic antidepressants
INH/insulin
Sympathomimetics

Camphor/cocaine
Amphetamines
Methylxanthines
PCP/phenol/propanolol
Benzodiazepine withdrawal
Ethanol withdrawal
Lithium/lindane
Lidocaine/lead

Beta blockers are contraindicated in cocaine toxicity; unopposed alpha stimulation may increase blood pressure.

MECHANISM OF TOXICITY

Multiple receptor types with varying pharmacology (discussed in toxidromes section)

CLINICAL SIGNS OF TOXICITY

- CNS depression
- Hypothermia, bradycardia, hypotension
- Miosis
- Histamine release may contribute to hypotension.
- Respiratory depression
- Noncardiogenic pulmonary edema
- Decreased GI motility—obstipation/constipation

Causes of miosis: **COPS**
Cholinergics/clonidine
Opiates/organophosphates
Phenothiazines/pilocarpine/pontine bleed
Sedative–hypnotics

MANAGEMENT

- Respiratory support using bag-valve mask or endotracheal intubation (respiratory depression is the major cause of mortality with opiates)
- Naloxone in incremental doses (titrate to response) (naloxone is pure antagonist at all three opiate receptors)
- Charcoal and WBI for body-packers
- Patients given naloxone may not leave until effects of naloxone have worn off (so that they do not pass out again in the street).
- Giving naloxone: Dilute 0.4 mg naloxone in 10 cc saline, then administer IV 1 cc at a time to full spontaneous respirations. Do not give more than needed, or you will have an angry, combative patient.

Amphetamines

EXPOSURE

- Long history of use and abuse as stimulants and nasal decongestants
- Currently used in the management of narcolepsy, attention deficit–hyperactivity disorder, and short-term weight reduction
- Methamphetamine (crystal, ice): High-potency stimulant effect
- MDMA (ecstasy, X, Adam): Serotonin effects, intensifies emotions
- Ephedrine: Amphetamine-like structure, used to ward off drowsiness

MECHANISM OF TOXICITY

- Release of catecholamines (dopamine and NE) from presynaptic nerve terminals
- Blocks reuptake of catecholamines (presynaptic)
- At higher doses, causes release of serotonin

CLINICAL SIGNS OF TOXICITY

- Hyperadrenergic: Tachycardia, hypertension, myocardial infarction, dysrhythmias
- CNS effects: Agitation, seizures, coma, ischemia/hemorrhage, psychosis (hallucinations, etc.) with serotonergic amphetamines
- Increased metabolism: Hyperthermia, dehydration, rhabdomyolysis

Toxic causes of hypertension: **CT SCAN**
Cocaine
Theophylline

Sympathomimetics
Caffeine
Amphetamines/anticholinergics
Nicotine

MANAGEMENT

- Decontamination using activated charcoal for oral ingestions

- Benzodiazepines for sedation and anticonvulsant
- External cooling and aggressive rehydration for hyperthermia
- Phentolamine or nitrates for control of severe hypertension

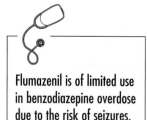

Causes of hypothermia:
COOLS
CO
Opiates
Oral hypoglycemics
Liquor (alcohols)
Sedative–hypnotics

Sedative–Hypnotics

A diverse group of drugs that cause sedation and hypnosis, used for:

- Insomnia
- Anxiety
- Seizures
- Alcohol withdrawal
- Anesthesia

EXPOSURE

- Benzodiazepines
- Barbiturates
- GHB (gamma-hydroxybutyrate)
- Others

MECHANISM OF TOXICITY

- Benzodiazepines/barbiturates both work by potentiating GABA:
  - GABA is the primary inhibitory neurotransmitter in the CNS.
  - $GABA_A$ receptor in cell membrane controls chloride ion flow.
  - Receptor has separate binding sites for benzodiazepines and barbiturates.
- GHB:
  - GHB is an endogenous metabolite of GABA.
  - Banned in the United States but available abroad
  - Used as a "date-rape drug" secondary to euphoria, aphrodisiac, and amnesia

CLINICAL SIGNS OF TOXICITY

- Sleepiness and sedation
- Muscle relaxation
- May induce general anesthesia
- May be associated with respiratory depression
- Tolerance may develop rapidly.
- Benzodiazepine overdose:
  - Isolated benzodiazepine overdose is rarely associated with death.
  - May potentiate other CNS depressants (ethanol, opioids, etc.)
  - Cardiorespiratory depression usually only seen with parenteral administration
- Barbiturate overdose:
  - Barbiturate overdose has a significant incidence of morbidity/mortality.
  - Confusion/lethargy progresses to coma with hypothermia, cardiovascular collapse, and respiratory arrest.

Sedative–hypnotics are frequently used in suicide attempts, especially in combination with alcohol. Patients should not receive regular prescriptions from the emergency department.

MANAGEMENT

- Control airway, breathing, and circulation (ABCs).
- Volume replacement and pressors as required for hemodynamic stability
- Consider lavage (agents cause decreased gut motility) and charcoal.
- Alkalinization of urine promotes elimination of phenobarbital.

Flumazenil is of limited use in benzodiazepine overdose due to the risk of seizures.

372

- Hemodialysis/hemoperfusion has limited utility in removing drug.
- Antidote:
  - Flumazenil is competitive antagonist at benzodiazepine receptor site.
  - Most appropriate for reversing benzodiazepines administered IV by physicians (conscious sedation)
  - Should not be used in overdose setting, as it may unmask seizures

INDUSTRIAL TOXINS

Hydrocarbons

Compounds consisting primarily of carbon and hydrogen

EXPOSURE

- Household products:
  - Polishes
  - Pine oils
  - Glues
- Petroleum distillates:
  - Kerosene
  - Gasoline
- Abused solvents (inhalants):
  - Nail polish remover
  - Paints, paint stripper
  - Typewriter correction fluid

MECHANISM OF TOXICITY

- The number of carbons determines physical state:
  - 1 to 4 = gas, low viscosity
  - 5 to 19 = liquid, low viscosity
  - 20 to 60 = solids, high viscosity
- Structures:
  - Aliphatics: Saturated straight/branched chain hydrocarbons
  - Aromatic: Unsaturated, contain at least one benzene ring
  - Alkene: Contain at least one carbon–carbon double bond
  - Cycloparaffins: Saturated hydrocarbons in closed rings
  - Halogenated: Chloride-containing hydrocarbons

CLINICAL SIGNS OF TOXICITY

- Pulmonary toxicity:
  - Most common organ system affected
  - Due to aspiration with direct toxic effects and disruption of surfactant
  - Associated with cough, rales, bronchospasm, tachypnea, pulmonary edema
  - Forty to 88% will have pneumonitis on chest film.
- CNS toxicity:
  - Seizures and/or coma
- GI toxicity:
  - Ulcers
  - Hematemesis

- Hydrocarbons with low viscosity and low surface tension are more likely to be aspirated.
- Halogenated hydrocarbons are associated with myocardial sensitization.

Typical scenario:
A 3-year-old boy presents with cough and tachypnea after being found in the kitchen. He smells like pine cleaner. *Think: Aspiration of hydrocarbon with pulmonary toxicity.*

Typical scenario:
A 15-year-old boy presents after being found by his mother in the garage passed out with a rag soaked in paint stripper. *Think: Inhalation of halogenated hydrocarbon with cardiac toxicity.*

Associated with systemic toxicity: CHAMPS
Camphor
Halogenated hydrocarbons
Aromatic hydrocarbons
Hydrocarbons associated with **M**etals
Hydrocarbons associated with **P**esticides
Suicidal ingestions

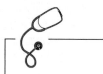

Most common caustic exposure: Household bleach (sodium hypochlorite)

Common acids:
- Sulfuric acid
- Formic acid
- Nitric acid
- Phosphoric acid
- Acetic acid
- Chromic acid
- Hydrofluoric acid

ACids cause Coagulation; aLkalies cause Liquefaction.

- Cardiac toxicity:
  - Myocardial sensitization and dysrhythmias
  - More common with halogenated hydrocarbons
- Dermatologic toxicity:
  - Dermatitis
  - Full-thickness burns reported

MANAGEMENT

- Control ABCs.
- Intubation, mechanical ventilation with positive end-expiratory pressure or jet ventilation for respiratory distress
- Avoid catecholamines if possible (myocardial sensitization).
- Gastric emptying is controversial:
  - May increase risk of aspiration
  - Consider if ingestion is > 30 mL.
  - Consider if hydrocarbon is associated with systemic toxicity.

Caustics

Acidic or alkaline substances capable of causing damage on contact with body surfaces

Acids

EXPOSURE

- Drain cleaners
- Disinfectants
- Rust removers
- Photography solutions

MECHANISM OF TOXICITY

- Acids cause coagulation necrosis.
- Dehydration of superficial tissues produces an eschar that limits tissue damage.
- Systemic absorption of strong acids causes acidosis, hemolysis, and renal failure.
- Acid exposure is associated with a higher mortality than alkali despite less local tissue destruction.

CLINICAL SIGNS OF TOXICITY

- Hematemesis, melena
- Abdominal pain
- Gastric perforation with peritonitis
- Gastric outlet obstruction
- Dermal burns

MANAGEMENT

- Control ABCs.
- Obtain blood gas to detect systemic absorption of acid.
- Obtain upright chest film to look for free air.
- Endoscopy of gastric mucosa

Alkalies

EXPOSURE

- Industrial cleaners
- Household bleach (sodium hypochlorite)
- Batteries
- Clinitest tablets

MECHANISM OF TOXICITY

- Cause liquefaction necrosis
- Lipids saponified, proteins denatured, causing deep local tissue injury
- Alkali exposure is associated with a lower mortality than acid despite more local tissue destruction.

CLINICAL SIGNS OF TOXICITY

- Orofacial burns
- Drooling, odynophagia
- Stridor, dyspnea
- Esophageal perforation, chest pain, mediastinitis
- Dermal burns

MANAGEMENT

- Control ABCs.
- Upright chest film to look for free air, button batteries
- For patients with alkali ingestions: If patient has orofacial burns, drooling, vomiting, stridor, or inability to drink sips of water, admit for endoscopy within 12 to 24 hours.
- Eye exposure: For both acid and alkali exposures to the cornea, irrigate with normal saline (2 to 10 L) until the pH is 7.5. Alkaline eye exposures may result in continued local tissue destruction and always require ophthalmology consultation.
- Endoscopic or bronchoscopic removal of ingested batteries is required.
- Surgical intervention if indicated
- Supportive care

Dermal exposure to hydrofluoric acid, found in rust removers, can result in systemic absorption, hypocalcemia, hypomagnesemia, and death. Treat with supportive care, calcium gluconate paste to dermal burn, and IV calcium.

Acid exposure is associated with a higher mortality than alkali due to systemic absorption of acid.

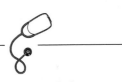

Common alkalies:
- Sodium hydroxide
- Lithium hydroxide
- Ammonium hydroxide
- Sodium hypochlorite

PESTICIDES

Organophosphates

EXPOSURE

- Pesticides
- Animal care
- Household products
- Chemical warfare

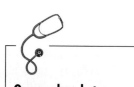

Why endoscope?
- Safe 12 to 24 hours after exposure
- May identify surgical candidates
- Grades injuries and predicts risk of strictures
- Patients who develop strictures are far more likely to develop neoplasm at stricture site than those without exposure.

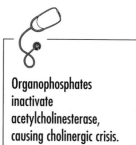

Organophosphate chemical warfare agents:
GA: Tabun
GB: Sarin
GC: Soman
VX

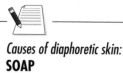

Organophosphates inactivate acetylcholinesterase, causing cholinergic crisis.

Causes of diaphoretic skin:
SOAP
Sympathomimetics
Organophosphates
Aspirin (salicylates)
PCP

MECHANISM OF TOXICITY

- Irreversibly binds to cholinesterase, inactivating it by phosphorylation
- Acetylcholinesterase in RBC/CNS, pseudocholinesterase in serum
- Phosphorylation ("aging") takes place between 24 and 48 hours postexposure. Once aging is complete, enzyme must be resynthesized (takes weeks).
- Accumulation of ACh in synapse causes cholinergic crisis.

CLINICAL SIGNS OF TOXICITY

- Muscarinic effects: "SLUDGE" symptoms
- Nicotinic effects:
  - Diaphoresis
  - Hypertension
  - Tachycardia
- Neuromuscular effects:
  - Fasciculations
  - Muscle weakness
- CNS effects:
  - Anxiety
  - Tremor
  - Confusion
  - Seizures
  - Coma
- Long-term effects:
  - Delayed neurotoxicity
  - Delayed polyneuropathy
  - Transient paralysis 24 to 96 hours after exposure

MANAGEMENT

- Supportive care (including airway)
- Atropine reverses CNS and muscarinic effects (may require multiple doses).
- Pralidoxime (2-PAM) regenerates acetylcholinesterase (must be given before 24 to 36 hours, before "aging" is complete).

Carbamates

Structurally related to organophosphates, carbamates also work by inhibiting cholinesterase.

EXPOSURE

- Insecticides
- Wartime pretreatment (carbamate pyridostigmine given in Gulf War)

MECHANISM OF TOXICITY

- Inhibit cholinesterase via carbamoylation, a transient and reversible process

CLINICAL SIGNS OF TOXICITY

- Similar to organophosphates: "SLUDGE," nicotinic and neuromuscular effects

- CNS effects not prominent
- All effects transient

MANAGEMENT

- Supportive care as with organophosphates
- Atropine for reversal of muscarinic symptoms
- 2-PAM usually not necessary (carbamate inhibition is transient)

ENVIRONMENTAL/OCCUPATIONAL TOXINS

Methemoglobin

EXPOSURE

- *Environmental:* Nitrates (well water, food, chemicals/dyes)
- *Medications:* Local anesthetics, dapsone, Pyridium, nitroglycerine
- *Hereditary:* Deficiency of reducing enzymes or abnormal Hgb

MECHANISM OF TOXICITY

Oxidation of Hgb
- Normal Hgb has Fe^{2+} group (able to bind oxygen). Oxidant stress causes $Fe^{2+} \rightarrow Fe^{3+}$ (methemoglobin).

Inability to Transport Oxygen
- Ferric ion (Fe^{3+}) in methemoglobin is unable to bind oxygen.
- Methemoglobin shifts oxygen dissociation curve to left (impairs release).
- With severe oxidant stress, methemoglobin begins to accumulate.

CLINICAL SIGNS OF TOXICITY

General Signs
- Cyanosis with normal pO_2 that doesn't respond to supplemental oxygen
- "Chocolate-brown" color of blood (compare with normal blood color)
- Confirmation of methemoglobin level by co-oximetry

Mild
- Methemoglobin level < 20%
- Cyanosis present

Moderate
- Methemoglobin level 20 to 50%
- Cyanosis, dyspnea, headache, fatigue

Severe
- Methemoglobin level 50 to 70%
- Seizures/coma, myocardial ischemia, acidosis

Death
- Methemoglobin level > 70%

Measurement of O_2 in methemoglobinemia:
- Pulse oximetry trends toward 85% (measures color).
- pO_2 from ABG measures dissolved oxygen and may be normal. Calculated O_2 saturation will also be normal.
- Accurate measurement by co-oximetry

MANAGEMENT

- Supportive care
- Antidote therapy: Methylene blue:
  - Indicated for patients with moderate to severe symptoms or level > 20%
  - An electron carrier that allows methemoglobin → Hgb
  - Utilizes NADPH pathway to reduce itself back to methylene blue
  - Can't use in patients with glucose-6-phosphate dehydrogenase deficiency (can't generate NADPH)
  - Pulse oximetry will drop transiently due to bluish discoloration of blood.
- Exchange transfusions and hyperbaric oxygen for refractory cases

CO

CO is responsible for the most deaths due to poisoning in the United States.

EXPOSURE

- *Combustion:* Fires, vehicle exhaust, home generators
- *Metabolism:* Methylene chloride (paint remover) is metabolized to CO in the liver.

MECHANISM OF TOXICITY

- Binds to Hgb with ~250 times greater affinity than oxygen
- Shifts oxygen–Hgb dissociation curve to left (decreases release of O_2)
- Binds to myoglobin in heart and skeletal muscle
- Binds to and inactivates cytochrome oxidase
- Associated with CNS ischemic reperfusion injury

CLINICAL SIGNS OF TOXICITY

Mild
- Headache, nausea, vomiting

Moderate
- Chest pain, confusion, dyspnea,
- Tachycardia, tachypnea, ataxia

Severe
- Palpitations, disorientation
- Seizures, coma, hypotension, myocardial ischemia, dysrhythmias, pulmonary edema, ARDS, rhabdomyolysis, renal failure, multiorgan failure, disseminated intravascular coagulation

MANAGEMENT

Elimination
- CO dissociates from Hgb at different rates depending on FiO_2:
  - Room air (21% O_2) ~4 hours
  - 100% O_2 (1 ATM) ~90 minutes
  - 100% O_2 (3 ATM) ~23 minutes

Fetal Hgb binds to CO with even greater affinity than adult Hgb.

Typical scenario:
A couple and their son present to the emergency department with flulike symptoms and mild confusion 1 day after using a home generator in the garage. *Think: CO poisoning.*
- Multiple victims
- Initial flulike symptoms
- Exposure to products of combustion

- Hyperbaric O_2 (HBO):
  - Enhances pulmonary elimination of CO as above
  - Displaces CO from myoglobin and cytochromes in peripheral tissues
  - Decreases reperfusion injury
  - May decrease delayed neurologic sequelae in some patients
- Indications for HBO:
  - Evidence of end-organ ischemia (syncope, coma, seizure, focal neurologic deficits, myocardial infarction, ventricular dysrhythmias)
  - CO–Hgb level > 25% (> 15% in pregnancy, children)
  - Severe metabolic acidosis
  - Unable to oxygenate (pulmonary edema)
  - No improvement with 100% O_2

Cyanide

Among the most potent and potentially lethal toxins

EXPOSURE

Inhalation
- Smoke from fires involving chemically treated wool, silk, rubber, polyurethane

Ingestion or Cutaneous Exposure
- Accidental or intentional ingestion of chemical baths used in photography, jewelry making, and electroplating
- Food and drug tampering (poisoning)
- Ingestion of plants or fruits containing cyanogenic compounds

Iatrogenic
- Nitroprusside contains cyanide.

MECHANISM OF TOXICITY

- Inhibits cytochrome oxidase at cytochrome aa_3 of the electron transport chain
- Causes cellular hypoxia and lactic acidosis
- Blocks production of adenosine triphosphate

CLINICAL SIGNS OF TOXICITY

- CNS dysfunction: Headache, seizures, coma
- Cardiovascular dysfunction: Bradycardia, decreased inotropy, hypotension
- Pulmonary edema
- Hemorrhagic gastritis

MANAGEMENT

- Supportive care (manage airway, fluids)
- Decontamination
- Antidote therapy:
  - Administration of nitrites generates methemoglobin.
  - Methemoglobin draws cyanide groups from cytochrome oxidase.
  - Thiosulfate transfers sulfur group to cyanomethemoglobin.
  - Thiocyanate (relatively harmless) is excreted in urine.

Treat coexistent CO poisoning in fires (further compromises O_2 supply).

"Classic" signs of cyanide toxicity such as bitter almond odor and cherry-red skin color are unreliable.

- Cyanide antidote (Lilly antidote kit):
  - Amyl nitrite pearls—crush and inhale
  - Sodium nitrite—give IV over 20 minutes
  - Sodium thiosulfate—IV (after nitrites)
  - Monitor excessive methemoglobin production during antidotal therapy.

Environmental Emergencies

AIR

LOW-PRESSURE DYSBARISM

DEFINITION

Impaired gas exchange at altitude

ALTITUDE CLASSIFICATION

- High altitude: 5,000 to 11,500 feet
- Very high altitude: 11,500 to 18,000 feet
- Extreme altitude: > 18,000 feet

SIGNS AND SYMPTOMS

High Altitude
- Decreased exercise performance
- Increased ventilation at rest

Very High Altitude
- Maximal SaO < 90%, PaO_2 < 60 mm Hg
- Stress and sleep hypoxemia

Extreme Altitude
- Severe hypoxemia and hypocapnia
- Acclimatization impossible

HIGH-ALTITUDE ACCLIMATIZATION

DEFINITION

The body's adjustment to lower ambient oxygen concentrations

PHYSIOLOGY

- Carotid body hypoxemia stimulates increase in ventilation, which leads to decreased $PaCO_2$ and increased PaO_2.
- Without adequate O_2, hyperventilation leads to acute respiratory alkalosis.
- Renal response is to excrete more bicarbonate, returning the pH to normal.
- Increased erythropoietin within 2 hours of ascent gives rise to an increased red cell mass in days to weeks, hence a minimal and subclinical decreased O_2-carrying capacity.

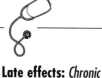

Late effects: *Chronic mountain polycythemia:*
- Headache
- Sleep difficulty
- Mental slowness
- Impaired circulation

ACUTE MOUNTAIN SICKNESS (AMS)

DEFINITION

Syndrome of several constitutional complaints related to hypobaric hypoxemia and its physiologic consequences

SIGNS AND SYMPTOMS

- At 24 hours: Hangover (lassitude, anorexia, headache, nausea, vomiting)
- Then oliguria, peripheral edema, retinal hemorrhages
- Finally high-altitude pulmonary edema (HAPE), high-altitude cerebral edema (HACE), death

Associated high-altitude symptoms:
- Snow blindness (ultraviolet keratitis)
- Pharyngitis
- Retinopathy

RISK FACTORS

- Childhood
- Rapid ascent
- Higher sleeping altitudes
- Chronic obstructive pulmonary disease
- Decreased vital capacity
- Cold
- Heavy exertion
- Sickle cell disease

Patients with sickle cell disease require supplemental oxygen for high-altitude exposures.

TREATMENT

- Oxygen
- Descent
- Acetazolamide
- HBO chamber
- Nonsteroidal anti-inflammatory drugs for headache
- Prochlorperazine for nausea and vomiting

Other helpful tips:
- Avoidance of alcohol and overexertion
- High-carbohydrate diet

Definitive treatment for all high-altitude syndromes is descent. Descent may be simulated with a Gamow bag, which is a portable hyperbaric oxygen (HBO) chamber.

HAPE

DEFINITION

Noncardiogenic pulmonary edema seen at altitude associated with decreased vasoconstriction, increased pulmonary hypertension, and capillary leak

SIGNS AND SYMPTOMS

- Dry to productive cough
- Tachypnea
- Tachycardia
- Peripheral cyanosis
- Fatigue
- Orthopnea
- Rales

TREATMENT

- Oxygen to keep SaO > 90%
- Immediate descent to lower altitude
- HBO chamber
- Continuous positive airway pressure
- Consider nifedipine if descent or HBO is not available.
- Minimize exertion.
- Keep warm (cold stress elevates pulmonary artery pressures).
- Consider morphine/furosemide.

HACE

DEFINITION

Progressive neurologic deterioration in someone with AMS

SIGNS AND SYMPTOMS

- Altered mental status
- Ataxia
- Cranial nerve palsy
- Seizure
- Stroke-like symptoms
- Coma (usually not permanent)
- Headache
- Nausea, vomiting

TREATMENT

- Oxygen to keep SaO > 90%
- Immediate descent to lower altitude
- Dexamethasone
- Loop diuretic
- HBO chamber

Best prevention for AMS is graded ascent with enough time at each altitude step for acclimatization.

HAPE is the most life threatening of AMS syndromes.

Early diagnosis of HAPE is key, because it is reversible in the early stages. Patients need not develop any signs of AMS before developing HAPE. Early presentation may be just a dry cough.

MEDICATIONS USED FOR HIGH-ALTITUDE ILLNESS

Drug	Mechanism of Action	Indications
Acetazolamide	■ Decreases the formation of bicarbonate by inhibiting the enzyme carbonic anhydrase ■ Diuretic action counters the fluid retention of AMS. ■ Decreases bicarbonate absorption in the kidney, resulting in a metabolic acidosis that stimulates hyperventilation (to blow off excess CO_2) ■ This compensatory hyperventilation is normally turned off as soon as the pH reaches close to 7.4. ■ By maintaining a constant forced bicarbonate diuresis, acetazolamide causes the central chemoreceptors to continually reset, permitting the hyperventilation to continue, thereby countering the altitude-induced hypoxemia.	■ Abrupt ascent to over 10,000 feet ■ Nocturnal dyspnea ■ AMS ■ History of altitude illness (used as prophylaxis)
Dexamethasone	■ Decreases vasogenic edema ■ Decreases intracranial pressure ■ Antiemetic ■ Mood elevator	■ HACE
Oxygen	■ Low-flow oxygen improves sleeping problems by ameliorating the normal hypoxemia that occurs during sleep.	■ AMS ■ HAPE ■ HACE
HBO	■ Improves hypoxemia for all altitude illness ■ In nitrogen narcosis, raises ambient pressure and PaO_2 in order to convert nitrogen bubbles back to solution and restore O_2 to deprived areas while the body eliminates the problem gas	■ AMS ■ HAPE ■ HACE ■ Nitrogen narcosis
Nifedipine	■ Decreases pulmonary artery pressure	■ HAPE when descent or oxygen are unavailable
Morphine, furosemide	■ Reduce pulmonary blood flow and decrease hydrostatic force, resulting in less fluid available for extravasation	■ HAPE

HIGH-PRESSURE DYSBARISM

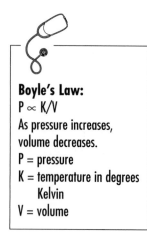

Boyle's Law:
$P \propto K/V$
As pressure increases, volume decreases.
P = pressure
K = temperature in degrees Kelvin
V = volume

Descent Barotrauma

DEFINITION

Barotrauma associated with descent or dive in body spaces that cannot equalize pressure; also known as the "squeeze"

SIGNS AND SYMPTOMS

- Middle ear squeeze (barotitis media):
  - Eustachian tube dysfunction
  - Ear fullness or pain
  - Nausea and vertigo
  - Hemotympanum

- External ear squeeze:
  - Due to occlusion of external ear canal with cerumen
  - Bloody otorrhea
  - Petechiae in canal
- Inner ear squeeze:
  - Rare
  - Associated with rapid descent
  - Tinnitus, vertigo, hearing loss
  - Nausea, vomiting
- Sinus squeeze:
  - Sinus pain or pressure
  - Usually frontal and maxillary
  - Can have epistaxis
  - Associated with preexisting sinus inflammation or blockage
- Lung squeeze:
  - Occurs in divers who hold their breath going down
  - Hemoptysis
  - Shortness of breath
  - Pulmonary edema
- Equipment squeeze:
  - Conjunctival/scleral/periorbital petechiae under face mask
  - Petechiae on skin under suit

TREATMENT

- All types of squeeze:
  - Cease dive.
  - Equilibrate spaces in advance (remove foreign body, use decongestants).
- Give antibiotics for:
  - Frontal or sphenoid sinus squeeze
  - Otitis externa
  - Tympanic membrane rupture
- Inner ear fistula requires surgical repair.

Most types of descent barotrauma resolve with ascent and rest.

Ascent Barotrauma

DEFINITION

Barotrauma caused by expansion of gas on ascent in body spaces that cannot equilibrate

SIGNS AND SYMPTOMS

- Reverse ear squeeze:
  - Tympanic membrane rupture
  - Ear pain
  - Bloody otorrhea
  - Occurs with rapid ascent
- Pulmonary barotrauma:
  - Dissection of air into pulmonary tissue with failure to exhale during ascent
  - Associated with:
    - Pneumomediastinum
    - Pneumopericardium
    - Local subcutaneous emphysema

Risk factor for reverse ear squeeze is upper respiratory tract congestion/infection.

- Pulmonary interstitial emphysema
- Pneumothorax

TREATMENT

- All types of ascent barotrauma:
  - Rest.
- Reverse ear squeeze:
  - Ear, nose, and throat consult
- Pulmonary barotrauma:
  - Oxygen
  - Observation
  - Most resolve without intervention.

DAE:
Occurs within 10 minutes of surfacing

Typical scenario:
A 24-year-old male diver syncopizes upon ascent to the surface. *Think: DAE.*

Dysbaric Air Embolism (DAE)

DEFINITION

Arterial air embolism associated with ruptured alveoli; enters left heart through pulmonary veins and may occlude an area of systemic circulation

SIGNS AND SYMPTOMS

- Coronary artery emboli:
  - Chest pain
  - Dysrhythmias
- Central nervous system (CNS) emboli:
  - Focal neurologic deficit
  - Aphasia
  - Seizure
  - Dizziness
  - Headache
  - Confusion
  - Visual field loss

TREATMENT

- HBO
- Avoid air transport (ascent).

Decompression Sickness

Decompression sickness:
Also known as "the bends"

DEFINITION

Illness due to nitrogen bubbles in the blood, which form on decompression (ascent)

SIGNS AND SYMPTOMS

Type 1: Skin, Lymphatic, Musculoskeletal "Bends"
- *Skin:* Pruritus, redness, mottling
- *Lymphatic:* Lymphedema
- *Musculoskeletal:* Periarticular joint pain

Type 2: Cardiovascular, Respiratory, CNS "Bends"
- *Cardiovascular:* Tachycardia, acute coronary syndrome

- *Respiratory:* Dyspnea, cough, pulmonary edema, pneumothorax, hemoptysis
- *CNS:* Focal neurologic deficit, back pain, urinary retention, incontinence

TREATMENT

- Transport immediately to HBO chamber
- Supine position
- Intravenous (IV) fluids
- 100% O_2
- Avoid air evacuation.
- Steroids controversial

Nitrogen Narcosis

DEFINITION

- The partial pressure of nitrogen in inspired tank air is increased at depth and as it accumulates in the tissues; the inert gas exerts an anesthetic effect on the diver.
- Becomes a problem at 70- to 100-foot dives

SIGNS AND SYMPTOMS

- Euphoria, disinhibition, overconfidence, poor judgment
- Slow reflexes
- Fine sensory discrimination loss
- At greater depths: Hallucinations, coma, death

TREATMENT

Ascend at a reasonable rate with assistance.

WATER

NEAR DROWNING/IMMERSION SYNDROME

DEFINITION

- *Drowning:* Death from an immersion
- *Near drowning:* Survival after an immersion

PATHOPHYSIOLOGY

- Mechanism of injury is suffocation from aspiration and associated laryngospasm.
- Fresh water (lakes, rivers, pools, baths): Hypotonic liquid disrupts surfactant and causes intrapulmonary shunting and fluid retention.
- Sea water (oceans and some lakes): Hypertonic liquid draws intravascular fluid into alveoli and causes intrapulmonary shunting.

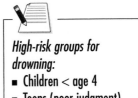

High-risk groups for drowning:
- Children < age 4
- Teens (poor judgment)
- Elderly (tubs)
- Alcohol and drug users

Risk factors for near drowning:
- **Hypoglycemia**
- **Head trauma**
- **Seizure**

They're not dead until they're warm and dead (see hypothermia).

SIGNS AND SYMPTOMS

- Vary significantly:
  - Mild cough and shortness of breath
  - Full cardiac arrest due to pneumonia/pneumonitis
- Once stable, hospital course can also vary, depending on:
  - Aspiration (usually contaminated water)
  - Physiologic reserve of victim

TREATMENT

- Rapid and cautious rescue
- C-spine immobilization
- Control airway, breathing, and circulation (ABCs).
- Rewarm as needed (see section on hypothermia).
- Treat associated injuries.
- Obtain chest x-ray, arterial blood gas, finger-stick glucose, electrolytes, toxicology screen, C-spine x-rays.
- No role for empiric steroids or antibiotics

PROGNOSIS

- Cerebral anoxic injury begins within a few minutes of no oxygen.
- Some authorities believe resuscitation should not be initiated if immersion > 10 minutes.
- Scattered case reports of survival without neurologic deficit in up to 24% of children requiring cardiopulmonary resuscitation

MARINE LIFE TRAUMA AND ENVENOMATION

The emergency physician must be familiar with the fauna of ocean and lake environments in order to diagnose and treat injuries and illnesses inflicted by them.

Type of Injury

- Marine life can be grossly divided into those that have stingers to cause injury and those that have nematocysts.
- A nematocyst is a microscopic "spring-loaded" venom gland, discharged by physical contact or osmotic gradient.
- The gland found on tentacles contracts when touched, striking victim repetitively, leaving whiplike scars.
- Gland remains active after the animal dies or tentacle rips off.

Stingers

- Stingrays
- Starfish
- Scorpion fish
- Sea urchins
- Catfish
- Lionfish
- Cone shells

Treatment of Stinger Injury

- Immerse wound in nonscalding hot water (45°C) for 90 minutes (or until pain is gone) to break down venom.
- X-ray to find and remove stings.
- Aggressive cleaning, antibiotics

Nematocysts

- Portuguese man-of-war
- Corals
- Fire corals
- Anemones
- Sea wasps
- Jellyfish

Treatment of Nematocyst Injury

- ABCs
- Inactivate nematocysts by immersing them in vinegar (5% acetic acid).
- Do not use tap water (causes venom discharge by osmotic gradient).
- Immobilize limb.
- IV access and fluids
- Antivenin: 1 ampule diluted 1:10 IV (20,000 U/ampule)
- Antihistamines/epinephrine/steroids for anaphylaxis
- Shave off remaining nematocysts.
- Pain control
- Tetanus prophylaxis

The main difference in treatment between a stinger and nematocyst injury is that you use water for a stinger and vinegar for a nematocyst.

Shark Attacks

- Sharks attack humans only when they can't see well enough to tell them apart from seals and sea lions, unless you invade their territory and start bleeding and flailing around haphazardly.
- Great white, mako, hammerhead, blue, bull, reef, and tiger sharks make up the majority of species reported to attack.
- If attacked, a force of ~18 tons per square inch and razor-sharp teeth digging into a limb or torso can quickly be a fatal blow if the victim doesn't immediately seek medical attention.

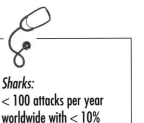

Sharks:
< 100 attacks per year worldwide with < 10% mortality

Blue-Ringed Octopus Envenomation

- Found off Australian coast
- Bites when handled and antagonized
- Beak injects venom containing tetrodotoxin (TTX), a paralyzing neurotoxin that blocks voltage-gated Na^+ channels
- Signs and symptoms: Paresthesias, diffuse flaccid paralysis, respiratory failure, local erythema

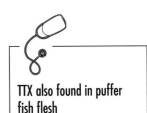

TTX also found in puffer fish flesh

Gila Monster and Mexican Beaded Lizard

- Normally timid, bite those who handle them
- Venom: Phospholipase-A, hyaluronidase, arginine esterase, and a kallikrein-like hypotensive enzyme secreted by glands in lower jaw

- Animal sometimes continues to bite/chew; the longer it holds on, the more venom gets in.
- Signs and symptoms:
  - Crush and puncture wounds, may have teeth in wound
  - Burning pain, radiates up extremity, lasts 8 hours, edema and cyanosis
  - Rare systemic effects: Weakness, fainting, hypotension, sweating
- Treatment:
  - Remove animal (if still attached)
  - Remove teeth, clean copiously and aggressively, broad-spectrum antibiotics, tetanus
  - Observation for systemic effects

Amphibians

- Colorado River toad, Columbian poison-dart frogs, and several species of newt and salamander secrete toxins in their skin and internal organs:
  - Batrachotoxin: Opens Na^+ channels irreversibly
  - Tetrodotoxin: Blocks Na^+ channels irreversibly
  - Bufotalin: Cardiac toxin, acts like digitalis
  - Samandarine: Opens CNS Na^+ channels irreversibly
- Treatment is supportive.

SNAKE ENVENOMATION

Crotalidae Family (Pit Vipers)

Includes rattlesnakes, massasauga, copperheads, and water moccasins (see Table 19-1)

SIGNS AND SYMPTOMS

Local (see Table 19-2)
- Burning pain (severity related to amount of venom)
- Edema spreading proximally
- Local petechiae, bullae, and skin necrosis

Systemic
- Nausea
- Fever
- Metallic taste
- Weakness
- Sweating
- Perioral paresthesias
- Hypotension
- Fasciculations
- Compartment syndrome (rare)
- Pulmonary edema
- Anaphylaxis
- Shock, intravascular coagulation, hemorrhage, and death

TABLE 19-1. Characteristics of Poisonous versus Nonpoisonous Snakes

Poisonous	Nonpoisonous
Triangle-shaped head	Rounded head
Elliptical pupil	Round pupil
Pit between eye and nostril	Absence of pit
Fangs	Absence of fangs

Elapidae Family (Coral Snakes)

- Includes the corals, cobras, kraits, and mambas
- Venom is a neurotoxin.

SIGNS AND SYMPTOMS

- Painless bite site
- Weak/numb within 90 minutes
- Euphoria
- Drowsiness
- Tremors
- Salivation
- Slurred speech
- Diplopia

Color pattern recognition (for U.S. snakes only):
- **Red-on-yellow . . . kill a fellow**
- **Red-on-black . . . venom lack**

TABLE 19-2. Snake Bite Grading System

Grade	Pit Viper	Coral Snake
0	• Fang marks • No pain • No systemic symptoms • **Don't give antivenin**	• No envenomation • Minimal fang scratches or punctures • Minimal local swelling • No systemic symptoms in 24 hours • **Give 3 vials antivenin**
I	• Fang marks • Mild pain/edema • No systemic symptoms • **Give 0–5 vials antivenin (50 mL)**	• Fang scratches or punctures • Minimal local swelling • Systemic symptoms present, but no respiratory paralysis • **Give 3 vials antivenin**
II	• Fang marks • Severe pain • Moderate edema • Mild systemic symptoms • **Give 10 vials antivenin (100 mL)**	• Severe envenomation • Respiratory paralysis occurs within 36 hours • **Give 5–10 vials antivenin**
III	• Fang marks • Severe pain/edema • Severe symptoms (hypotension, dyspnea) • Evidence of systemic coagulopathy • **Give 15–20 vials (150–200 mL)**	

- Flaccid paralysis
- Respiratory failure

TREATMENT FOR ALL SNAKE BITES

- ABCs
- Reassure patient.
- Immobilize extremity.
- Horse antivenin for bite grades I, II, and III (pit vipers)
- Antivenin for all coral snake bites (regardless of symptoms)
- Local wound care
- Tetanus prophylaxis
- Prophylactic antibiotics not recommended

SPIDERS

Brown Recluse Spider

Loxosceles reclusa

DEFINITION

Identified by violin design on its back

EXPOSURE

- Found in midwestern, mid-atlantic, and southern states
- Inhabits warm, dry places—typically woodpiles, cellars, and abandoned buildings
- Venom: Proteases, alkaline phosphatase, lipase, complement-system substances

SIGNS AND SYMPTOMS

- Necrosis at bite site due to local hemolysis and thrombosis associated with ischemia:
  - Mild red lesion, may be bluish/ischemic
  - Varying degrees of pain, blistering, necrosis within 3 to 4 days
  - May take weeks to heal
- Systemic symptoms:
  - Fever
  - Chills
  - Nausea
  - Myalgias, arthralgias
  - Hemolysis, petechiae
  - Seizure
  - Renal failure
  - Death

> Loxoscelism is a reaction to *Loxosceles* spider venom proportional to amount of venom exposure.

TREATMENT

- Monitor ABCs.
- Daily wound care
- Analgesia
- Tetanus prophylaxis
- Antibiotics if wound becomes infected

Black Widow Spider

Latrodectus mactans

DEFINITION

- Identified by red-orange hourglass on abdomen
- Female two times size of male, has design, is only one that can envenomate humans

EXPOSURE

- Found throughout the United States (except Alaska)
- Inhabits warm, dry, protected places, typically woodpiles, cellars, barns, under rocks, etc.
- Venom: Neurotoxic protein causing acetylcholine and norepinephrine release at synapses

SIGNS AND SYMPTOMS

- Local pinprick sensation, red, swollen
- Then slow progression of painful muscle spasm of large groups
- Lasts a few hours, resolves spontaneously
- Systemic signs:
  - Hypertension
  - Coma
  - Shock
  - Respiratory failure
  - Death (more often in children)

TREATMENT

- Pain control and muscle relaxants (narcotics and benzodiazepines)
- Tetanus, local wound care
- Antivenin available for severe reactions (1 to 2 vials IV over 30 minutes)

Abdominal muscle spasm of black widow spider bite may mimic peritonitis.

Patients who should get antivenin:
- Extremes of age
- Pregnant
- Underlying medical conditions (check for hypersensitivity/allergy with skin test prior to administration)

SCORPION

Bark scorpion (*Centruroides exilicauda*)

DEFINITION

- Has venom gland and stinger in last segment of tail

EXPOSURE

- Found in Arizona, California, Nevada, and Texas
- Bark scorpion inhabits areas around trees.
- Other species usually under rocks, logs, floors, boots
- Victims usually children and campers/hikers
- Venom activates Na^+ channels, damaging parasympathetic, somatic, and sympathetic nerves.
- Other proteins may cause hemolysis, hemorrhage, and local tissue destruction.

SIGNS AND SYMPTOMS

- Severe and immediate pain (erythema and swelling are species dependent)
- Then tachycardia, increased secretions, fasciculations, nausea, vomiting, blurred vision, dysphagia, roving eye movements, opisthotonos, respiratory failure, syncope, death (rare)

TREATMENT

- ABCs
- Sedation with benzodiazepines
- No opiates, may potentiate venom
- Tetanus prophylaxis, local wound care
- Antivenin: Unlicensed, available in Arizona only, derived from goat serum—skin test first, use for extremes of age, severe reactions (1 to 2 vials), observe for 24 hours (especially children)

BEES AND WASPS (APIDS AND VESPIDS)

DEFINITION

- Apids: Honeybees, bumblebees
- Vespids: Wasps, hornets, yellow jackets
- "Africanized" honeybees: Much more aggressive but venom contains same substances
- Yellow jackets cause most allergic reactions.

EXPOSURE

- Venom: Mostly proteins and peptides (phospholipase-A, hyaluronidase, histamine, serotonin, bradykinin, dopamine), also lipids and carbohydrates
- Systemically, toxicity from venom or anaphylaxis can occur within minutes.

SIGNS AND SYMPTOMS

- Most commonly local: Burning pain, erythema, edema at sting site, lasting ~24 hours
- Local/systemic delayed reaction up to 1.5 to 2 weeks later
- Toxicity: Vomiting, diarrhea, fever, drowsiness, syncope, seizure, muscle spasm, and rarely neuritis, nephritis, vasculitis
- Anaphylaxis possible

TREATMENT

- ABCs:
    - Airway can be compromised early (ask about prior bee stings).
- For any systemic signs:
    - Epinephrine 1:1000 0.3 to 0.5 mL SQ in adults, 0.01 mL/kg in children
    - Antihistamine (e.g., 50 mg diphenhydramine IV)
    - Steroid (e.g., 125 mg methylprednisolone IV)
    - Beta-2 agonist for wheezing (e.g., albuterol nebulizer treatment)
    - Admit and observe

> *Apids* sting only once — stinger detaches in skin, bee then dies.
> *Vespids* can sting again and again — stinger has no retroserrate barbs.

EXPOSURE

- *Soleneopsis invicta*—"unvanquished ant," Brazilian import to the United States in 1930s
- The ant bites with its mandibles, then stings with its venom apparatus in its hindquarters.
- Venom:
  - Contains 99% insoluble alkaloid, causing hemolysis, membrane depolarization, local tissue destruction, and activation of complement pathway
  - Approximately 10 to 16% of population have fire ant hypersensitivity and are susceptible to anaphylaxis.
  - No cross-reactivity with that of bees

SIGNS AND SYMPTOMS

- Immediate intense burning pain locally
- Becomes sterile pustule in 6 hours
- With multiple stings in sensitized individuals, nausea, sweating, dizziness, and anaphylaxis can occur.

TREATMENT

- ABCs
- Local cleaning
- Analgesia, ice
- For systemic reactions: Treat as for bee sting.

TERRESTRIAL ANIMAL TRAUMA

Dogs

- 80 to 90% of reported animal bites
- Usually lacerations, crush injury, punctures, and avulsions
- Wounds are infection and tetanus prone, bacteria from animal oral flora (not human skin):
  - Aerobes: *Streptococcus, Staphylococcus aureus, Pasteurella multocida* (20 to 30%), *Staphylococcus intermedius, Eikenella corrodens*
  - Anaerobes: *Bacteroides* spp., *Actinomyces* spp., *Fusobacterium* spp., *Peptostreptococcus* spp.

SIGNS AND SYMPTOMS

- Ask about ownership of dog and behavior.
- If stray and cannot be observed, initiate rabies immunization.

TREATMENT

- ABCs as appropriate
- Local wound care: Aggressive irrigation, debridement; loose suturing or leave open for delayed primary closure
- Tetanus prophylaxis

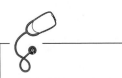

Dog bites:
Wound location frequency:
Upper extremity >>
lower extremity >>
head and neck (kids) >>
trunk

Cat and dog bite infection rules of thumb:
- Infection in < 24 hours: *P. multocida.* Rx: penicillin, if penicillin allergic, tetracycline, or erythromycin
- Infection in > 24 hours: *Staph* or *Strep* Rx: Dicloxacillin or cephalexin

HIGH-YIELD FACTS

Environmental Emergencies

TABLE 19-3. Closure and Prophylaxis for Bites

Animal Bite/Sting	Close?	Main Offending Organism	Antibiotics?
Dog	Yes, except if crush injury or bite to hand	*Capnocytophaga canimorsus*	Yes
Cat	No	*Pasteurella multocida*	Yes
Rodent	No	Multiple	No
Monkey	No	Herpesvirus	Acyclovir for high-risk bites
Human	Yes, except if closed fist injury	*Eikenella corrodens*	Yes

- Prophylactic antibiotics for the immunocompromised and frail (amoxicillin/clavulanic acid for outpatient, ampicillin/sulbactam inpatient) (see Table 19-3)

Cat Bites

- 5 to 18% of reported animal bites in United States
- More likely to contain *P. multocida* in wound

SIGNS AND SYMPTOMS

- Punctures (57 to 86%)
- Abrasions (9 to 25%)
- Lacerations (5 to 17%)

TREATMENT

See dog bites.

Humans

- Behavior at times animal-like
- Clenched fist injuries (CFIs) from punches in the face have high incidence of poor wound healing and complications.
- Bites to areas other than the hand have similar rates of infection as nonbite lacerations.
- Human oral flora is polymicrobial:
  - Aerobes: *Streptococcus viridans*, *S. aureus*, *Haemophilus* spp., *E. corrodens*
  - Anaerobes: *Bacteroides* spp., *Fusobacterium* spp., *Peptostreptococcus* spp.

TREATMENT

- CFIs: Copious irrigation, debridement, tetanus, penicillin, and second-generation cephalosporin for *Staphylococcus* coverage. Diabetics should get an aminoglycoside.
- Immobilize, daily dressing changes, elevate extremity

Cat bites:
Wound location: Upper extremity >> head and neck > lower extremity > trunk

E. corrodens: A gram-negative rod of the normal human oral flora, distinguished by being susceptible to penicillin but resistant to penicillinase-resistant penicillins, clindamycin, metronidazole, cephalosporins

FIRE

DESCRIPTION OF DEPTH

First Degree
- Superficial burn, epidermis only, mild–moderate erythema, heals without scar

Second Degree
- Superficial partial thickness, epidermis and part of dermis (follicles and glands spared), blisters and erythema, very painful, heals with or without scar in 2 to 3 weeks
- Deep partial thickness, epidermis and deeper dermal layers (follicles and glands), blisters, erythema, some charring, painful, heals in 3 to 4 weeks with some scarring

Third Degree
- Full thickness, epidermis, dermis, subcutaneous fat; pale, charred, painless, leathery; surgical skin grafts necessary for healing; moderate–severe scarring

Fourth Degree
- Skin, fat, muscle, bone involvement; severe, life-threatening injury

DESCRIPTION OF SIZE

- Estimate size with rule of nines (Figure 19-1)
- Size of patient's palm roughly 1% of their total body surface area (TBSA)

CATEGORIZATION

Minor Burns
- < 15% TBSA for ages 10 to 50
- < 10% TBSA for ages < 10 or > 50
- < 2% TBSA full thickness, any age, no other injury

Moderate Burns
- 15 to 25% TBSA second degree for ages 10 to 50
- 10 to 20% TBSA second degree for ages < 10 or > 50
- 2 to 10% TBSA full thickness, any age
- No perineal, facial, foot, hand, or circumferential limb burns

Major Burns
- > 25% TBSA second degree for ages 10 to 50
- > 20% TBSA second degree for ages < 10 or > 50
- > 10% TBSA full thickness, any age
- Hand, foot, perineal, circumferential limb, major joint, electrical burns
- Associated inhalation injury or other trauma in elderly, infants, poor-risk patients

> *Typical cause of burns:*
> **First degree: Sunburn**
> **Second degree: Hot liquids**
> **Third degree: Hot liquids, steam, hot oil, flame**
> **Fourth degree: Flame, hot oil, steam**

> *Poor-risk burn patients:*
> **Those with diabetes, heart and lung disease, age < 10 or > 50**

HIGH-YIELD FACTS

Environmental Emergencies

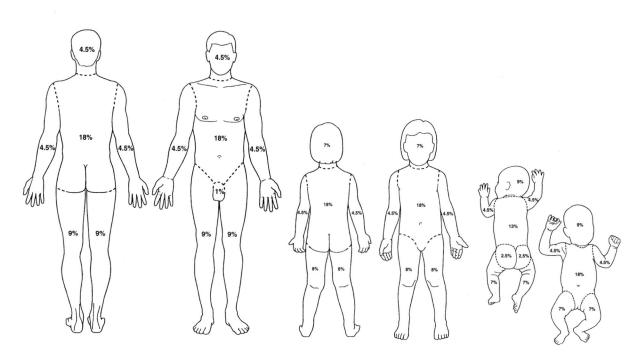

FIGURE 19-1. Rule of nines for adults, children, and infants.

(Reproduced, with permission, from Stead L. *BRS: Emergency Medicine*. Philadelphia, PA: Lippincott Williams and Wilkins, 2000: 558.)

Parkland formula: 4 mL/kg/% TBSA burned; one half over first 8 hours from time of burn, and remaining one half over next 16 hours. Ringer's lactate is fluid of choice.

Children have increased TBSA relative to their weight, increased evaporative water loss, and therefore increased fluid requirements.

TREATMENT

- Prehospital: Transport to nearest burn-capable hospital, preferably within 30 minutes.
- Emergency department (ED): Ask age, medical history, tetanus status, what burned, was there an explosion/blast injury, were there toxic substances, enclosed space?
- Fiberoptically evaluate airway for edema and injury, or intubate and protect the airway prior to respiratory failure.
- Humidified 100% O_2
- Fluid resuscitation according to Parkland formula
- Beware of overaggressive fluid resuscitation leading to excessive pulmonary and peripheral edema.
- Foley catheter to monitor urine output (maintain 1 cc/kg/hr)
- Primary and secondary surveys: Treat all associated injuries appropriately.
- Management of the burn wound:
  - Within 30 minutes: "Put out the fire"—cool water
  - Always cover with clean, sterile, saline-soaked dressings to small areas.
  - Protect against hypothermia: Cover with sterile sheets.
  - Escharotomy for full-thickness or circumferential burns
  - Analgesia with morphine
  - Blisters: Best left intact until consulting service can evaluate (skin is protective); incise and drain sterilely all those not on palms and soles if delayed transfer or consultation.
  - No role for prophylactic antibiotics

- Antibiotic skin cream/ointment application only if delay of transfer to burn unit or delay in arrival of consulting service for many hours; silver sulfadiazine or bacitracin
- Tetanus prophylaxis

CRITERIA FOR TRANSFER TO BURN UNIT

- > 10% TBSA in ages < 10 or > 50
- > 20% TBSA for all ages
- Burns to face, eyes, ears, hands, feet, genitalia, perineum, or major joints
- > 5% TBSA third-degree burn
- Electrical and chemical burns
- Inhalational injury
- Children

CHEMICAL BURNS

General

- Determine what chemical is by history and physical examination.
- Remove patient from agent, then remove agent from patient.
- If wet agent, dilute with water.
- If dry agent, wipe off first.
- Remove clothing.
- Assess size and depth of burn.

Any chemical burn to the eye is the number 1 eye emergency and needs immediate irrigation! (Test ocular pH before and after irrigation; goal is 7.3 to 7.7, ideally 7.45.)

Hydrofluoric Acid (HF)

- Penetrates tissues like alkalies and releases F$^-$, which immobilizes intracellular Ca^{2+} and Mg^{2+}, poisoning enzymes

TREATMENT

- Dilute with water for 30 minutes.
- Detoxify: Local intramuscular/subcutaneous/transdermal, IV, or intra-arterial 5 to 10% calcium gluconate solution

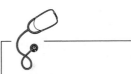

HF is found in glass etching, dyes, high-octane gas, and germicides.

Phenol (Carbolic Acid)

- Causes local coagulation necrosis, protein denaturation, and systemic life-threatening complications

TREATMENT

- Dilute with water.
- Isopropyl alcohol decreases local absorption and necrosis.

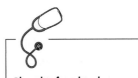

Phenol is found in dyes, deodorants, agriculture, and disinfectants.

Lime (Calcium Oxide)

- Desiccates
- Converted to alkali by water (calcium hydroxide)

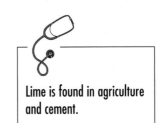

Lime is found in agriculture and cement.

TREATMENT

Brush off, then dilute.

Lyes [KOH, NaOH, Ca(OH)$_2$, LiOH]

- Strong alkalies burn more deeply and longer, leading to liquefaction necrosis.
- High tissue absorption
- If swallowed, aggressively manage airway and have surgical intervention available. Dilute aggressively.

TREATMENT

Dilute with water.

Metals (Industrial, Molten)

Water can cause severe exothermic reaction.

TREATMENT

- Cover hot metal fragments with mineral oil.
- Brush off or excise fragments.

Hydrocarbons

- Tar causes deep thermal burns.
- Dissolve tar, don't peel it off (takes skin too).

TREATMENT

- Dilute gasoline with water.
- Aggressively cool tar.
- Use Neosporin (polysorbate) to remove tar.

> Tar is found in gasoline and hot tars.

> Do not try to remove tar with acetone. It will make the tar stick to the skin even more and continue burning.

> Ohm's law: $V = I \times R$
> Joule's law: $E = I^2 \times R \times$ time

ELECTRICAL BURNS

PHYSICS OF ELECTRICITY

- I = current (amps), R = resistance (ohms), E = energy (joules), V = voltage (volts)
- As current flows through a resistor (tissue), energy is deposited as heat; the ↑er R, the ↑er E (burn)
- Current flows through path of least resistance.
- High voltage ≥ 1,000 V (> 600 V clinically)
- U.S. household circuits = 110 V (220 V entering home)
- AC (alternating current) 60 Hz (cycles/second)
- Tasers = 50,000 V, 10 to 15 pulses per second

SIGNS AND SYMPTOMS

- On scene: Look for source, entrance/exit wounds, extent of cutaneous injury (may reflect internal)

- Underlying internal damage far exceeds skin burns (rule of nines need not apply).
- Blood vessels, nerves, and muscle damaged most (leads to compromised vasculature, vasospasm, rhabdomyolysis, paralysis, neuropathies)
- Children biting electric cords: Risk of delayed hemorrhage from labial artery at mouth edges
- Delayed cataracts with ocular involvement

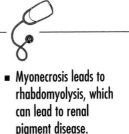

- Myonecrosis leads to rhabdomyolysis, which can lead to renal pigment disease.
- Alkalinize urine (IV 44 mEq NaHCO$_3$ in 1 L of IV fluid).

TREATMENT

- Scene safety
- ABCs, support respirations
- Advanced cardiac life support (ACLS) protocol as appropriate
- IV access and fluids—20 cc/kg bolus
- Treat thermal burns.
- Tetanus prophylaxis
- Admit if poor risk, pregnant, high voltage, or systemic injury.

Lightning Injury

PHYSICS OF LIGHTNING

- 10 million to 2 billion V
- Unidirectional impulse of current
- Temperature 14,432 to 90,032°F
- Hot, humid days
- Strikes metal or tall objects
- Electricity flows over the body (flashover) as well as through, causing pathognomonic fern-shaped mark on the skin caused by electron showering.

DEFINITIONS

- Direct strike: Lightning versus person
- Contact strike: Lightning versus object person is touching
- Side flash: Lightning versus object near person, then flash from object
- Ground current: Lightning versus ground near person, then up person's foot
- Stride potential/step voltage: Lightning versus ground near person, then up one foot and down the other; temporarily cold, numb, paretic, pulseless legs

SIGNS AND SYMPTOMS

- Fernlike pattern to skin (cutaneous streaking) (Figure 19-2)
- Ruptured tympanic membranes
- Often unconscious
- Cardiac arrhythmias

TREATMENT

- ABCs, secure airway
- ACLS protocol as appropriate
- Reverse triage if multiple injured: Care for "dead" first—they recover if supported.
- Immobilize C-spine.

Typical scenario:
A 29-year-old man is found lying down in a big open field outdoors, not breathing and pulseless. His clothes are tattered, he has no shoes, but has blood in his ear canals. He is awake but confused. You notice fernlike burns on his skin. *Think: Lightning injury.*

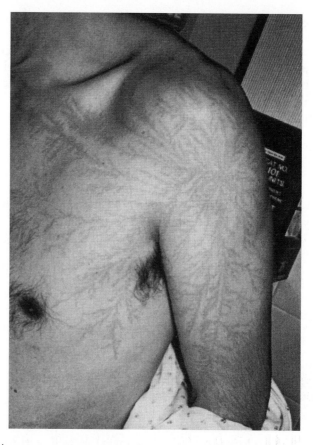

FIGURE 19-2. Characteristic cutaneous streaking pattern of lightning injury.
(Reproduced, with permission, from Tintinalli JE, Kelen GD, Stapczynski JS. *Emergency Medicine: A Comprehensive Study Guide*, 5th ed. New York: McGraw-Hill, 2000: 1300.)

- Tetanus prophylaxis
- Electrocardiogram (ECG) and cardiac monitor
- Urinalysis, complete blood count, creatine kinase (CK) and CK-MB, lytes, blood urea nitrogen (BUN)/creatinine
- Treat any bony fractures; admit for observation.

HEAT ILLNESS

Heat Transfer

- Radiation:
  - 65% of normal body cooling
  - Heat transfer from electromagnetic waves
- Convection:
  - 10 to 15% of normal body cooling
  - Heat transfer from cooler water vapor in air current
- Conduction:
  - 2% of normal body cooling
  - Heat transfer from direct physical contact
- Evaporation:
  - 15 to 25% of normal body cooling
  - Heat transfer from evaporated sweat/breath

Heat Exhaustion

DEFINITION

Syndrome of vague constitutional symptoms associated with salt and water depletion, and heat exposure or heavy exertion

SIGNS AND SYMPTOMS

- Dizziness or fatigue with normal mental status
- Nausea/vomiting
- Headache
- Positional hypotension/syncope
- Mildly elevated temperature
- Diaphoresis
- Heat-related illnesses: Prickly heat, heat cramps, or heat tetany

TREATMENT

- Remove from heat.
- Rest.
- IV hydration with normal saline, oral hydration with sports drinks
- Check and correct electrolytes.
- Observe for resolution of symptoms.

Heatstroke

DEFINITION

Rapid rise in core temperature (> 104.9°F) associated with:
- Altered mental status
- Symptoms of heat exhaustion
- Anhydrosis
- Loss of temperature regulation

SIGNS AND SYMPTOMS

- CNS abnormalities:
    - Ataxia
    - Combativeness
    - Hallucination
    - Seizure
    - Posturing
    - Hemiplegia
    - Coma
- Renal failure:
    - Decreased Ca^{2+}
    - Hypo- or hypernatremia
    - Decreased PO_4^-
    - Hypo- or hyperkalemia
- Coagulation:
    - Increased bleeding times
    - Consumptive coagulopathy and disseminated intravascular coagulation
- Liver failure:
    - Abnormal liver function tests
    - Increased creatine phosphokinase (CPK) and rhabdomyolysis
- Hypotension
- Death

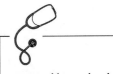

Associated heat-related symptoms:
- Heat syncope (postural hypotension)
- Prickly heat (maculopapular rash under clothed areas)
- Heat tetany (carpopedal spasm, hyperventilation)
- Heat cramps (muscle cramping due to electrolyte loss)

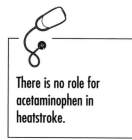

There is no role for acetaminophen in heatstroke.

TREATMENT

- Rule out other causes of fever and altered mental status (sepsis, thyrotoxicosis, meningitis, etc.).
- Remove from heat sources.
- Control ABCs, O_2, monitor, rectal temperature
- Use cooling techniques; avoid rebound hypothermia.
- Correct electrolyte abnormalities.
- Check complete blood count, urinalysis, CPK, prothrombin time, partial thromboplastin time, BUN/creatinine, and ECG.
- Benzodiazepines for shivering

COOLING TECHNIQUES

Evaporation

- Water mist and blowing fans
- Heat dissipated by evaporation
- Rapid
- Easiest in the ED

Immersion

- Tub of water and ice
- Heat dissipated by conduction
- Impractical
- Can't monitor patient

Ice Packing

- Ice bags to groin and axillae
- Heat dissipated by conduction
- Easy
- Slow
- Poorly tolerated

Cool Lavage

Gastric
- Via nasogastric tube
- Heat dissipated by conduction
- Invasive
- Slow
- Poorly tolerated

Peritoneal
- Via peritoneal catheter
- Heat dissipated by conduction
- Invasive
- Very rapid
- Questionable sterility

DEFINITION

Autosomal dominant pseudocholinesterase deficiency

SIGNS AND SYMPTOMS

- Hyperthermia
- Rhabdomyolysis
- Muscle rigidity
- Not related to exogenous heat sources
- Pathophysiology is distinct from neuroleptic malignant syndrome.

TREATMENT

- Dantrolene 2 to 3 mg/kg IV q6h
- No more succinylcholine

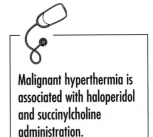

Malignant hyperthermia is associated with haloperidol and succinylcholine administration.

Chilblains

DEFINITION

- Local injury from dry cold at nonfreezing temperatures
- Most commonly affects extremities and ears

SIGNS AND SYMPTOMS

- Local edema
- Nodules or blisters
- Erythema or cyanosis
- Rarely ulcers or bullae

TREATMENT

- Reversible with gentle rewarming
- Moisturizer
- Avoidance of the cold

Trench Foot

DEFINITION

- Nonfreezing injury from wet cold
- Due to prolonged immersion in standing water
- Causes direct soft-tissue injury and nerve damage

SIGNS AND SYMPTOMS

- Numbness/tingling, permanent numbness possible
- Pallor, mottling
- Lack of pulses

HIGH-YIELD FACTS

Environmental Emergencies

- Rest, elevation, local skin care
- Avoidance of the cold

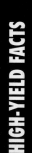

Frostnip: Mild reversible, superficial frostbite

Frostbite

DEFINITION

- Freezing injury when skin temperatures fall below 32°F from body trying to maintain normal core temperature (prefreeze state)
- Ice crystals form in extracellular space (freeze state).
- Tissue loss
- Most commonly occurs on extremities and face

SIGNS AND SYMPTOMS

- Throbbing, shooting pain in joints
- Numbness, tingling
- Edema
- Blisters (clear or hemorrhagic)
- Eschars (develop over a few days)

TREATMENT

- Active rewarming in warm water (104 to 108°F)
- Tetanus, analgesia
- Aspirate clear blisters.
- Limb elevation
- Topical aloe vera
- Treat for associated hypothermia (see below).

Hypothermia

DEFINITION

- Core temperature < 95°F
- Usually due to prolonged overwhelming cold exposure; can occur in any season

SIGNS AND SYMPTOMS

At risk for hypothermia:
- Extremes of age
- Alcohol users
- Homeless
- Altered mental status (including psychiatric disorders)
- Trauma victims
- Underlying chronic illness
- Hypoglycemia
- Sepsis

Mild Hypothermia (90 to 95°F)
- Shivering
- Excitation
- Tachypnea
- Tachycardia
- Apathy
- Poor judgment
- Dysarthria
- Ataxia

Moderate Hypothermia (82 to 90°F)
- Shivering ceases
- Stupor
- Bradycardia

- Dysrhythmias (often atrial fibrillation)
- Dilated pupils

Severe Hypothermia (< 82°F)
- Coma
- Hypotension
- Decreased cardiac output
- Areflexia
- Decreased respiratory rate
- Dysrhythmias (often ventricular fibrillation, agonal, or asystole)
- May appear dead

TREATMENT

All Patients
- Remove wet clothing.
- Get rectal temperature.
- Get ECG (Figure 19-3).
- Look for and treat concomitant illness (alcohol, hypoglycemia, trauma).

Mild Hypothermia
- Passive rewarming with blankets

Moderate and Severe Hypothermia
- Active rewarming
- Handle with care: Sudden manipulation can precipitate cardiac dysrhythmias.
- Cardiac monitoring

Cardiac Dysrhythmias
- Treat cardiac dysrhythmias as per ACLS protocol.
- Remember, the best treatment for cardiac dysrhythmias in hypothermia is rewarming.
- Severely hypothermic patients who appear dead can have normal or near-normal neurologic outcomes: **Continue resuscitation until warm!**

Special note for trauma patients: Patients who arrive with hypothermia and obvious head trauma may have improved neurologic outcome if hypothermia is maintained. Consult with neurosurgeons.

Tympanic membrane temperature measurements are not reliable below 94°F. *Get a rectal temperature!*

Methods of active rewarming (in order of invasiveness):
- Warmed blankets
- Mechanical warming blanket
- Warmed IV fluids
- Warmed bladder irrigation
- Warmed gastric lavage
- Warmed peritoneal irrigation
- Warmed cardiopulmonary bypass

HIGH-YIELD FACTS

Environmental Emergencies

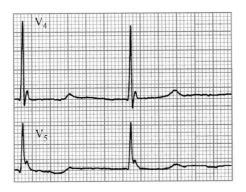

FIGURE 19-3. Osborn (J) wave of hypothermia.

Emergency Medical Services

Note: Contents of this chapter are not tested on the Emergency Medicine (EM) clerkship exam and may be skipped when studying for the test. The purpose of this chapter is to provide an understanding and appreciation of what goes on prior to a patient's arriving at the emergency department (ED).

HISTORY OF EMERGENCY MEDICAL SERVICES (EMS)

- Prior to 1970, the primary role of EMS providers was to provide rapid transportation to the nearest hospital.
- During the early 1960s, several national agencies began investigating issues and problems relating to highway safety. These investigations revealed for the first time how poor emergency services actually were.
- In 1965, the President's Commission of Highway Safety recommended a National Accident Response Program to decrease death and injury from highway accidents.
- In 1973, Congress enacted the Emergency Medical Services System Act, which authorized and funded the Department of Health, Education, and Welfare to designate more than 300 regional EMS systems throughout the country.
- Over the last three decades, EMS has become a crucial and integral component of emergency care. Coordinated and professional prehospital care can help make the difference between life and death.

PRIVATE VERSUS PUBLIC

- Within both the private and public sectors, EMS providers are paid and volunteer professionals.
- All certified and/or licensed EMS providers are expected to function only within their prospective scope of practice.

Private

- Many local EMS systems are privately owned and operated and provide emergency care where local government has not assumed responsibility.

- The provider usually does dispatching.
- A contracted physician or a local physician board usually provides medical direction.
- They more frequently provide interfacility transport than do public systems.

Public

- Public EMS systems—those not incorporated into public fire departments—are formed as their own structure and are known as municipal third-party systems.
- They are operated by county or municipal governments and are supported and endorsed by local city counsels or commissioners.
- An advisory council or medical control committee oversees administration and basic operations.
- Dispatching is provided by a separate public safety organization or by an individual EMS system provider.

SPECIALTY CARE CENTERS

Types of specialty centers:
- Trauma
- Hyperbaric
- Burn
- Envenomation
- Perinatal
- Spinal
- Pediatric
- Poison
- Cardiac
- Psychiatric

- Patients must be triaged and transported to an appropriate level facility.
- Every EMS system must be able to identify local hospitals capable of administering specialty services including level I, level II, and level III care.
- When available, direct transport to the specialty center from the prehospital setting is desirable.
- If unavailable, interhospital transfer can be utilized once the patient is stabilized at the initial receiving facility.

EMS FIELD PERSONNEL

First Responder (FR)

- Usually a police officer, firefighter, or EMS provider, arriving on scene within minutes, prior to arrival of any ambulance
- Quickly assesses the patient(s) situation and determines if additional personnel or additional resources are required
- Can provide vital initial information to approaching EMS providers
- May begin cardiopulmonary resuscitation (CPR), assist in airway management, control hemorrhaging, and provide spinal immobilization until EMS is on scene

Emergency Medical Technician—Basic (EMT-B)

- Minimum level required to staff a basic life support (BLS) ambulance
- Provides more thorough assessment of patient than FR and provides transportation to health care facility

Emergency Medical Technician—Intermediate (EMT-I)

- Provides a more comprehensive assessment of the patient over the EMT-B, when paramedic services are not available
- Scope of practice varies from state to state.
- Most systems allow placement of IV, administration of some medications, adjunctive airway devices, and defibrillation.

Emergency Medical Technician—Paramedic (EMT-P)

- Most advanced of the prehospital providers
- Capable to provide advanced cardiac life support (ACLS) to all prehospital emergencies
- Can provide defibrillation and endotracheal intubation
- Can perform invasive procedures such as needle decompression of a pneumothorax, needle or surgical cricothyrotomy, and transthoracic cardiac pacing
- Can administer a variety of medications, IV fluids, and all ACLS medication
- Medical direction is required for many paramedics.

UNIVERSAL PRECAUTIONS

- The Federal Occupational Safety and Health Administration mandates that all EMS personnel are compliant regarding observance of all universal precautions.
- Every EMS provider must be protected against exposure to blood and other bodily fluids from all patient care.

Gloves, masks, eye goggles, and gowns must be carried on every EMS vehicle.

TRANSPORT OPTIONS

Ground Vehicles

- Minimum crew of driver and EMT-B/I/P
- Scene response, safety, and cost are directly related to regional areas.
- Most frequently the choice for interfacility transport. ED physician or nurse may accompany in some cases in which ACLS transportation is required but unavailable.

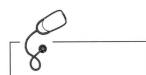

BLS call: Minimum of a driver and EMT-B
ALS (advanced life support) call: Minimum of a driver and EMT-P

Air Transport

PERSONNEL

- Primary crew member: Pilot
- Registered nurses/flight nurses
- Paramedics
- Respiratory therapists
- Physicians

Nurse—paramedic team is most common.

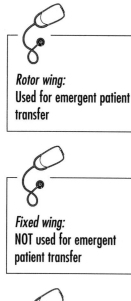

Rotor wing:
Used for emergent patient transfer

Fixed wing:
NOT used for emergent patient transfer

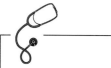

Pilot holds primary responsibility for safety of flight.

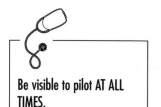

Be visible to pilot AT ALL TIMES.

ROTOR-WING AIRCRAFT/HELICOPTER

- 125- to 175-mph ambulances
- Not limited by traffic or road conditions
- Flight range 150 to 200 miles
- Three to four times more expensive than fixed-wing transport
- Requires only 60 × 60-foot landing zone
- Limited by weather conditions

FIXED-WING AIRCRAFT

- 120- to 500-mph ambulances
- Flights not as restricted secondary to inclement weather
- Loading and unloading of patient is usually difficult because of door height and size.
- Much faster than rotor wing and less expensive per mile
- Require local airport with adequate runway, and ambulance service at both ends

AVIATION SAFETY STANDARDS

- Regulated by Commission on Accreditation of Air Medical Services
- Fixed-wing aircraft must comply with Federal Aviation Administration
- All flight personnel must be instructed in the emergency operations of the aircraft.

LANDING ZONE SAFETY

- Always approach aircraft from front.
- Most dangerous area of a helicopter is the tail rotor, which is virtually invisible when in motion.
- Landings and takeoffs are the most likely times for an accident to occur.

GUIDELINES FOR TRAUMA SCENE RESPONSE

See Figure 20-1.

RELATIVE CONTRAINDICATIONS TO AIR TRANSPORT

Cardiac Patients

- Hypoxia present at altitude can cause a compensatory increase in pulse and respiratory rate, increasing myocardial oxygen demand (MVO_2), and may result in cardiac decompensation. Further increase on MVO_2 demands may be caused by an increase in catecholamine release during flight.
- Patient should not fly < 2 weeks after a myocardial infarction (MI) or < 8 weeks following a complicated MI.
- Severe uncontrolled hypertension, severe congestive heart failure, symptomatic valvular disease, uncontrolled dysrhythmias, and unstable/ischemic angina at rest

Respiratory Patients

- The decreased PaO_2 at altitude may exacerbate/complicate chronic obstructure pulmonary disease or recent cardiac surgery.
- Increased risk of tension pneumothorax seen with congenital pulmonary cysts, severe bullous emphysema, and pneumothorax
- Risk of thickening secretions from dryness at altitude is associated with cystic fibrosis.

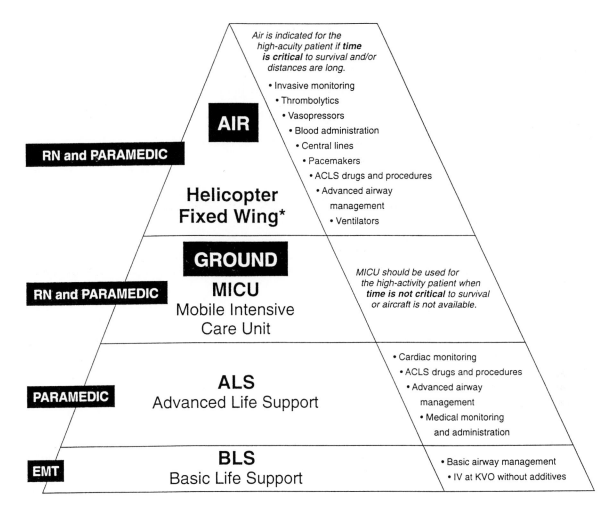

FIGURE 20-1. Guidelines for trauma scene response.
(Reproduced, with permission, from Tintinalli JE, Kelen GD, Stapczynski JS. *Emergency Medicine: A Comprehensive Study Guide,* 5th ed. New York: McGraw-Hill, 2000: 13.)

Neurologic/Psychiatric Patients

- Recent cerebrovascular accident
- Uncontrolled epilepsy
- Recent skull fracture
- Brain tumors
- Uncontrolled violent behavior
- Claustrophobia/aerophobia

Eye, Ear, Nose, and Throat Patients

- Recent ophthalmologic surgery
- Sinusitis, otitis
- Recent facial fracture

Miscellaneous

- Pregnancy > 36 weeks' gestation (hypoxia)
- Neonates in first 24 to 48 hours of life
- Unstable premature infants
- Sickle cell disease (hypoxia can lead to sickle crisis)

- Uncontrolled diabetes mellitus
- Recent casting of extremity or abdominal surgery
- Diving 12 to 24 hours before flight (risk of air embolism)

ABSOLUTE CONTRAINDICATIONS TO AIR TRANSPORT

- High probability of death during flight
- Active contagious disease
- Immobility

Hemorrhage Control

- Bandages
- Abdominal dressings
- Tape
- Sandbags
- Tourniquets
- Sterile gloves
- Goggles, face masks
- Gown

Spinal Immobilization

- Sized cervical collars
- Backboard
- Head immobilizers
- Straps

Extremity Immobilization

- Slings, swathes, hard and air splints
- Lower extremity traction splints maintain traction and distal pulses.

Pneumatic Antishock Garments (PASGs)

- Designed to counteract hypovolemic shock
- Helps control internal bleeding
- Stabilizes numerous fractures
- Works by providing pressure to lower extremities, pelvis, and abdomen, which reduces vascular compartment size, and increasing blood pressure, as well as serving as an air splint for fractures
- IV correction of volume loss should be initiated prior to slow deflation of garment.
- Electrocardiograms, x-rays, Foley catheter insertion, and other routine tests can be performed with the garment inflated.

Labor and Delivery

- Several pairs of sterile gloves
- Towels

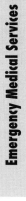

Abrupt removal of PASGs may cause severe shock.

HIGH-YIELD FACTS

Emergency Medical Services

- 4×4 gauze pads
- Small rubber bulb syringe
- Cord clamps or hemostats
- Umbilical cord tape
- Surgical scissors
- Baby blanket
- Sanitary napkins
- Placenta container

Resuscitation

- Cannulas
- Masks
- Intubation supplies
- Ambu bag
- Defibrillator
- Automatic external defibrillators
- Cardiac monitor
- IV supplies, IV fluids
- CPR board

Drugs

- Respiratory medications
- Glucose, insulin
- Antiemetics
- Cardiac medications: Blood pressure medications, angina, antiarrhythmics, all ACLS protocol medications, naloxone

> Only ALS personnel can administer ALS medications.

COMMUNICATION SYSTEM

Initiation

911 is the priority number to initiate the EMS system.

Dispatch

- Approximately 15 to 20% of all 911 calls are true emergencies.
- Dispatcher is usually located at the central communication center.
- Must follow dispatch protocols based on priority or criteria, dispatching appropriate ambulance (BLS/ALS), and any additional local resources required (police, firehouse, FR, local utility companies, animal control)
- Pre-EMS arrival instructions

Field Communications

- Two-way radios, both in the ambulance and handheld by EMS crew, provide communications between on-scene personnel, on-scene ambulances, and dispatcher.
- Ambulance radios can also contact their local ED to communicate vital patient information prior to arrival, enhancing ED's response.

- Cellular phones are also used to maintain contact with on-scene crew, ED, and medical control.

- For optimal and safe prehospital care, the EMS system requires medical direction.
- This medical control, or observation of EMS care, can be done directly or indirectly.
- The medical director is responsible for indirect control of the EMS system. Direction and accountability are maintained by a contractual agreement, securing authority over patient care protocols and any administrative matters.

Indirect Medical Control

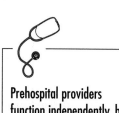

Prehospital providers function independently, but under the license of the medical director.

- Development of patient care protocols and guidelines for care
- Development of medical accountability
- Development of ongoing education
- Instruct all EMS personnel on standing orders, triage guidelines, and patient care according to state regulations and level of certification.
- EMS providers provide care based on recognized standards and protocols set forth by the medical director.
- Initiate and maintain quality assurance of prehospital care. Provide guidance in patient care or any controversial issues.

Direct Medical Control

- "Real-time" direction, usually done by radio or telephone
- Dedicated medical control physicians, nurses, or paramedics function as medical control and are held accountable for their ordered interventions.

On-Scene Physician (OSP)

- Prehospital personnel must insist on proof of licensure to prove that OSP is a medical doctor.
- Does not have any authority at the scene
- Will be immediately informed that medical control is accountable for all patient care
- If OSP wishes to assume control, he or she must assume all responsibility for patient care and should accompany the patient to the hospital, after medical control is notified.

- There is no one definition of a disaster that encompasses all possible disasters.
- In general, a disaster can be described as an event that overwhelms re-

sponse capabilities, and outside emergency assistance is required to respond to the event.

- The sheer number of casualties alone does not determine a disaster, nor does it have to have many casualties at all. For example, a flood or a hurricane can be considered a disaster, yet there may not be many people wounded.
- A multicasualty incident (MCI) is not necessarily a disaster if the receiving hospital(s) is (are) prepared for and can adequately handle all pending emergencies from the incident.
- A disaster can also be defined as internal or external.
- The most useful disaster classification divides disasters into levels of preparedness.

Level I

A disaster in which local resources are adequate to handle all casualties, once local disaster plan has been initiated

Level II

A disaster that overwhelms local resources and requires assistance from neighboring jurisdictions

Level III

A disaster that exceeds even local and neighboring resources, requiring state and/or federal assistance

Types of Disasters

- Natural: Hurricane, tornado, earthquake, flood, storm
- Explosions and fires
- Transportation or terrorist incidents: Train/plane crashes
- Toxic: Hazardous waste spill, bioterrorism

Mass Gatherings

- Any collection of > 1,000 people at any one site or location
- Producer or promoter of any mass gathering event has a responsibility for the safety and security of its participants, spectators, and all employees.
- Medical director plays a key role in the development of treatment protocols and procedures.
- Interdisciplinary coordination must be planned out prior to event, for most effective response.

Fire, rescue, hazardous material team, public health department, law enforcement, and security need to be planned for in advance.

Incident Command System (ICS)

The ICS is a standard emergency management system used throughout the United States to provide a flexible command and control structure on which to organize a response.

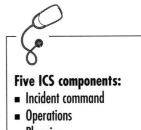

Five ICS components:
- Incident command
- Operations
- Planning
- Logistics
- Finance

417

Disaster Preparedness and Planning

Roles, responsibilities, and working relationships among those responsible for disaster operations should be clarified in the planning process, to diminish any confusion or chaos that might result from a disaster.

ESSENTIAL QUESTIONS

- What types of disasters are most likely to occur in the community?
- What are the disaster planning requirements of local, state, and federal agencies, as well as the Joint Commission on the Accreditation of Healthcare Organizations (JCAHO)?
- What are the responsibilities and capabilities of the hospital, with and without additional local resources used?

HAZARD ANALYSIS

- Emergency planners need to consider the most probable event to occur in their community and plan for a multidisciplinary response accordingly.
- Both in-house and locally coordinated drills are run to actually test the emergency response, critique their response, and make appropriate changes as necessary.

COMMUNITY DISASTER TEAM

See Table 20-1.

PLANNING HOSPITAL RESPONSE

- The JCAHO requires that hospitals have a written disaster plan for the timely care of all casualties arising from both internal and external disasters.

INTERNAL DISASTER PLAN

- Every hospital department must participate in the planning and in-house drills of such possible disasters.

TABLE 20-1. Community Disaster Team

Community Agency	Responsibilities
EMS provider	Patient triage in the field, stabilization, transfer to definitive care facility
Fire service Police service	Overall scene command, victim rescue, hazard control, traffic management, scene security
Emergency manager	Communications, personnel and equipment support, liaison with state and federal agencies
Public works	Support equipment and personnel, structural safety expertis
Chief executive officer	Management of overall operation, assurance of public safety, communication with public, direction of requests for outside assistance to appropriate state and federal authorities

Reproduced, with permission, from Tintinalli JE, Kelen GD, Stapczynski JS. *Emergency Medicine: A Comprehensive Study Guide*, 5th ed. New York: McGraw-Hill, 2000: 24.

- The plan must clearly define circumstances in which it is to be activated.
- Identify the command structure, noting defined authority and responsibilities.
- Describe a specific response strategy to each possible incident.
- Estimate impact on safety and hospital function.
- Provide evacuation plan.
- List critical numbers for hospital and community agencies.
- Map out vital supplies/equipment: Fire extinguishers, water valves, oxygen shut-off valves, drugs, emergency equipment

EXTERNAL DISASTER PLAN

- Generally assumes that the disaster has no direct impact on hospital functioning
- A member of the EM department, usually the medical director, takes on a leadership role in the planning and implementation of all external disaster plans.
- Specific plans are designed in conjunction with community organizations to provide an organized response for the management of any casualties arising from the event.

HOSPITAL DISASTER PLAN

- Based on standard operating procedures of all hospital personnel
- Activation of disaster plan
- Assessment of the hospital's capacity
- Establishment of a command center
- Communication
- Supplies
- Hospital administrative and treatment areas
- Training and drills

Phases of a Disaster Response

ACTIVATION

Initial Call and an Organized Response
- *Phase 1:* Notification and initial response when event first discovered
- *Phase 2:* Organization of command and scene assessment

IMPLEMENTATION

Management of Hazards and Victims
- *Phase 3:* Search and rescue
- *Phase 4:* Victim extrication, triage, stabilization, and transport
- *Phase 5:* Scene management

RECOVERY

Critique Response and Provide Support to Rescuers
- *Phase 6:* Scene withdrawal
- *Phase 7:* Return to normal operations
- *Phase 8:* Debriefing

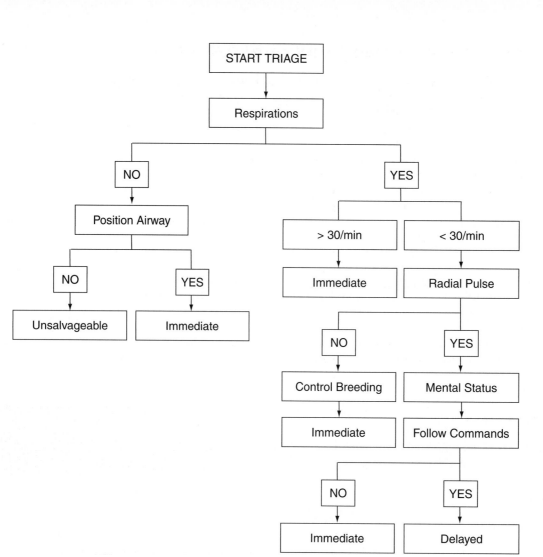

FIGURE 20-2. Simple triage and rapid treatment algorithm.
(Reproduced, with permission, from Tintinalli JE, Kelen GD, Stapczynski JS. *Emergency Medicine: A Comprehensive Study Guide,* 5th ed. New York: McGraw-Hill, 2000: 27.)

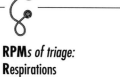

RPMs *of triage:*
Respirations
Perfusion
Mental status

Disaster Triage

- Disaster scene triage requires a rapid assessment of emergent health care needs.
- In the field, rescue personnel often use a simple triage and rapid assessment treatment technique that depends on a quick assessment of respiration, perfusion, and mental status (Figure 20-2).

SPECIAL CONCERNS

- Age (children < 12, adults > 55)
- Multiple injuries
- Preexisting illness/disease

FIELD TRIAGE CATEGORIES

See Table 20-2.

TABLE 20-2. Field Triage Categories

Red	Yellow	Green	Black
First priority Most urgent Life-threatening shock or hypoxia is present or imminent, but patient can be stabilized and, if given immediate care, will probably survive.	Second priority Urgent Injuries have systemic implications or effects, but patient is not yet in life-threatening shock or hypoxia; although systemic decline will ensue, given appropriate care, patient seems able to withstand a 45- to 60-minute wait without immediate risk.	Third priority Nonurgent Injuries are localized and without immediate systemic implications; with a minimum of care, patient generally does not deteriorate for up to several hours.	Dead No distinction can be made between clinical and biologic death in a mass-casualty incident, and any unresponsive patient who has no spontaneous ventilation or circulation is classified as dead; some classify in this category catastrophically injured patients who have a poor chance for survival regardless of care.

Reproduced, with permission, from Tintinalli JE, Kelen GD, Stapczynski JS. *Emergency Medicine: A Comprehensive Study Guide*, 5th ed. New York: McGraw-Hill, 2000: 29.

Hospital Disaster Response

The ED is the most crucial part of a hospital's initial response to an external disaster.

INITIAL RESPONSE

- Call is received about a disaster or potential MCI.
- Verification of the incident must be made, following policy.
- Once verified, administration notifies ED that external disaster plan is in effect.
- Prepare ED for incoming wounded; triage, transfer, or discharge patients presently in ED.

Black = dead
Red = really sick
Yellow = urgent
Green = stable

RESOURCE MANAGEMENT

- Full inventory of hospital's resources must be available, including equipment, space, and personnel within the institution.
- Director of the ED or a designee should have a list of all appropriate personnel to be called into work or placed on standby notice.
- Protocol for utilizing volunteers is crucial.

COMMAND STRUCTURE

- Clear chain of command, previously planned, must be initiated.
- Command center must be located and set up to control all communications and command functions.

COMMUNICATIONS

- Direct lines of communication must be established.
- *Phone system is usually the first system compromised*, either by disaster itself, or by influx of nonessential calls (e.g., public, media, staff).
- Secondary system must also be in place; two-way radios are often used.

HIGH-YIELD FACTS

Emergency Medical Services

- Traffic control is maintained by local law enforcement.
- Hospital security play a key role in the ED by diverting nonessential vehicles and monitoring flow of persons into ED (e.g., public, media, nonessential staff).

MEDIA AND PUBLIC

- Predesignated individual must coordinate all media interactions.
- Media must be directed to an area away from patient care area.
- A hospital administrator must closely supervise pressroom or public relations specialist, who is in direct contact with the command center.
- Staff must not talk to media and should refer all questions to the public relations specialist or administrator.
- Family members should not be allowed into patient care areas!
- Crisis teams of nurses, social workers, and clergy should be utilized for family members of those involved in the disaster.

BLOOD BANK

- As many as 50 units of blood should be on hand.
- Nearby hospitals may be a resource for additional blood.
- A source of volunteer donors should also be readily accessible and rapidly mobilized.
- Other potential sources of blood include friends and family members of patients, staff, and those patients with minor injuries.

ED Disaster Response

TRIAGE TEAM

- Upon arrival at the ED, immediate priorities consist of identification of patients and a reassessment of the triage category assigned in the field.
- Triage team usually consists of an ED physician, ED nurse, and admitting clerk, who are responsible for triaging *every patient* that comes into the ED.
- Triage team should *never* become involved with direct patient care, except for basic steps like opening an airway or applying pressure to active bleeding.

ADMITTING CLERK

- Admitting clerk's role is to complete triage tags and attach to victims, collect valuables and clothing for bagging, and maintain a triage casualty log.
- Proper tagging and identification of triage patients is essential to accurate ED documentation and for supplying both families and the media with accurate information.

EXCEPTIONS TO ROUTINE ED EVALUATION AND TREATMENT

- Triage always starts with the ABC's, followed by routine labs, examinations, and radiographic studies.
- However, in a disaster situation, protocols shift to helping the greatest number of patients, using the least amount of resources, and prioritizing those with the best chance for survival.

- Patients in cardiac arrest do not usually receive ALS and CPR, so that other critically injured patients with a better chance of survival can be treated with available resources.
- Radiographic studies:
  - Limited to those patients for whom the test results will change therapeutic intervention
  - Films of closed or nondisplaced potential fractures can be safely delayed for 24 to 48 hours, so that indicated films such as cervical spines and pelvic and femur fractures can be done.
  - A chest film is indicated on patients complaining of chest pain, dyspnea, or abnormal chest wall motion.
- Laboratory:
  - Limited to patients for whom the test result will change therapeutic intervention (e.g., urine dipsticks can test for blood and may be useful in detecting renal or urinary tract injuries)
  - All other lab work should be considered accessory.

WOUND CARE

- In disasters, patients are cut by flying glass, metal, or any number of highly contaminated objects.
- All wounds should be flushed excessively.
- If any laceration appears contaminated, it should be debrided and left open for delayed primary closure.
- Trapped victims with prolonged extrications may suffer from compartment syndrome.
- Tetanus prophylaxis should be administered if indicated.

MEDICAL-LEGAL CONCERNS OF EMS

Judicial

- *Negligence:* Every individual should act in a manner in which a reasonable person with the same or similar knowledge and training would act under the same or similar circumstances.
- *Gross negligence:* Willful and wanton
- Vicarious liability/respondent superior: Medical directors are held accountable for the alleged actions of EMS personnel, inadequate training or supervision, and improper certification.

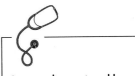

Negligence includes both improper acts and failure to act.

Responsibility to Act

Both the EMS system and the medical director have the responsibility to respond to and act appropriately to the public, upholding the standards the systems itself presents to the public.

Gross negligence is reckless disregard for safety.

Refusal of Care

- A conscious, competent adult has the right to refuse medical treatment, even at the risk to his or her well-being.
- EMS personnel and medical control can determine if the patient has the capacity to refuse care.

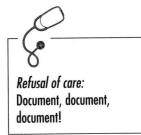

Refusal of care: Document, document, document!

- Patient must be informed of the risks involved with the refusal of care.
- Documentation is extremely important and should include that patient understands care being offered and all of the possible outcomes stemming from the patient's refusal to consent to treatment.
- Against medical advice release form should be signed, but can be easily challenged in court.

Impaired Patients

- EMS providers are entitled to use only reasonable force to defend themselves.
- Every effort must be attempted to appropriately restrain the patient without inflicting any harm.
- When necessary, law enforcement should be involved for proper management of an impaired patient.
- Thorough documentation of the incident, including all measures taken to comfort, calm, and eventually gain control, must be completed.

"Do Not Resuscitate" (DNR) Orders

Once CPR is initiated, it is extremely difficult to justify a termination.

- DNR orders must be clear and verified as being current.
- Online medical direction can assist with decisions.
- Authority of family members to terminate CPR varies from state to state.
- Regardless of DNR order, when on scene, EMS personnel should document scene, present family members, witnesses, and any vital signs or lack thereof.

Documentation

- Appropriate documentation is always required.
- Special importance lies in motor vehicle accidents, assaults, slip and fall, alleged rape, child abuse, refusal of treatment or transport, and physician on scene, which may involve subsequent litigation.

Confidentiality

- EMS records are deemed to be part of the patient's medical record.
- EMS system and all EMS personnel are bound to maintain strict patient confidentiality regarding patient name, medical condition, treatment, and any information regarding the incident.
- All patient records must be preserved without disclosure unless ordered by a court of law, or with a signed release form from the patient directly.

Ethics, Medicolegal Issues, and Evidence-Based Medicine

PRINCIPLES OF MEDICAL ETHICS

Beneficence — To act in the best interest of one's patient

Nonmaleficence — To do one's patient no harm: This includes protecting one's patient from personnel not qualified to deliver appropriate care due to lack of training, experience, or impairment.

Privacy and confidentiality — Physicians have a duty to protect the confidentiality of patient information. Disclosure of sensitive information is appropriate only when such disclosure is necessary to carry out a stronger conflicting duty, such as a duty to protect an identifiable third party from serious harm or to comply with a just law.

Autonomy — The ability to function independently and to make decisions about one's care free from the undue influence or bias of others

- All patients are considered autonomous if they have the ability to understand the situation as evaluated with competency examination by psychiatrist (capacity) and are not a danger to self or others (suicidal, homicidal, demented, delirious).
- Physicians have a duty to respect the health care preferences of their patients.

Justice — The principle of equal and fair allocation of benefit

- Provision of emergency medical treatment should not be based on gender, age, race, socioeconomic status, or cultural background.
- No patient should ever be abused, demeaned, or given substandard care.

> The "duty to warn" was established by the Tarasoff case. In this case, a physician caring for a patient who made homicidal statements about another person was found liable for her death because he failed to protect or warn her, or to report the situation to police.

425

Advance Directives

- Oral or written instructions from a patient to family members and health care professionals about health care decisions
- May include living wills; designation of a health care proxy; specific instructions about which therapies to accept or decline, including intubation, surgery or medical treatments, and Do Not Attempt Resuscitation orders
- A Do Not Resuscitate order applies only to advanced cardiac life support resuscitation and does not include intubation and ventilation unless specifically addressed.

Medical Decision Surrogates

Also known as a health care proxy; appointed by the patient

PHYSICIAN IMPAIRMENT

Physicians have a duty to report an impaired or incompetent colleague to the chief of staff or appropriate regulatory agency. Many states have mechanisms in place whereby anonymous reporting can be done. Physicians who conscientiously fulfill this responsibility should be protected from adverse political, legal, or financial consequences. Action toward the impaired physician may include internal discipline and/or remedial training. It does not necessarily mean the physician will lose his or her license to practice medicine.

MEDICAL RECORD DOCUMENTATION GUIDELINES

General Principles

- Medical record should be legible and complete.
- Rationale for ordering laboratory and other ancillary tests should be documented.
- Patient's emergency department course, including response to any treatment, should be documented.
- Documentation in record should support Current Procedural Terminology and ICD-9-CM codes submitted on insurance form and billing statement.

Key Elements of Chart

- Reason for encounter (chief complaint)
- History, physical exam (including addressing of any abnormal vital signs)
- Assessment, clinical impression, or diagnosis
- Care plan
- Date and legible identity of observer

Battery	Unwanted touching
Malpractice	Four elements:
	■ Duty
	■ Breach of duty
	■ Causation
	■ Harm
Emergency Medical Treatment and Active Labor Act	Federal law that says all persons presenting to an emergency department have the right to:
	■ A medical screening exam to determine if they have a medical emergency
	■ Receive necessary stabilizing treatment for any medical emergency including active labor in a pregnant woman
	■ Transfer to appropriate facility once the patient is stable

PRACTICE MANAGEMENT CONCEPTS

Cost Containment

The practice of conscientiously limiting medical expenses without sacrificing the medical care of the patient. The factor most directly in the control of the physician is the judicious use of laboratory and radiographic tests.

MANDATORY REPORTING

Child Abuse

All human services professionals, including physicians, are required by all 50 states to report known or *suspected* child abuse. There is no penalty for the reporting of cases that turn out not to be cases of abuse.

Communicable Diseases

The following infectious diseases were designated as notifiable at the national level in the United States, as of 1997:
- Acquired immune deficiency syndrome
- Anthrax
- Botulism
- Brucellosis
- Chancroid
- *Chlamydia trachomatis*, genital infections
- Cholera
- Coccidioidomycosis
- Cryptosporidiosis
- Diphtheria

- Encephalitides
- *Escherichia coli* O157
- Gonorrhea
- *Haemophilus influenzae*, invasive
- Hansen disease (leprosy)
- Hantavirus pulmonary syndrome
- Hepatitis
- Legionellosis
- Lyme disease
- Malaria
- Measles
- Meningococcal disease
- Mumps
- Pertussis
- Plague
- Poliomyelitis
- Psittacosis
- Rabies, animal and human
- Rocky Mountain spotted fever
- Rubella
- Salmonellosis
- Shigellosis
- *Streptococcus pneumoniae*, invasive drug-resistant disease
- Syphilis
- Tetanus
- Toxic shock syndrome
- Trichinosis
- Tuberculosis
- Typhoid fever
- Yellow fever

PRINCIPLES OF EVIDENCE-BASED MEDICINE

Evidence-based medicine is the practice of incorporating the best available evidence from the medical literature for a diagnostic test or treatment into daily patient care. It is an active process that requires five steps:

1. Identify a clinical problem.
2. Formulate a question.
3. Search for the best evidence.
4. Appraise the evidence.
5. Apply the information to the clinical problem.

A thorough search of the medical literature requires a computer or Internet search of MEDLINE, through OVID, Grateful Med, or Pub Med. All relevant articles should be considered. The best evidence is most often provided by meta-analysis or randomized clinical trials.

Sensitivity

(People with disease who tested positive)/(All people with disease)
true positive (TP)/(TP + false negative [FN])
Low rate of false negatives gives high value.

The more sensitive a test, the less likely the test is to fail to detect a positive result.

Specificity

(People without disease who tested negative)/(All people without disease)
true negative (TN)/(TN + false positive [FP])
Low rate of false positives gives high value.

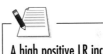

The more specific a test, the less likely the test is to fail to detect negative result.

Positive Predictive Value

(People with disease who tested positive)/(All people who tested positive)
TP/(TP + FP)
All positive variables

Negative Predictive Value

(People without disease who tested negative)/(All people who tested negative)
TN/(TN + FN)
All negative variables

Likelihood Ratio (LR)

Measures the fixed relationship between the chance of given test result in a patient with the disorder and the chance of the same test result in a patient without the disorder

LR for a positive test result = Sensitivity/(1 − specificity)
LR for a negative test result = (1 - sensitivity)/Specificity

A high positive LR increases the pretest likelihood that a patient has a disease.

Confidence Interval (CI)

Measures the range of values in which the true value studied (treatment difference, proportion, or probability) resides. Even if a study shows a benefit or harm of a given intervention, if the CI crosses zero, no treatment difference may exist. A study result with a CI that excludes zero is statistically significant.

Number Needed to Treat

Measures the number of patients with a given disease that a clinician would need to treat with the tested therapy in order to see one beneficial event or prevent one adverse event

SOURCES OF MEDICAL EVIDENCE

Meta-analysis

Evaluates the data of many trials that address the same question and attempts to combine the information: These studies are best used when the clinical problem is infrequent and large randomized trials cannot be done.

Randomized Controlled Clinical Trial (RCT)

The selected population is randomized to receive either the treatment in question or a placebo, and the outcome is measured. The ideal RCT is triple-blinded, meaning that the treating physician, the patient, and the investigators do not know which treatment has been given until the analysis is complete. These studies can establish cause and effect.

Cohort Study

The selected population is identified as being exposed or not exposed and is monitored for subsequent effects. These studies are used when the exposure cannot be assigned for logistical or ethical reasons.

Case Control Study

Populations with and without a given outcome are selected, and historical (retrospective) data are collected on exposure to a given agent or treatment.

Awards and Opportunities for Students Interested in Emergency Medicine

www.emra.org

www.saem.org

www.aaem.org

Web Site Resources for Students Interested in an EM Residency

Who Can Join EMRA?

Any medical student who is interested in emergency medicine as a career choice. EMRA's by-laws require that all members also be members of the American College of Emergency Physicians (ACEP).

Why Join EMRA?

EMRA membership provides a number of member benefits that will help you understand how emergency medicine fits into the provision of health care to the nation's citizens. Here's a short list of what you receive when you join.

- *EM Resident*—A bimonthly newsletter featuring articles, opinions, and information that affects emergency medicine residents and students. Each issue also features job placement information.
- *Top 30 Problems in Emergency Medicine*—This book is designed as a quiz and reference book you can keep in your pocket and test yourself on during down time or refer to during a case. References to other books, medical journals, and publications are provided as sources that can be accessed for more information on a specific topic. Topics include: rapid sequence intubation, useful formulas and mechanical ventilation, ATLS, infectious disease and emergency dosages.
- *Guide to Antibiotic Use in the Emergency Department*—This handy pocket reference is a great guide you can keep for easily accessible help in determining type and dosages of the most common antibiotics used in the emergency department.

- *Emergency Medicine in Focus*—This handy guide gives vital information of preparing for, applying to, and being successful in an emergency medicine residency and career.
- **Representation to Other Key Medical Organizations**—EMRA sends representatives to such medical specialty organizations as the ACEP, the American Academy of Emergency Medicine, the Society for Academic Emergency Medicine, and the American Medical Association so your views and concerns can be presented directly to members of these important organizations.
- **Medical Student Forum Admission**—Membership gains you free addmission to EMRA's annual Medical Student Forum held in conjunction with ACEP's Scientific Assembly.
- **The Residency Fair**—This is a key opportunity to meet residency directors and get information about specific residency programs. Free to you, this meeting is held during ACEP's Scientific Assembly.

What Does the EMRA Medical Student Committee (MSC) Do?

The MSC has developed goals and objectives that are in addition to EMRA's specific goals and objectives. The MSC focuses strictly on the medical students who indicate they are working toward a specialty in emergency medicine. The MSC:

- Educates medical students about the specialty of emergency medicine and its importance to the practice of medicine in this country.

- Provides information to those students interested in emergency medicine regarding career options and emergency medicine training programs.
- Develops a network of physician advisors for third- and fourth-year medical students who may not have access to role models in emergency medicine.
- Establishes a peer network for medical students aspiring to careers in emergency medicine and allows them the opportunity to assume leadership roles in organized emergency medicine.
- Provides ACEP and Society for Academic Emergency Medicine (SAEM) with a resource for dissemination of materials and information to medical students and training institutions.

What Are EMRA's Key Spheres of Influence?

EMRA is active within the house of medicine and, most particularly, in established liaison relationships with other emergency medicine–related organizations.

Listed below are some of the organizations that EMRA interacts with routinely in order to ensure that your voice as an emergency medicine resident is heard in the larger community of organized medicine and organized emergency medicine.

- ABEM–EMRA has an ongoing opportunity to work with the American Board of Emergency Medicine on a variety of issues.
- ACEP–EMRA holds four voting positions on ACEP's Council, as well as voting representation on the college's

432

Academic Affairs Committee and a number of other ACEP committees. EMRA also has a reporting representative at all ACEP Board meetings.

- AMA/AOA–EMRA maintains liaison relationships with students and house staff organizations such as the American Medical Association Resident Physician Section (AMA/RPS) and the American Osteopathic Association (AOA).
- SAEM–EMRA has an ongoing relationship with the SAEM and has a reporting representative at SAEM Board meetings.
- Other voting relationships —EMRA elects a voting member to the Residency Review Committee for Emergency Medicine (RRC/EM) and appoints a representative to the Emergency Medicine Foundation (EMF) Board of Directors.

ACEP/EMRA
Mentorship Program

The American College of Emergency Physicians (ACEP) has joined with EMRA (Emergency Medicine Residents' Association) to create a mentorship program in which seasoned emergency physicians and emergency medicine residents with similar interests can meet and learn from each other.

If you are interested in joining the mentorship program, please contact Sonja Montgomery of ACEP at *smontgomery@acep.org*, or 800-798-1822, ext. 3202.

EMRA LOCAL
ACTION GRANTS

In order to promote the involvement of emergency medicine residents in community service and other activities that support the specialty of emergency medicine, EMRA has instituted a Local Action Grant Program. Grants will be available to any EMRA member (**medical students,** residents, fellows) or any emergency medicine interest group whose principal applicant is an EMRA member. Recipients will be selected to receive an award of up to $500. Grants will be awarded at the spring membership meeting at SAEM's Annual Meeting. The deadline for nominations is March 1.

Regions Hospital Student EM CD Now Downloadable

The Regions EM student program is now available for download from the Internet. It contains an overview of the student program, student responsibilities, an example of our feedback card system, presentation and documentation guidelines for students, a study guide for readings, case studies, and procedural workshops on suturing, splinting, use of the slit lamp and clearing the cervical spine. Each student that rotates at Regions (MN) receives this CD. You can download this from *http://www.healthpartners.com/regions/em/homepage/index.html*.

EMRA Medical
Student Award

The EMRA Medical Student Award recognizes a student who displays a significant interest in emergency medicine. More importantly, this student "goes out of his or her way" for patients and colleagues. This student demonstrates a service-oriented attitude even when faced with difficult situations and stresses. The recipient receives a plaque and $250. This award is presented annually at the Spring Awards Reception held during SAEM's Annual Meeting and EMRA will notify the recipient's Dean of the honor. The deadline for nominations is March 1. To apply for this award, send an informal, anecdotal essay of 500 words or less that demonstrates the student's commitment to service. The application must also include the applicant's name, address, phone number and e-mail address, the name and address of the student's medical school and name of the school's dean.

Catalog of EM medical student electives may be found at: *http://www.saem.org/rotation/contents.htm*

Emergency Medicine Medical Student Interest Group Educational Grants

SAEM recognizes the valuable role of emergency medicine interest groups (EMIG's) for medical students interested in emergency medicine as a career. The Society will offer grants of up to $500 each to established or developing EMIG's located at medical schools with or without emergency medicine residencies. Grant monies can be used for supplies, consultation and seed money to support activities such as skills laboratories (suturing, casting, airway etc), lectures, or workshops. Grant proposals should focus on educational activities or projects related to undergraduate education in emergency medicine.

Individuals or institutions interested in applying for a grant should submit an application to the SAEM office. The deadline for submission is August 15 of the grant year with a funding date of October 1. Grants will be reviewed by a subcommittee of the Undergraduate Education Committee.

Medical Student Excellence in Emergency Medicine Award

This award is offered annually to each medical school in the United States and Canada. It is awarded to the senior medical student at each school who best exemplifies the qualities of an excellent emergency physician, as manifested by excellent clinical, interpersonal, and manual skills, and a dedication to continued professional development leading to outstanding performance on emergency medicine rotations. The award, presented at graduation, conveys a one-year membership in SAEM, which includes subscriptions the SAEM monthly journal, *Academic Emergency Medicine*, the SAEM Newsletter, and an award certificate.

Announcements describing the program and applications are sent to the Dean's Office at each medical school in February. Coordinators of emergency medicine student rotations then select an appropriate student based on the student's intramural and extramural performance in emergency medicine. Each school must submit the name of their recipient no later than June 1. The list of winners is published in a summer issue of the SAEM Newsletter.

Over 110 medical schools currently participate in this award. Contact SAEM at saem@saem.org if your school would like to participate.

MEDICAL STUDENT MEMBERSHIP IN SAEM

Medical students interested in emergency medicine are invited to become members of SAEM. Membership benefits include a reduced registration fee to attend the SAEM annual meeting; a subscription to *Academic Emergency Medicine*, the monthly SAEM journal; and a subscription to the SAEM Newsletter (6 issues per year). Annual dues are $75 (includes journal subscription) or $50 (not including journal subscription).

MEDICAL STUDENT EM RESEARCH GRANTS

SAEM and the Emergency Medicine Foundation sponsor annual grants of up to a maximum of $2,400 over 3 months for medical students. Applications can be obtained from EMF. The deadline is in late January every year.

AAEM: AMERICAN ACADEMY OF EMERGENCY MEDICINE

AAEM is one of the smaller EM organizations whose mission is to support fair and equitable practice environments for EM physicians. They offer medical students membership, an e-mail contact list, and a "medical student forum" feature in their monthly newsletter.

AAEM.ORG

PUBLISH IN JEM!

The Journal of Emergency Medicine is looking for medical student authors to submit contributions on topics of interest to medical students such as residency application, away clerkships, resources for students, book/Web site reviews, or interviews. If interested, please contact the Student Representative on the AAEM/RES Board of Directors.

virtualer.com

Site offers links to many Web pages related to emergency medicine. Connect to tutorials, image libraries, professional organizations, job searches, free medline searches, and more!

trauma.orhs.org

A Web site dedicated to trauma and critical from Orlando Regional health care system. It features a trauma and emergency surgery e-mail discussion group and weekly trauma case studies.

embbs.com

Features photographic case reports with clinical pearls from *Academic Emergency Medicine*, the official journal of the Society of Academic Emergency medicine.

mdchoice.com

Site features interesting radiology (CT and plain film) cases.

erl.pathology.iupui.edu

Site featuring dermatopathology cases from the University of Indiana. Excellent photos of all the derm conditions you need to know in EM.

CDC.org

Presents a wealth of information including clinical guidelines, up-to-date info on most major diseases, and an excellent search engine with links to other governmental agencies.

NCEMI.ORG

Web site of the National Center for Emergency Medicine Informatics. Presented as a daily newspaper page with question of the day, and ECG, x-ray photo and cartoon of the week. Summarizes important abstracts in EM. Has several excellent to other EM sites. Has many clever medical calculators and facts and formulae.

emedicine.com

This Web site has online textbooks in emergency medicine and most other primary specialties for use free of charge. These textbooks have four levels of peer review and are continually updated. Opportunities for authorship in one of the many textbooks are available.

medschool.com

Founded by the original creator of the First Aid series, Dr. Vikas Bhushan, this site has multiple weekly features such as pearl, question, and image of the week; medical humor; book and Web site reviews, online chat forums, a premed resource center, a USMLE study center, and a way to ask faculty questions directly. A must visit site!

SAEM Medical Student Emergency Medicine Symposium

Each year during the SAEM annual meeting, an Emergency Medicine Medical Student Forum is held. This session is designed to help the medical student understand the residency and career options that exist in emergency medicine, develop an optimal senior year schedule, evaluate residency programs, and navigate the residency application process. The medical student also learns to recognize and begin management of common and potentially life-threatening problems that present to the emergency department. A Medical Student/Resident Visual Diagnosis Photography Contest is also held at the SAEM annual meeting. Small prizes are awarded and winners are acknowledged in the SAEM Newsletter.

Future Annual Meetings:
May 19–22, 2002, St. Louis
May 29–June 1, 2003, Boston
May 16–19, 2004, Orlando

RESIDENCY APPLICATION GUIDE ONLINE

This guide by the University California at San Francisco may be found at *http://www.som.ucsf.edu/education/student/orgs/emig/appguide/index.htm*.

Catalog of emergency medicine residencies may be found at *http://www.saem.org/rescat/contents.htm*.

CLASSIFIED

435

EM Residency Formats

U.S. allopathic programs are structured in three different formats:

1–4 programs: There are 14 of these 4-year programs.

2–4 programs: There are 22 of these 3-year programs (3 years after a separate 1-year internship).

1–3 programs: There are 86 of these 3-year programs (3 years including the internship year).

There are also Canadian and osteopathic programs.

Combined programs with internal medicine, pediatrics, and family medicine also exist, and these are generally 5 years in length.

Articles of Interest That Can Be Found at saem.org

- Pro vs Con: Four vs Three— Pro: Four Years are Optimal versus Con: Three Years are Enough
- Medical Students and Research
- Taming the Residency Application Process
- Bibliographic Citation Guidelines for EM Residency Applicants
- ERAS Made Easy . . . or how your life has been made better by the AAMC!
- EM Resident Career Satisfaction
- Advice to Students Seeking an Academic Career in Emergency Medicine
- Advice to Students Beginning a Medical Student Rotation in Emergency Medicine
- The 2000 NRMP Match in Emergency Medicine
- Emergency Medicine as a Career Choice
- Top Ten Questions Regarding the Organization of Your Senior Year
- Emergency Medicine Clubs
- 10 Things To Do Before Applying To An Emergency Medicine Residency.
- Selection Criteria for Emergency Medicine Residency Applications
- Does Interview Date affect Match List Position in the Emergency Medicine National Residency Matching Program Match?

Index

Amylase, 120, 180
Amyl nitrite pearls, 380
Amyloidosis, 78
Anaerobes, 238
Anal fissure
    definition, 186
    etiology, 186
    treatment, 186
    See also Rectum/anus
Analgesics
    acute pancreatitis, 182
    anal fissure, 186
    endometriosis, 236
    headache, 84
    hemorrhoids, 186
    opioids, 348
    osteoarthritis, 276
    septic arthritis, 269
    sickle cell anemia, 223
    varicella zoster, 308
Anemia
    abdominal pain, 189
    aplastic, 215
    diverticular disease, 185
    glucose-6-phosphate dehydrogenase, 224
    heart failure, high-output, 149
    hemolytic, 33, 219
    hydatidiform mole, 250
    macrocytic, 32
    megaloblastic, 215
    pernicious, 32
    sickle cell anemia, 189, 223
    sinus tachycardia, 138
    thrombocytopenia, 214, 215
    thrombotic thrombocytopenic purpura, 218
Anesthesia, 274, 325–326, 372
Angina
    aortic insufficiency, 155
    aortic stenosis, 154
    dilated cardiomyopathy, 144
    hypertrophic cardiomyopathy, 147
    mitral regurgitation, 157
    nitrates, 125
    prehospital equipment, 415
    sick sinus syndrome, 142
    stable, 132
    supraventricular tachycardia, 140
    unstable, 132
    variant, 132
Angiocatheter, 20–21
Angiodysplasia, 185
Angioedema, 309–310
Angiography
    acute chest syndrome, 222
    aortic rupture, traumatic, 63
    carotid or vertebral artery dissection, 90
    mesenteric ischemia, 174
    neck trauma, 53
    pulmonary embolus, 118
Angiotensin, 178, 242
Angiotensin-converting enzyme (ACE), 25, 128, 151
Anhydrosis, 403
Animal trauma, terrestrial
    cats, 396
    dogs, 395–396
    humans, 396
    See also Marine life trauma and envenomation
Anion gap, 30, 287, 367
Anisocoria, 46
Ankles, 327, 333–334
Ankylosing spondylitis, 155
Anorexia
    acute mountain sickness, 382
    acute pancreatitis, 181
    appendicitis, 183
    diverticular disease, 185
    foreign body ingestion, esophageal, 166
    hepatitis, 177
    lower GI bleed, 186
    tuberculosis, 122
Anoscopy, 186
Anoxic brain damage, 72

Antacids, 168, 170
Antalgic gait, 280, 282
Antecubital fossae, 43
Anterior cord syndrome, 56
Anterior epistaxis
    diagnosis, 113
    etiology, 113
    packing, procedure for anterior nasal, 113–114
    treatment, 113
Anterior triangle, 51
Antibacterials, 299
Antibiotics
    acute bacterial endocarditis, 149
    acute mastoiditis, 110
    acute sinusitis, 107
    appendicitis, 183
    barotrauma, descent, 385
    Bartholin's gland abscess, 238
    brain abscess, 97
    brown recluse spider, 392
    burns, 399
    candidiasis, 234
    cavernous sinus thrombosis, 108
    cellulitis, 267, 301
    cholangitis, 180
    decubitus ulcers, 320
    disseminated intravascular coagulation, 221
    endometritis, 254
    erysipelas, 302
    extremity trauma, 69
    impetigo, 301
    inflammatory bowel disease, 173–174
    marine life trauma and envenomation, 390
    mitral regurgitation, 157
    myocarditis, 151
    myxedema coma, 294
    neutropenic sepsis, 226
    osteomyelitis, 269
    otitis media, 109
    pancreatic abscess, 182
    paronychia, 265, 266
    pelvic inflammatory disease, 240
    peptic ulcer disease, 171
    peritonsillar abscess, 111
    pneumonia, 116
    septic abortion, 247
    septic arthritis, 269
    small bowel obstruction, 176
    spontaneous bacterial peritonitis, 179
    tenosynovitis, 266
    See also Metronidazole; Penicillin
Anticholinergics
    gastroesophageal reflux disease, 167
    inflammatory bowel disease, 172
    Ogilvie's syndrome, 184
    toxicology, emergency
        antipsychotics, 364
        gastric lavage, 350
        toxidromes, 347
    tricyclic antidepressants, 360
Anticholinesterase, 98
Anticoagulants
    antiplatelet therapy, 216
    atrial fibrillation, 140
    dysfunctional uterine bleeding, 237
    hypertrophic cardiomyopathy, 147
    lower GI bleed, 185
    platelet dysfunction, chemically induced, 216, 217
    posterior epistaxis, 114
    pulmonary embolus, 119
    stroke, 78, 80
    subdural hematoma, 88
    thrombophlebitis, 164
Anticonvulsants
    fosphenytoin, 100
    headache, 84
    phenytoin, 100
    toxicology, emergency
        carbamazepine, 365
        phenytoin, 364–365
        valproic acid, 365
    See also Phenytoin

Antidepressants
    toxicology, emergency
        anticholinergics, 347
        antipsychotics, 363–364
        lithium, 363–364
        monoamine oxidase inhibitors, 362
        selective serotonin reuptake inhibitors, 361–362
        tricyclic, 101, 171, 184, 217, 348
    See also individual drug
Antidiarrheals, 172
Antidiuretic hormone (ADH), 291
Antidysrhythmics, 126–127
Antiemetics, 91–93, 182, 415
Antifreeze, 367, 368
Antifungal agents, 96
Antihistamines
    bees and wasps, 394
    benign paroxysmal positional vertigo, 91
    erythema multiforme, 313
    labyrinthitis, 92
    Ménière's disease, 92
    overview, 299
    pityriasis rosea, 318
    post-traumatic vertigo, 93
    Stevens–Johnson syndrome, 313
    toxicology, emergency
        anticholinergics, 347
        antipsychotics, 364
        selective serotonin reuptake inhibitors, 362
    tricyclic antidepressants, 360
    urticaria, 310
    vestibular neuronitis, 93
Antihypertensives, 160
Antihyperthyroid medications, 292
Antimalarials, 224
Antimicrobials, 152
Antineoplastic therapy, 228
Antinuclear antibody (ANA), 280
Antiparasitics, 299–300
Antiparkinsons, 347
Antiplatelet therapy, 80, 125, 216, 219
Antipsychotics
    toxicology, emergency
        anticholinergics, 347
        clinical signs of toxicity, 364
        exposure, 363
        management, 364
        mechanism of toxicity, 364
Anti-Rh IgG (RhoGAM), 225, 246
Antithrombin, 164, 221
Antitrypsin, 121
Anti-tumor necrosis factor alpha, 174
Antivenin, 389, 393, 394
Antivertigo agents, 92–93
Antivirals, 300
Anus. *See* Rectum/anus
Anxiety
    amphetamines, 371
    foreign body ingestion, esophageal, 166
    glucose, 358
    monoamine oxidase inhibitors, 362
    opioids, 348
    organophosphates, 376
    pericarditis, 152
    pulmonary embolus, 118
    sedation, conscious, 329
    sedative–hypnotics, 372
    selective serotonin reuptake inhibitors, 361
    sinus tachycardia, 138
    sympathomimetics, 348
Aortic aneurysm
    abdominal, 158–159
    thoracic, 159–161
Aortic dissection, 123, 155
Aortic regurgitation/failure, 18
Aortic rupture, traumatic, 62–63
Aortic stenosis
    definition, 154
    diagnosis, 154–155
    etiology, 154
    signs and symptoms, 154
    treatment, 154–155